New Applications of Interpersonal Psychotherapy

New Applications of Interpersonal Psychotherapy

Edited by

Gerald L. Klerman, M.D.

Associate Chair for Research and
Professor of Psychiatry
Cornell University Medical College
Payne Whitney Psychiatric Clinic
New York, New York

Myrna M. Weissman, Ph.D.

Professor of Epidemiology in Psychiatry
Department of Psychiatry
College of Physicians and
Surgeons of Columbia University;
Director, Division of Clinical and Genetic Epidemiology
New York State Psychiatric Institute
New York, New York

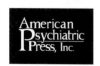

Washington, DC
London, England

Copyright © 1993 American Psychiatric Press
ALL RIGHTS RESERVED
Manufactured in the United States of America on acid-free paper
96 95 94 93   4 3 2 1
First Edition

American Psychiatric Press, Inc.
1400 K Street, N.W., Washington, DC   20005

Library of Congress Cataloging-in-Publication Data
New applications of interpersonal psychotherapy /   edited by Gerald L.
Klerman, Myrna M. Weissman. — 1st ed.
    p.   cm.
Includes bibliographical references and index.
ISBN 0-88048-511-6
    1. Depression—Treatment. 2. Psychotherapy. I. Klerman, Gerald
L., 1928– . II. Weissman, Myrna M.
    [DNLM: 1. Depression—therapy. 2. Interpersonal Relations.
3. Psychotherapy—methods. WM 420 N5303]
RC537.H486 1993
616.85′270651—dc20
DNLM/DLC   92-48959
for Library of Congress   CIP

British Library Cataloguing in Publication Data
A CIP record is available from the British Library.

Contents

Section Three:
Interpersonal Psychotherapy for
Other Psychiatric Disorders

Dedication

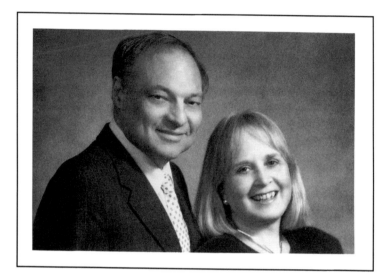

To my beloved husband

. . . they leave many of their tasks unfinished, their plans unfulfilled, their dreams unrealized. It would be more than we could bear, but for the faith that our little day finds its permanence . . . and our work its completion in the unfolding of Your purpose for humanity.

. . . We recall the joy of their companionship. We feel a pang, the echo of that intenser grief when first their death lay before our stricken eyes. Now we know that they will never vanish, so long as heart and thought remain within us. By love are they remembered, and in memory they live.

. . . grant that their memory may bring strength and blessing. May the nobility in their lives and the high ideals they cherished endure in our thoughts and live on in our deeds. May we, carrying on their work, help to redeem Your promise that life shall prevail.

Gates of Prayer
Central Conference of American Rabbis
New York, New York, 1975

Gerald L. Klerman died on April 3, 1992 after this book was completed but before it was published. This book is a small legacy of my husband's career, which spanned such major universities as Harvard, Yale, and Cornell, and the most influential government position for psychiatry in the United States in the 1980s as head of the Alcohol, Drug Abuse, and Mental Health Administration. These positions were a forum to carry out research in the treatment, epidemiology, and psychopathology of the major mental illnesses; to develop public policy that would enhance the quality and delivery of care to psychiatric patients; and to train a generation of future investigators. He believed that the patient had the right to the "right" treatment and that the "right" treatment should be grounded in empiricism, not in ideology.

His early career was strongly rooted in psychopharmacological research. He began his residency when chlorpromazine was introduced, and under Jonathan Cole, M.D., he coordinated the first multicentered trial of antipsychotic drugs while completing his military service at the National Institute of Mental Health in Bethesda, Maryland. He was one of the original members of the American College of Neuropsychopharmacology (ACNP). In the 1980s, after leaving government, he directed a cross-national collaborative study of the treatment of panic disorder that involved 12 countries. As a side effect of this study, a common diagnostic language was developed among the participating young investigators from France, Germany, Italy, Spain, Great Britain, Australia, Brazil, Mexico, Colombia, and Canada.

His interest in pharmacological research did not distract from the fact that he felt psychotherapy was important in the treatment of psychiatric patients. He loved doing and teaching psychotherapy. While he believed that psychotherapy was a powerful tool, he did not think it was a universal solvent. It depended upon the patient's diagnosis and the type of psychotherapy. He was disappointed that some of the potentially most powerful psychotherapies did not have a sufficient empirical basis. He believed that psychotherapy was as much an art form as surgery. In both, the practitioners needed to be highly trained as well as skilled in the specific techniques, but the final outcome of the procedures across practitioners could be tested.

He certainly did not believe that interpersonal psychotherapy (IPT) was the best or only treatment for all psychiatric conditions or even for all depressions. He saw it as a formalization of procedures often used in time-limited treatment with depressed patients. He was delighted that the efficacy of IPT had been shown in research studies conducted outside the enthusiastic home of its originators.

This book has a heavy note of sadness, as it will appear after his death. Little can temper my personal sadness. Since the book represents work in progress, new directions, developments of Gerry's ideas, and a new generation of investigators, many of whom were trained by him, it is a wonderful professional legacy.

Myrna M. Weissman, Ph.D.
New York, New York
July 1992

Contributors

Kathleen Carroll, Ph.D.
Assistant Professor of Psychiatry
Department of Psychiatry
Yale University School of Medicine;
Director of Psychotherapy Research
Substance Abuse Treatment Unit
Yale University School of Medicine
New Haven, Connecticut

Kathleen F. Clougherty, M.S.W.
Research Associate in Psychiatry
Cornell University Medical Center
New York, New York

Cleon Cornes, M.D.
Associate Professor of Psychiatry
Department of Psychiatry
University of Pittsburgh School of Medicine
Pittsburgh, Pennsylvania

Christopher G. Fairburn, M.D.
Wellcome Trust Senior Lecturer
Department of Psychiatry
Oxford University
Warneford Hospital
Oxford, United Kingdom

Ellen Frank, Ph.D.
Associate Professor of Psychiatry and Psychology
Department of Psychiatry
University of Pittsburgh School of Medicine
Pittsburgh, Pennsylvania

Nancy Frank, A.C.S.W.
Pittsburgh, Pennsylvania

Stanley D. Imber, Ph.D.
Professor of Psychiatry and Psychology
Department of Psychiatry
University of Pittsburgh School of Medicine
Pittsburgh, Pennsylvania

Laura S. Josephs, Ph.D.
Clinical Instructor of Psychology in Psychiatry
Cornell University Medical Center
New York, New York

Gerald L. Klerman, M.D.
Associate Chair for Research and Professor of Psychiatry
Cornell University Medical College
Payne Whitney Psychiatric Clinic
New York, New York

David J. Kupfer, M.D.
Professor of Psychiatry
Department of Psychiatry
University of Pittsburgh School of Medicine
Pittsburgh, Pennsylvania

Michael J. Madonia, M.S.W.
Project Coordinator
Department of Psychiatry
University of Pittsburgh School of Medicine
Pittsburgh, Pennsylvania

John C. Markowitz, M.D.
Assistant Professor of Psychiatry
Cornell University Medical College
New York, New York

Barbara J. Mason, Ph.D.
Associate Professor
Department of Psychiatry
University of Miami School of Medicine
Miami, Florida

Mark D. Miller, M.D.
Assistant Professor of Psychiatry
Department of Psychiatry
University of Pittsburgh School of Medicine
Pittsburgh, Pennsylvania

Donna Moreau, M.D.
Assistant Professor of Clinical Psychiatry in Child Psychiatry
College of Physicians and Surgeons of Columbia University;
Clinical Director of Children's Anxiety and Depression Clinic
Babies Hospital
New York, New York

Susan M. Morris, L.S.W.
Department of Psychiatry
University of Pittsburgh School of Medicine
Pittsburgh, Pennsylvania

Laura H. Mufson, Ph.D.
Assistant Professor of Clinical Psychology in Psychiatry
College of Physicians and Surgeons of Columbia University;
Research Scientist,
Division of Clinical and Genetic Epidemiology
New York State Psychiatric Institute
New York, New York

Samuel W. Perry, M.D.
Professor of Psychiatry
Cornell University Medical Center
New York, New York

Charles F. Reynolds III, M.D.
Professor of Psychiatry
Department of Psychiatry
University of Pittsburgh School of Medicine
Pittsburgh, Pennsylvania

Bruce J. Rounsaville, M.D.
Associate Professor of Psychiatry
Department of Psychiatry;
Director of Psychosocial Research
Substance Abuse Treatment Unit
Yale University School of Medicine
New Haven, Connecticut

Herbert C. Schulberg, Ph.D.
Professor of Psychiatry, Psychology, and Medicine
Department of Psychiatry
University of Pittsburgh School of Medicine
Pittsburgh, Pennsylvania

C. Paul Scott, M.D.
Clinical Associate Professor of Psychiatry
Department of Psychiatry
University of Pittsburgh School of Medicine;
St. Margaret Memorial Hospital Family Practice Residency
Pittsburgh, Pennsylvania

Myrna M. Weissman, Ph.D.
Professor of Epidemiology in Psychiatry
Department of Psychiatry
College of Physicians and Surgeons of Columbia University;
Director, Division of Clinical and Genetic Epidemiology
New York State Psychiatric Institute
New York, New York

Preface

Interpersonal psychotherapy (IPT) is a brief psychological treatment specified in a manual initially developed and tested for depressed outpatients.[1] In the last few years, several adaptations of IPT have appeared. This book compiles these adapted approaches so that clinicians can be aware of new adaptations that have been tested and researchers can gain knowledge of the new adaptations that are available and require testing.

We believe that the best interests of patients with mental disorders are served by the availability of a range of treatments and that the psychotherapies are among them. We also believe that all treatments should be subjected to testing through controlled clinical trials and that the findings from these trials provide the best evidence to guide clinical practice.

For psychotherapy, we see the specification of the procedures in a manual as a first step in the process of testing. We welcome the development of manuals that specify new treatments and, particularly, the new adaptations of interpersonal psychotherapy. However, we do not equate the availability of manuals with the demonstration of their efficacy.

We are well aware of the demonstrated efficacy of many medications for depression and other psychiatric disorders. We have tested several in clinical trials and have prescribed them in practice. Since the introduction of effective psychopharmacological medications in the 1960s and 1970s, there has been a growing presumption that all patients who meet DSM-III (or DSM-III-R) criteria for major depression should receive antidepressant medication. We do not interpret the findings from controlled trials as supporting that presumption. For a substantial proportion of depressed patients—those clinically judged to be mild to moderately symptomatic—the evidence from clinical trials, particularly the large multisite National

---

[1] G. L. Klerman, M. M. Weissman, B. J. Rounsaville, et al.: *Interpersonal Psychotherapy for Depression.* New York, Basic Books, 1984.

Institute of Mental Health Treatment of Depression Collaborative Research Program, indicates that short-term focused psychotherapy, such as IPT, is equivalent in efficacy to imipramine.

For severely depressed patients, including depressed patients who are delusional or have been hospitalized, have recurrent episodes, or are bipolar, antidepressant medication is required. Even so, the combination of medication and psychotherapy often yields better clinical outcomes than either treatment alone.

In many, but not all, cases, medication will act more quickly and consistently than psychotherapy on the reduction of the depressed patient's symptoms. However, many depressed patients will not or cannot take medications, particularly women who want to become pregnant or are nursing; elderly persons, in whom medical problems or the use of some medication for chronic medical illnesses is a contraindication for psychotropic drugs; or adolescents, for whom the efficacy of psychotropic drugs has not yet been established. Moreover, many depressed patients have social and interpersonal problems as the source or a consequence of their illness that do not simply resolve when these patients are feeling better. We are not ideologically bound to any one form of treatment for mental disorders. For many patients, combinations of drugs and psychotherapy may be the best treatment. Such recommendations for clinical practice should be supported by appropriate evidence.

This book is primarily intended for professionals involved in psychotherapy, in its clinical practice, and in its research and evaluation. For the practitioner, the book describes the new applications of IPT in different formats or for clinical conditions that have not previously been the target for IPT. Hopefully, this information will assist clinicians in planning their treatment programs for patients with these conditions and adjust current practices in light of new developments.

For the researcher involved in research on treatment in general and in psychotherapy in particular, this book will illustrate the application of new techniques and designs in psychotherapy research to different facets of depression other than the acute depressive states for which IPT was first developed. The application of these approaches allows the efficacy of IPT to be assessed in disorders other than depression, such as bulimia nervosa and heroin addiction. Hopefully, these innovative techniques will enhance the efficacy of psychotherapy by increased specification of treatment and generation of evidence for effectiveness.

In Section One the authors describe the background and concepts of IPT, although the reader will need to refer to the Klerman et al. (1984) manual for full details. Recent advances in the understanding of the epidemiology, genetics, and treatment of depression are described because an integral part of the first phase of IPT for depression is educating the patient about the illness. Finally, the scientific status of psychotherapy and its testing are reviewed in order to place the data on IPT in perspective. In Section Two, new adaptations of IPT for depression are described, including IPT as maintenance treatment for recurrent depression; in a conjoint format for couples with marital disputes where one partner is depressed; for depressed adolescents; for elderly persons; for depressed HIV-seropositive patients; for patients with dysthymia; and for depressed medical patients in primary care. In Section Three, the authors describe the extension of IPT to other disorders, including a simpler counseling format for stress and distress, for drug abuse, and for bulimia nervosa.

We hope that the reader does not find the mixed nature of the information and variability in the chapters disconcerting. Some chapters provide a review of efficacy data on new indications for IPT, and others present adaptations of IPT for new populations and disorders without efficacy data. This unevenness and inconsistency reflect the status of the work. We felt that it would be useful to provide information on new adaptations before the efficacy studies are complete (e.g., in the case of IPT for depressed adolescents or with HIV-seropositive patients) as a way of stimulating the field. Of course, without the efficacy data, the value of the adaptation is uncertain.

We are grateful for the financial support of the National Institute of Mental Health for most of this research over the years, and, more recently, to the John D. and Catherine T. MacArthur Foundation, the NARSAD Foundation, and the Anne Pollock Lederer Foundation. We were honored to receive the Foundation Funds Prize for Research in Psychiatry at the 1978 annual meeting of the American Psychiatric Association in Atlanta, Georgia, and the Anna Monica Foundation Award, presented in 1986 in Basel, Switzerland, for the efficacy studies, which form the scientific basis of this treatment.

The ideas have been developed and the research conducted over the years in several supportive universities and hospitals: Yale University

School of Medicine, Department of Psychiatry and the Connecticut Mental Health Center, New Haven, Connecticut (Myrna M. Weissman and Gerald L. Klerman); Harvard Medical School, Department of Psychiatry, the Massachusetts General Hospital, and the Harvard Community Health Plan, Boston, Massachusetts (Gerald L. Klerman); Cornell Medical School, the Payne Whitney Clinic, New York, New York (Gerald L. Klerman); and the College of Physicians and Surgeons of Columbia University, Department of Psychiatry and Epidemiology, and the New York State Psychiatric Institute, New York, New York (Myrna M. Weissman).

Many colleagues generously gave their comments and advice. Many students committed their training to learning these methods and carrying out these studies. Their names are found in the chapters included and in the many articles referenced, which they coauthored and which form their scientific legacy.

All case material has been altered to protect confidentiality.

Gerald L. Klerman, M.D.
Myrna M. Weissman, Ph.D.
New York, New York, 1992

SECTION

ONE

Overview

CHAPTER 1

Interpersonal Psychotherapy for Depression: Background and Concepts

Gerald L. Klerman, M.D.
Myrna M. Weissman, Ph.D.

In this chapter we review the concept, development, and testing of *interpersonal psychotherapy* (IPT) for depressed adults and introduce its recent adaptations.

Background

Interpersonal psychotherapy was developed initially as a time-limited weekly psychotherapy for the ambulatory, nonbipolar, nonpsychotic depressed patient. The goals of IPT are to reduce the symptoms of depression and to improve the quality of the patient's current interpersonal functioning. These goals are achieved in the initial formulation of IPT by weekly face-to-face sessions between the patient and the therapist in which the following occur:

1. The depression is explicitly diagnosed.
2. The patient is educated about depression and its causes, and the various treatments available.
3. The interpersonal context of depression and its development are identified.
4. Strategies for dealing with the context evolve and are attempted by the patient.

Initially, techniques were developed for the management of depressed patients with grief and loss, interpersonal deficits, interpersonal (usually marital) role disputes, and role transitions. Later adaptations have been modified or have added to these areas. IPT can be administered after appropriate training by experienced psychiatrists, psychologists, and social workers. It can be used alone or with medication.[1]

Interpersonal psychotherapy has evolved over nearly 25 years of treatment and research experience with ambulatory depressed patients. The development began in 1968 as part of a clinical trial for depressed outpatients that was designed to test approaches to preventing relapse following reduction of acute symptoms of depression with pharmacotherapy. By the mid-1960s, it was clear that the new antidepressants were effective in reducing acute depressive symptoms. Sleep, appetite, and mood usually improved in 2 to 4 weeks. However, the relapse rate was high, and it was unclear how long medication should continue and whether there was any advantage to adding psychotherapy. The intent in specifying the psychotherapy in the first clinical trial was to ensure consistency between therapists. Our intent was not to develop a new psychotherapy but to describe what we believed was reasonable and current practice with depressed patients and might be considered for inclusion under the rubric of short-term supportive psychotherapy.

To standardize the treatment so that clinical trials could be undertaken, the concepts, techniques, and methods of IPT were specified and operationally described in a manual. The manual, which has undergone a number of revisions, was published in a book (Klerman et al. 1984). A

---

[1] These adaptations will be described in detail by their respective authors in Sections Two and Three of this volume.

training program for experienced psychotherapists of different disciplines providing the treatment for these clinical trials was developed (Weissman et al. 1982).[2]

Theoretical Sources

Interpersonal psychotherapy derives from a number of sources. The ideas of Adolf Meyer, whose psychobiological approach to understanding psychiatric disorders placed great emphasis on the patient's relation to his or her environment, constitute the most prominent theoretical sources for IPT (Meyer 1957). Meyer viewed psychiatric disorders as an expression of the patient's attempt to adapt to his or her environment. An individual's response to environmental change is determined by prior experiences, particularly early experiences in the family and the individual's affiliation with various social groups. Among Meyer's associates, Harry Stack Sullivan stands out for his general theory of interpersonal relationships and for his writings linking clinical psychiatry to the emerging social sciences (Sullivan 1953).

In addition, a major source of theoretical understanding derives from the work of the English child psychoanalyst John Bowlby and his emphasis on attachment and bonding (Bowlby 1969). Whereas previous psychodynamic theories emphasized depressive states as reflective of aggressive and libidinous drives, Bowlby drew attention to the large body of sociobiological and animal research, particularly in primates and mammals, on the importance of attachment and bonding. This perspective has particular significance for humans. Given the long period of extrauterine life required for development of independence and maturity, the human infant requires considerable protection and other activities from the mothering figure. This sets the stage for further evolution of emotional life, with an impact on cognitive, behavioral, and social activities.

---

[2] There is, to our knowledge, no ongoing training program for practitioners, although workshops are available from time to time. There are plans in process for formal training programs. We are planning to prepare video training tapes, and some of the investigators who have adapted IPT have videotapes available. Klerman et al.'s (1984) book can serve as a guide for the experienced clinician who wants to learn IPT for depressed patients, and the reader is referred to this book for the full details of the treatment and the background to development.

Empirical Sources

The empirical basis for understanding and treating depression with IPT includes the following:

- Studies associating stress and life events with the onset and clinical course of depression
- Longitudinal studies demonstrating the social impairment of depressed women during the acute depressive phase and the following symptomatic recovery
- Studies by Brown and Harris (1978) that demonstrate the role of intimacy and social supports as protection against depression in the face of adverse life stress
- Studies by Pearlin and Lieberman (1979) that show the impact of chronic social and interpersonal stress, particularly marital stress, on the onset of depression
- The works of Bowlby (1969) and Henderson et al. (1978), who emphasize the importance of attachment bonds or, conversely, show that the loss of social attachments can be associated with the onset of depression
- Epidemiological data that show a strong association between marital disputes and major depression (Weissman 1987)

Clinical Depression as Conceptualized in Interpersonal Psychotherapy

Interpersonal psychotherapy makes no assumptions about the causes of depression, which remain for scientific investigation to fully identify and verify. However, IPT does assume that the development of clinical depression occurs in a social and interpersonal context and that the onset, response to treatment, and outcomes are influenced by the interpersonal relations between the depressed patient and significant others.

Clinical depression is conceptualized as having three component processes:

1. *Symptom formation,* involving the development of the depressive affect and the signs and symptoms, which may derive from psychobiological and/or psychodynamic mechanisms

2. *Social functioning,* involving social interactions with other persons that derive from learning based on childhood experiences, concurrent social reinforcement, and/or current personal efforts at mastery and competence
3. *Personality,* involving more enduring traits and behaviors—the handling of anger and guilt and overall self-esteem—that constitute the person's unique reactions and patterns of functioning and that also may contribute to a predisposition to symptom episodes

Interpersonal psychotherapy, as it was originally developed, attempts to intervene in the first two processes. However, because of the brevity of the treatment, the low level of psychotherapeutic intensity, and the focus on the current depressive episode, no claim is made that IPT will have an impact on the enduring aspects of personality, although personality functioning is assessed.

Interpersonal psychotherapy develops directly from an interpersonal conceptualization of depression. It does not, however, assume that interpersonal problems "cause" depression, but rather that, whatever the cause, the current depression occurs in an interpersonal context. The therapeutic strategies of IPT are designed to help the patient master that context. IPT facilitates recovery from acute depression by relieving depressive symptoms and by helping the patient become more effective in dealing with current interpersonal problems that are associated with the onset of symptoms. Symptom relief begins with helping the patient understand that the vague and uncomfortable symptoms are part of a known syndrome, which responds to various treatments and has good prognosis. Psychotropic drugs may be used in conjunction with IPT to alleviate symptoms more rapidly.

Treating the depressed patient's difficulties in interpersonal relations proceeds by exploring the four problem areas commonly associated with the onset of depression: grief, role disputes, role transition, and interpersonal deficit. The middle phase of IPT focuses on the patient's particular interpersonal problem area as it relates to the onset of depression.

An essential feature of IPT for depression is the intentional avoidance, during the treatment of the acute symptomatic episode, of issues related to personality functioning and character pathology. Our clinical experience suggests that more than minimum attention to issues of personality and character will result in delay of recovery and prolongation of the depressive episode.

There are many ways of conceptualizing any psychotherapy. We have conceptualized IPT at three levels: 1) strategies for specific tasks, 2) techniques, and 3) therapeutic stance. IPT is similar to many other therapies at the level of techniques and stance but is distinct at the level of strategies.

The strategies of IPT occur in three phases of treatment. During the first phase, the depression is diagnosed within a medical model and explained to the patient. The major problem associated with the onset of the depression is identified, and an explicit treatment contract to work on this problem area is made with the patient. Then, during the intermediate phase of treatment, work on the major current interpersonal problem areas is accomplished. The termination phase is not unique to IPT in that feelings about termination are discussed, progress is reviewed, and the remaining work is outlined. As in other brief treatments, the arrangements for termination are explicit and are followed closely.

The IPT structure, including techniques and stance, is outlined in Table 1–1. Readers are referred to the book *Interpersonal Psychotherapy for Depression* (Klerman et al. 1984) for details.

Comparison of Interpersonal Psychotherapy With Other Psychotherapies

The procedures and techniques of many psychotherapies have much in common. Many therapies emphasize helping the patient develop a sense of mastery and reducing social isolation. The psychotherapies differ, however, as to whether the patient's problems are defined as lying in the far past, the immediate past, or the present. *IPT focuses primarily on the patient's present. It differs from other psychotherapies in its specified duration, its attention to current depressive symptoms, and its focus on the current depression-related interpersonal context.* Given this frame of reference, IPT includes a systematic review of the patient's current relations with significant others.

Interpersonal psychotherapy was originally developed as a brief treatment. However, an adaptation with long duration (i.e., 3 years) but non-

Table 1–1.	Outline of interpersonal psychotherapy

I. The initial sessions
  A. Dealing with depression
    1. Review depressive symptoms.
    2. Give the syndrome a name.
    3. Explain depression and the treatment.
    4. Give the patient the "sick role."
    5. Evaluate the need for medication.
  B. Relation of depression to interpersonal context
    1. Review current and past interpersonal relationships as they relate to current depressive symptoms. Determine with the patient the following:
      a. Nature of interaction with significant persons
      b Expectations of patient and significant persons from each other and whether these were fulfilled
      c. Satisfying and unsatisfying aspects of the relationships
      d. Changes in the relationships that the patient wants to make
  C. Identification of major problem areas
    1. Determine the problem area related to current depression and set the treatment goals.
    2. Determine which relationship or aspect of a relationship is related to the depression and what might change in it.
  D. Explanation of the IPT concepts and contract
    1. Outline your understanding of the problem.
    2. Agree on treatment goals (i.e., which problem area will be the focus).
    3. Describe procedures of IPT, including "here and now" focus and the need for patient to discuss important concerns; review of current interpersonal relations; and practical aspects of treatment, such as length, frequency, times, fees, and policy for missed appointments.
II. Intermediate sessions: the problem areas
  A. Grief
    Goals
    1. Facilitate the mourning process.
    2. Help the patient reestablish interest and relationships to substitute for what has been lost.
    Strategies
    1. Review depressive symptoms.
    2. Relate symptom onset to death of significant other.
    3. Reconstruct the patient's relationship with the deceased.
    4. Describe the sequence and consequences of events just prior to, during, and after the death.

Table 1–1.   Outline of interpersonal psychotherapy *(continued)*

5. Explore associated feelings (negative as well as positive).
6. Help patient consider possible ways of becoming involved with others.

B. Interpersonal disputes

Goals
1. Identify dispute.
2. Choose plan of action.
3. Modify expectations or faulty communication to bring about a satisfactory resolution.

Strategies
1. Review depressive symptoms.
2. Relate symptoms' onset to overt or covert dispute with significant other with whom patient is currently involved.
3. Determine stage of dispute:
   a. Renegotiation (Calm down participants to facilitate resolution.)
   b. Impasse (Increase disharmony in order to reopen negotiation.)
   c. Dissolution (Assist mourning.)
4. Understand how nonreciprocal role expectations relate to dispute:
   a. What are the issues in the dispute?
   b. What are differences in expectations and values?
   c. What are the options?
   d. What is the likelihood of finding alternatives?
   e. What resources are available to bring about change in the relationship?
5. Are there parallels in other relationships?
   a. What is the patient gaining?
   b. What unspoken assumptions lie behind the patient's behavior?
6. How is the dispute perpetuated?

C. Role transitions

Goals
1. Facilitate mourning and acceptance of the loss of the old role.
2. Help the patient to regard the new role as more positive.
3. Help the patient to restore self-esteem by developing a sense of mastery regarding demands of new roles.

Strategies
1. Review depressive symptoms.
2. Relate depressive symptoms to difficulty in coping with some recent life change.
3. Review positive and negative aspects of old and new roles.
4. Explore feelings about what is lost.
5. Explore feelings about the change itself.

Table 1–1.   Outline of interpersonal psychotherapy *(continued)*

---

   6. Explore opportunities in new role.
   7. Realistically evaluate what is lost.
   8. Encourage appropriate release of affect.
   9. Encourage development of social support system and of new skills called for in new role.
  D. Interpersonal deficits
     <u>Goals</u>
   1. Reduce the patient's social isolation.
   2. Encourage formation of new relationships.
     <u>Strategies</u>
   1. Review depressive symptoms.
   2. Relate depressive symptoms to problems of social isolation or unfulfillment.
   3. Review past significant relationships including their negative and positive aspects.
   4. Explore repetitive patterns in relationships.
   5. Discuss patient's positive and negative feelings about the therapist and seek parallels in other relationships.
III. Termination
   1. Explicitly discuss termination.
   2. Acknowledge that termination is a time of grieving.
   3. Help patient move toward recognition of independent competence.
IV. Specific techniques
   1. Exploratory
   2. Encouragement of affect
   3. Clarification
   4. Communication analysis
   5. Use of therapeutic relationships
   6. Behavior-change techniques
   7. Adjunctive techniques
V. Therapist's role
   1. Therapist is patient advocate, not neutral.
   2. Therapist is active, not passive.
   3. Therapeutic relationship is not interpreted as transference.
   4. Therapeutic relationship is not a friendship.

---

intensive (i.e., monthly) sessions for maintenance treatment for severe recurrent depression has been developed (Frank et al. 1989; also see Chapter 4). Even within this maintenance treatment format, IPT is time limited in that a specific time contract is made with the patient at the onset. Although long-term, more intensive, open-ended treatment may still by required for recognition of maladaptive interpersonal and cognitive patterns and for amelioration of dysfunctional social skills, evidence for the efficacy of long-term psychotherapy is not yet available. There are no published clinical trials indicating the efficacy of any psychotherapy for personality problems. Moreover, long-term intensive treatment may promote dependence and reinforce avoidance behavior. Psychotherapies that are short-term with specific goals or long-term but not intensive may minimize these adverse effects for some depressed patients.

Interpersonal psychotherapy is focused and not nondirective, addressing one or two problem areas in the patient's current interpersonal functioning. The focus is agreed on by the patient and the psychotherapist after initial evaluation sessions. The topical content of sessions is, therefore, not open ended.

Dealing with current, not past, interpersonal relationships, IPT focuses on the patient's immediate social context just before and as it has been since the onset of the current depressive episode. Past depressive episodes, early family relationships, previous significant relationships, and friendship patterns are assessed in order to understand overall patterns in the patient's interpersonal relations. The psychotherapist does not frame the patient's current situation as a manifestation of internal conflict or as a recurrence of prior intrafamilial maladaptive patterns, but rather explores the patient's current disorder in terms of interpersonal relations.

IPT and Psychodynamic Psychotherapy

In discussing the similarities between IPT and other forms of psychotherapy, the most frequently asked questions deal with the relationship of IPT to psychodynamic psychotherapy.

The term *psychodynamic psychotherapy* refers to a general approach to psychotherapy derived from psychoanalysis. The theoretical structure of psychoanalysis forms the background for the dynamic approach to psychiatry, with emphasis on the role of unconscious mental processes, early childhood experiences, and libidinous and structural changes in personality through childhood, adolescence, and adulthood. Psychodynamic psychotherapy has emerged as a derivative of the dynamic approach, modifying many of the therapeutic techniques of classical psychoanalysis for application to a variety of clinical conditions and personality difficulties. In contrast to psychoanalysis, in psychodynamic psychotherapy the patient does not lie on the couch and is usually seen one or two times a week. The essential features of psychodynamic psychotherapy include the following:

1. Primacy is given to transference reactions and their resolution in the psychotherapeutic process.
2. Symptoms and difficulties in social functioning are seen as derivative of deeper, more fundamental unresolved personality difficulties or character problems.
3. Efforts are made to uncover unconscious mental processes—wishes, fantasies, defenses—through use of free-association techniques, dreams, and exploration of fantasies.
4. Major effort is given to reconstruction of intrafamilial interpersonal relationships during infancy, childhood, and adolescence. Adult difficulties are seen as the recapitulation of unresolved issues in childhood.

In psychodynamic psychotherapy a clinical depression may be regarded as a regressive state precipitated by an experience interpreted by the patient as a loss. Thus, the symptoms of clinical depression bear many similarities to normal mourning, grief, and bereavement. However, as Freud has pointed out in his classic paper "Mourning and Melancholia" (1917[1915]/1957), there are important differences between melancholia, or clinical depression, and mourning. One difference is the permanent role of guilt in the psychic experience of the depressed patient, and this is related by Freud and other psychoanalysts to the important role of retroflection of hostility against the self. Rage, anger, and aggressive drive, unconsciously directed against the lost object, are turned against the self, which leads to self-reproach, despair, hopelessness, and, ultimately, suicide attempts and death. According to the psychodynamic view, the depressed patient has had an excessively strong superego (conscious) preceding the onset of a clinical depression, and this character feature contributes to the patient's sense of worthlessness, shame, guilt, self-reproach, and feelings of failure and inadequacy.

The interpersonal relations of the depressed individual, according to the psychodynamic view, are characterized by excess dependency, which has its origin in childhood. In this view, common depression is regarded not as a primary affect but rather as a derivative of hostility. Hostility and instinctual aggression are transformed by the activities of the superego-conscience and are experienced as depression, guilt, and self-reproach. The goals of psychodynamically oriented treatment for depression are to uncover these unconscious conflicts and to modify the rage and hostility so as to free the ego for a more independent, autonomous functioning. This may require long periods of intensive therapy, perhaps including periods of hospitalization if regression is severe or suicidal trends emerge.

In contrast, in the interpersonal approach to psychotherapy, depressive affect is regarded as a normal state, a biologically based emotional response common to all mammals, primates, and humans, having had significant evolutionary value in the development of the species, particularly given the immature state with which the human infant is born and the need for a prolonged period of protection, nurturance, and succor. Thus, dependency upon the mothering parental figure is a normal aspect of childhood and infant development, and autonomy and independence emerge only gradually. Disruption of attachment bonds in infancy and thereafter precipitates a characteristic pattern response that we identify as sadness or depression. The origins of clinical depression are not known with precision; there are probably several causes, including hereditary as well as experiential components. IPT, as stated before, focuses on rapid symptom reduction and the promotion of social adjustment and the facilitation of interpersonal relations.

IPT and Cognitive Therapy

Interpersonal psychotherapy and cognitive therapy, both of which have been developed specifically for depression, are time-limited therapies. Both have manuals specifying the procedures, and each modality has undergone testing in a number of controlled, clinical trials.

Interpersonal psychotherapy and cognitive therapy differ in theory and procedure. Cognitive therapy derives from the phenomenological school of psychology, which assumes that the individual's view of self determines behavior. Following from that, cognitive therapy for depression is based on the assumption that the affective response in depression is determined by the way an individual structures his or her experience ideationally (Beck 1976). As a result of an emergence of certain maladaptive cognitive themes, the depressed patient tends to regard himself or herself and his or her future in a negative way. Correction of negative concepts is expected to alleviate the depressive symptoms. For example, a person with an extremely low self concept can be treated by presenting a hierarchy of cognitive tasks and, through these tasks, demonstrating the invalidity of the patient's self-reproaches.

The cognitive therapist clarifies how the patient views things, the bases for these views, and their accuracies and consequences. The empirical testing for the patient is encouraged by the cognitive therapist through homework assignments, graded tasks, and clarification of assumptions. IPT does not engage the patient in graded tasks or homework but rather deals with the patient's negative self-images by attempting to understand his or her interpersonal context or by viewing the self-images as part of the symptoms picture, which will be alleviated as the interpersonal problems are resolved. In contrast, cognitive therapy challenges the negative self-images directly.

Conducting Research on Interpersonal Psychotherapy for Acute Depression

Specification of Treatment by Manual

Psychotherapy manuals that specify the main procedure of the psychotherapy being tested are now required for clinical trials of psychotherapy. These manuals enhance the consistency and reliability of psychotherapy procedures among psychotherapies and facilitate training. Manuals specify the aims, tasks, and sequence of procedures, and the tasks are operationalized; scripts and case examples may be supplemented by videotapes of actual sessions. The first manuals were designed by the behavior therapists (Lewisohn 1980). It was the ability of the behavioral investigators to specify intervention such as desensitization and implosion with precision that gave impetus to the field. Beck developed the first comprehensive manual specifically for the treatment (using cognitive therapy) of depression (Beck et al. 1979). Since then, many manuals have been developed.

Treatment manuals are not just applicable to psychotherapy. Fawcett and Epstein (1987) have developed a manual for the administration of pharmacotherapy. Rounsaville et al. (1988) have shown that IPT therapists were able to adhere to the manual over the course of the 16-week National Institute of Mental Health (NIMH) Treatment of Depression Collaborative Research Program. DeRubeis et al. (1982) and Hollon et al. (1984) have shown that blind raters were able to differentiate between IPT and cognitive therapies and clinical management (see Rounsaville et al. 1988 for review).

It should be emphasized that specifying the psychotherapy or differentiating between psychotherapies and procedures is a necessary requirement for studying their efficacy through controlled clinical trials, but it is not evidence or indication of efficacy. Psychotherapies that have very different procedures may have similar outcomes. This finding does not, however, necessarily negate the value of specifying the different procedures. The situation is comparable to pharmacotherapies in which drugs with somewhat different chemical structures may have similar effects on reducing depressive symptoms. Yet, individual patient variation, side effects, or timing of onset of action makes it advantageous to have more than one tricyclic antidepressant or serotonergic uptake blocker.

Selection of Psychotherapists for Research

A key to the success of training is the selection of the proper psychotherapist. In the NIMH Treatment of Depression Collaborative Research Program, the psychotherapist applicants were prescreened to meet certain preliminary selection criteria. The initial requirements included fully qualified psychiatrists or Ph.D. clinical psychologists (although social workers would have been suitable), with a minimum of 2 years of clinical experience following completion of their training; training in a psychodynamic framework; treatment of a minimum of 10 depressed patients in psychotherapy; and, finally, willingness to submit a videotape of their psychotherapy sessions with a depressed patient, using their customary treatment approach. Each prospective therapist was interviewed as part of a pre-screening procedure in which some assessment was made of his or her overall clinical experience, commitment to the approach, and general suitability (Chevron et al. 1983).

The psychotherapists' videotapes were reviewed by three independent evaluators who evaluated each therapist's potential, blind to his or her credentials and professional training. Agreement between independent evaluators was excellent, and the one variable that differentiated therapists from this already highly screened pool was experience. Psychotherapists with over 10 years of experience, regardless of discipline, were independently rated more highly by the three evaluators.

Efforts to identify the characteristics of the therapist that are most promising as predictors of patients' outcome in psychotherapy have not yielded replicated results. The results of this one study suggested that selection criteria should be specified and that attention should be paid to the therapist's level of experience.

Training of Psychotherapists for IPT Research

Standardized training programs based on manual-specific procedures for the psychotherapy being tested are also a requirement for efficacy studies of psychotherapies. The training programs that are developed for psychotherapy clinical trials are not designed to teach inexperienced persons how to become therapists, or to teach fundamental skills such as empathy, handling of transference, or timing. They are instead designed to modify practices of fully trained, competent therapists to conduct the psychotherapy under study as specified in the manual. The goal is to develop a shared language and a specified procedure in an agreed-upon sequence among the therapists participating in the trial.

If there is a careful selection of the therapist—namely, those experienced in psychotherapy and committed to the particular approach to be tested—then training can be brief. The sequence adopted in the NIMH Treatment of Depression Collaborative Research Program (Elkin et al. 1989), which has become a model for subsequent studies (Frank et al. 1990b), includes a brief didactic phase in which the manual is reviewed. This is followed by a longer, supervised practicum component during which the therapist treats patients under supervision, monitored by actual videotapes of the sessions (Rounsaville et al. 1986, 1988; Weissman et al.

1982). Rounsaville et al. (1986) subsequently demonstrated that therapists who performed well on their first supervised case did not require further intensive supervision.

Evaluating the Quality of the IPT Psychotherapist

Chevron and Rounsaville (1983) evaluated different methods for assessing psychotherapy skills during a clinical trial of IPT: didactic examinations, global ratings by trainers, supervised ratings based on psychotherapists' retrospective process notes, therapists' self-ratings, and independent evaluators' ratings of observation of actual psychotherapy sessions as video-recorded. The results showed poor agreement among the assessment of therapists' skills based on the different sources. More importantly, ratings based on the review of the videotape sessions were not correlated with those based on the process notes. Of the five types of ratings of psychotherapists' skill, only the supervisors' ratings of the actual videotape sessions were correlated with patient outcome. It was concluded that therapists' self-ratings may serve an important function in encouraging therapists to think about their work in terms of prescribed techniques and strategies, but these ratings may be biased. Supervisors' ratings that are based on the process notes seem to reflect patient improvement rather than therapists' expertise. Results of this study show the importance of using video- or audiotape review of actual therapy sessions in the clinical training. The results also raise questions about the customary reliance on process reporting as a sole basis on which to make judgments about a therapist's skills. Certification criteria for the therapist should be developed and applied, following the training period. An evaluation of whether the therapist has met these criteria and can be certified should be carried out.

In the NIMH Treatment of Depression Collaborative Research Program, certification was carried out by an independent evaluator, a highly experienced IPT therapist who viewed the videotapes of the training sessions and determined whether the therapist had met competence criteria. Independent monitoring of selected videotapes throughout the course of the clinical trial ensured that the quality and standards of the therapy were being maintained. If there was therapist drift, supervisory sessions were held. In all cases, the manual was the guide and was used as the standard to which the therapist adhered.

Efficacy of Interpersonal
Psychotherapy for Depression

Interpersonal psychotherapy has been evaluated in a number of studies for depression both as acute and as maintenance treatment. These controlled clinical trials provide the foundation for clinical practice utilizing IPT and for efforts to modify IPT for application to other clinical conditions.

Interpersonal psychotherapy has been tested alone and in comparison and in combination with tricyclics in six clinical trials with depressed patients—three of acute treatment (Elkin et al. 1989; Sloane et al. 1985; Weissman et al. 1979) and three of maintenance treatment (Klerman et al. 1974; Kupfer et al. 1989; Reynolds and Imber 1988; Weissman et al. 1974).

Five completed studies have included a drug comparison group (Elkin et al. 1989; Klerman et al. 1974; Kupfer et al. 1989; Reynolds and Imber 1988; Sloane et al. 1985; Weissman et al. 1979), and four have included a combination of IPT and drugs (Klerman et al. 1974; Kupfer et al. 1989; Reynolds and Imber 1988; Weissman et al. 1979).

Acute Treatment Studies

There have been two controlled trials of the use of IPT in the treatment of acute depressive episodes in adults: the New Haven–Boston Collaborative Study of the Treatment of Acute Depression and the NIMH Treatment of Depression Collaborative Research Program.

The New Haven–Boston Collaborative Study of the Treatment of Acute Depression

The first study of IPT for the treatment of acute depression was initiated in 1973. It was a 16-week treatment study of 81 ambulatory depressed patients, both men and women, using IPT and amitriptyline each alone and in combination against a nonscheduled psychotherapy treatment (DiMascio et al. 1979; Weissman et al. 1979). IPT was administered weekly by experienced psychiatrists. This study demonstrated that both active treatments, IPT and the tricyclic, were more effective than the control treatment and that combined treatment was superior to either treatment alone.

In addition, a 1-year follow-up study provided evidence that the therapeutic benefit of IPT was sustained for many patients. Patients who had received IPT either alone or in combination with drugs were functioning better than patients who had received either drugs alone or the control treatment (Weissman et al. 1981). At the 1-year follow-up, there was no effect of IPT on symptom relapse or recurrence. A fraction of patients in all treatments relapsed, and additional treatment was required.

National Institute of Mental Health Treatment of Depression Collaborative Research Program

A multicenter, controlled, clinical trial of drugs and two psychotherapies, cognitive therapy and IPT, in the treatment of acute ambulatory depression was initiated by the NIMH (Elkin et al. 1989). A group of outpatients ($N = 250$) were randomly assigned to four treatment conditions—cognitive therapy, IPT, imipramine, and a placebo–clinical management combination—for 16 weeks. Extensive efforts were made in the selection and training of the psychotherapists. Of the 250 patients who entered treatment, 68% completed at least 15 weeks and 12 sessions of treatment. Overall, the findings showed that all active treatments were superior to placebo in the reduction of symptoms over a 16-week period. The overall degree of improvement for all patients, regardless of treatment, was highly significant clinically, and over half of the patients were symptom free at the end of treatment.

More patients in the placebo–clinical management condition (in fact, twice as many as for IPT, which had the lowest attrition rate) dropped out or were withdrawn. At the end of 12 weeks of treatment, the two psychotherapies and imipramine were equivalent in the reduction of depressive symptoms on many measures. Imipramine had a more rapid initial onset of action and more consistent differences from placebo than either of the two psychotherapies.

Although many of the patients who were less severely depressed at intake improved with all treatment conditions, including the placebo group, more severely depressed patients in the placebo group did poorly. For the less severely depressed group, there were no differences among the treatments. Forty-four percent of the sample were moderately depressed at intake. For the more severe group (Hamilton Rating Scale for Depression [Ham-D] score of 20 or more at intake), patients in the IPT and the imipramine groups had better outcome scores than did the placebo group on the Ham-D. Of the psychotherapies, only IPT was significantly superior to placebo for the severely depressed group. For the severely depressed patients, IPT was as effective as imipramine on some outcome measures. The statistical approach used in these analyses was controversial, and reanalysis has been undertaken. Thus, more information on this study is forthcoming.

IPT as Maintenance Treatment for Depression

With increased knowledge of the natural history and clinical course of depression, it became apparent to the investigators that many patients have recurrences and relapses and require long-term treatment. There have been two randomized controlled trials evaluating the role of long-term IPT as maintenance treatment: the New Haven–Boston Maintenance Treatment Study and the Pittsburgh Study of Maintenance Treatment of Recurrent Depression.

The New Haven–Boston Maintenance Treatment Study

The first systematic study of IPT, begun in 1968, was of maintenance treatment (Klerman et al. 1974; Paykel et al. 1976). By today's standards this study would be considered a continuation study. The protocol was designed to determine how long treatment with tricyclic antidepressants should continue and what the role of psychotherapy was in maintenance treatment.

A group of acutely depressed outpatients ($N = 150$) who had responded to amitriptyline with symptom reduction were studied. Each patient received 8 months of maintenance treatment with pharmacotherapy alone, psychotherapy (i.e., IPT) alone, or a combination of both. The major findings of this study were that maintenance drug treatment prevented relapse (Klerman et al. 1974) and that the effect of IPT was on enhancing social functioning (Weissman et al. 1974). Moreover, the effects of psychotherapy were not apparent for 6 to 8 months. Because of the differential effects of the treatments being studied, the combination of drugs and psychotherapy was the most efficacious (Klerman et al. 1974; Paykel et al. 1976), and no negative interactions between drugs and psychotherapy were found.

The Pittsburgh Study of Maintenance Treatment of Recurrent Depression

In the early 1980s, the University of Pittsburgh group designed and initiated a long-term clinical trial to determine the efficacy of drugs (imipramine) and/or IPT in the prevention of relapse for severe recurrent depression (Frank et al. 1990b; see Chapter 4 for full details). The impetus for this study was the finding that there were a large number of patients with multiple recurrent episodes who were difficult to treat, had a high relapse rate, and frequently utilized medical and social services. In this study patients with recurrent depression (i.e., at least two previous episodes of major depression) who had responded to imipramine plus IPT were randomly assigned to one of five treatments for 3 years of maintenance treatment: 1) IPT alone, 2) IPT and placebo, 3) IPT and imipramine, 4) clinical management and imipramine, and 5) clinical management and placebo. Contrary to previous experience, imipramine was administered in the *highest* doses (over 200 mg), and IPT was administered monthly in the *lowest* dose ever used in clinical trials.

The major findings were that there were 1) a high rate of recurrence in 1 year for untreated control groups; 2) a clinically meaningful and statistically significant prevention of relapse and recurrence by both imipramine and IPT; 3) a nonsignificant trend toward value of combined treatment over either treatment alone. The value of this study was enhanced by the fact that it involved high-dose imipramine (over 200 mg/day) (previously considerably lower maintenance doses had been recommended) and the lowest dose of IPT ever used (i.e., monthly). This long-term study, along with several others using drugs with and without psychotherapy, clearly established the value of maintenance treatment in the prevention of relapse and recurrence in major depression.

New Applications
of Interpersonal Psychotherapy

Since IPT was developed, new applications have appeared and will be subjects in this volume. IPT has been tested in a conjoint format for depressed patients with marital disputes (Foley et al. 1989; see Chapter 5); for patients who are in distress but not clinically depressed (interpersonal counseling; see Klerman et al. 1987; Weissman and Klerman 1988; also see Chapter 11); for long-term maintenance treatment of patients with recurrent depression (Frank et al. 1989, 1990b; see Chapter 4); for elderly persons (Frank et al. 1988; Reynolds and Imber 1988; see Chapter 7); for depressed medically ill patients in primary care (see Chapter 10); for patients addicted to opiates (Rounsaville et al. 1983; see Chapter 12); for patients who abuse cocaine (Carroll et al. 1992; Rounsaville and Kleber 1985; Rounsaville et al. 1985); and for patients with bulimia (Fairburn 1988; Fairburn et al. 1991; see Chapter 13). In addition, IPT has been adapted for HIV-positive patients with depression (see Chapter 8); for depressed adolescents (Moreau et al. 1991); and for patients with dysthymia (see Chapter 9). Trials are underway or being planned for these populations.[3]

Conclusions

Most trials of IPT have been for the ambulatory depressed patient, as acute and as maintenance treatment. The findings for conjoint marital treatment, as well as for primary care patients in distress and for persons with bulimia, are promising, but the results are still based on small samples, as will be described in later chapters. The adaptation and testing of IPT for geriatric patients with recurrent depression, depressed adolescents, HIV-seropositive patients, and dysthymic patients are still underway. The findings on IPT as a treatment for persons who abuse drugs, either cocaine or opiates, are largely negative, although further testing in select samples from other sites may be warranted.

Although the positive findings of the clinical trials of IPT in the NIMH Treatment of Depression Collaborative Research Program and other studies described are encouraging, there are limitations. These studies of IPT, including those by our group and by the NIMH, were conducted on

---

[3] Not included in this volume because of their early stage of development is the new work by Frank et al. (1990a) at the Department of Psychiatry, University of Pittsburgh for bipolar patients; the work of M. O'Hara of the Department of Psychology at the University of Iowa, who is modifying IPT for the acute treatment of depressed women with postpartum depression; and the work of Laurie A. Gillies of the Clarke Institute of Psychiatry in Toronto, who is modifying IPT for personality disorder.

ambulatory depressed patients. Moreover, these results should not be interpreted as implying that all forms of psychotherapy are effective for treatment of depression or, alternatively, that only IPT is effective. One significant feature of recent advances in psychotherapy research is in the development of psychotherapies specifically designed for depression—that is, time-limited and of brief duration. Just as there are specific forms of medication, there are specific forms of psychotherapy. Just as it would be an error to conclude that all forms of medication are useful for treatment of all types of depression, so it would be an error to conclude that all forms of psychotherapy are efficacious for all forms of depression.

In regard to the findings for depression, we conclude that many, but not all, treatments may be effective for depression. The depressed patient's interests are best served by the availability and scientific testing of different psychological as well as pharmacological treatments to be used alone or in combination. Ultimately, clinical testing and experience will determine which is the best treatment for that particular patient.

References

Beck A: Cognitive Therapy and the Emotional Disorders. New York, International Universities Press, 1976

Beck AT, Rush AJ, Shaw BF, et al: Cognitive Theory of Depression. New York, Guilford, 1979

Bowlby J: Attachment and Loss, Vol 1: Attachment. London, Hogarth Press, 1969

Brown GW, Harris T: Social Origins of Depression: A Study of Psychiatric Disorder in Women. New York, Free Press, 1978

Carroll KM, Rounsaville BJ, Gawin FH: A comparative trial of psychotherapies for ambulatory cocaine abusers: relapse prevention and interpersonal psychotherapy. Am J Drug Alcohol Abuse 17:229–247, 1992

Chevron E, Rounsaville BJ: Evaluating the clinical skills of psychotherapists: a comparison of techniques. Arch Gen Psychiatry 40:1129–1132, 1983

Chevron E, Rounsaville B, Rothblum ED, et al: Selecting psychotherapists to participate in psychotherapy outcome studies: relationship between psychotherapist characteristics and assessment of clinical skills. J Nerv Ment Dis 171:348–353, 1983

DeRubeis RJ, Hollon SD, Evans MD, et al: Can psychotherapies for depression be discriminated? A systematic investigation of cognitive therapy and interpersonal therapy. J Consult Clin Psychol 50:744–756, 1982

DiMascio A, Weissman MM, Prusoff BA, et al: Differential symptom reduction by drugs and psychotherapy in acute depression. Arch Gen Psychiatry 36:1450–1456, 1979

Elkin I, Shea MT, Watkins JT, et al: National Institute of Mental Health Treatment of Depression Collaborative Research Program: general effectiveness of treatment. Arch Gen Psychiatry 46:971–983, 1989

Fairburn CG: The current status of the psychological treatments for bulimia nervosa. J Psychosom Res 32:635–645, 1988

Fairburn CG, Jones R, Peveler RC, et al: Three psychological treatments for bulimia nervosa: a comparative trial. Arch Gen Psychiatry 48:463–469, 1991

Fawcett J, Epstein P: Clinical management of imipramine and placebo administration. Psychopharmacol Bull 23:309–324, 1987

Foley SH, Rounsaville BJ, Weissman MM, et al: Individual versus conjoint interpersonal psychotherapy for depressed patients with marital disputes. International Journal of Family Psychiatry 10:29–42, 1989

Frank E, Frank N, Reynolds CF: Manual for the Adaptation of Interpersonal Psychotherapy to Maintenance Treatment of Recurrent Depression in Late Life (IPT-LLM). Pittsburgh, PA, University of Pittsburgh School of Medicine, May 1988

Frank E, Kupfer DF, Perel JM: Early recurrence in unipolar depression. Arch Gen Psychiatry 46:397–400, 1989

Frank E, Kupfer DJ, Cornes C, et al: Manual for the Adaptation of Interpersonal Psychotherapy to the Treatment of Bipolar Disorder (IPT-BP). Pittsburgh, PA, University of Pittsburgh, June 1990a

Frank E, Kupfer DF, Perel JM, et al: Three-year outcomes for maintenance therapies in recurrent depression. Arch Gen Psychiatry 47:1093–1099, 1990b

Freud S: Mourning and melancholia (1917[1915]), in The Standard Edition of the Complete Psychological Works of Sigmund Freud, Vol 14. Translated and edited by Strachey J. London, Hogarth Press, 1957, pp 237–260

Henderson S, Byrne DG, Duncan-Jones P, et al: Social bonds in the epidemiology of neurosis. Br J Psychiatry 132:463–466, 1978

Hollon SD, Evans MD, Elkin I, et al: System rating therapies for depression. Paper presented at the annual meeting of the American Psychiatric Association, Los Angeles, CA, May 1984

Klerman GL, DiMascio A, Weissman, et al: Treatment of depression by drugs and psychotherapy. Am J Psychiatry 131:186–194, 1974

Klerman GL, Weissman MM, Rounsaville BJ, et al: Interpersonal Psychotherapy for Depression. New York, Basic Books, 1984

Klerman GL, Budman S, Berwick D, et al: Efficacy of a brief psychosocial intervention for symptoms of stress and distress among patients in primary care. Med Care 25:1078–1088, 1987

Kupfer DJ, Frank E, Perel JM: The advantage of early treatment intervention in recurrent depression. Arch Gen Psychiatry 46:771–775, 1989

Lewisohn PM: A behavioral approach to depression, in The Psychology of Depression: Contemporary Theory and Research. Edited by Friedman RJ, Katz MM. Washington, DC, Wiley, 1980, pp 2–12

Meyer A: Psychobiology: A Science of Man. Springfield, IL, Charles C Thomas, 1957

Moreau D, Mufson L, Weissman MM, et al: Interpersonal psychotherapy for adolescent depression: description of modification and preliminary application. J Am Acad Child Adolesc Psychiatry 30:642–651, 1991

Paykel ES, DiMascio A, Klerman GL, et al: Maintenance therapy of depression. Pharmakopsychiatrie Neuropsychopharmakologie 9:127–136, 1976

Pearlin LI, Lieberman MA: Social sources of emotional distress, in Research in Community and Mental Health, Vol 1. Edited by Simmons R. Greenwich, CT, JAI Publishing, 1979, pp 217–248

Reynolds C, Imber S: Maintenance Therapies in Latelife Depression (DHHS Publ No MH-43832). Bethesda, MD, National Institute of Mental Health, 1988

Rounsaville BJ, Kleber HD: Psychotherapy/counseling for opiate addicts: strategies for use in different treatment settings. Int J Addict 20:869–896, 1985

Rounsaville BJ, Glazer W, Wilber CH, et al: Short-term interpersonal psychotherapy in methadone-maintained opiate addicts. Arch Gen Psychiatry 40:629–636, 1983

Rounsaville BJ, Gawin F, Kleber H: Interpersonal psychotherapy adapted for ambulatory cocaine abusers. Am J Drug Alcohol Abuse 11(3/4):171–191, 1985

Rounsaville BJ, Chevron ES, Weissman MM, et al: Training therapists to perform interpersonal psychotherapy in clinical trials. Compr Psychiatry 27:364–371, 1986

Rounsaville BJ, O'Malley S, Foley S, et al: Role of manual-guided training in the conduct and efficacy of interpersonal psychotherapy for depression. J Consult Clin Psychol 56:681–688, 1988

Sloane RB, Stapes FR, Schneider LS: Interpersonal therapy versus nortriptyline for depression in the elderly, in Clinical and Pharmacological Studies in Psychiatric Disorders. Edited by Burrows GD, Norman TR, Dennerstein L. London, John Libbey, 1985, pp 344–346

Sullivan HS: The Interpersonal Theory of Psychiatry. New York, WW Norton, 1953

Weissman MM: Advances in psychiatric epidemiology: rates and risks for major depression. Am J Public Health 77:445–451, 1987

Weissman MM, Klerman GL: Interpersonal Counseling (IPC) for Stress and Distress in Primary Care Settings. New York, College of Physicians and Surgeons, Columbia University and Cornell Medical School, March 1988

Weissman MM, Klerman GL, Paykel ES, et al: Treatment effects on the social adjustment of depressed patients. Arch Gen Psychiatry 30:771–778, 1974

Weissman MM, Prusoff BA, DiMascio A, et al: The efficacy of drugs and psychotherapy in the treatment of acute depressive episodes. Am J Psychiatry 136:555–558, 1979

Weissman MM, Klerman GL, Prusoff BA, et al: Depressed outpatients: results one year after treatment with drugs and/or interpersonal psychotherapy. Arch Gen Psychiatry 38:52–55, 1981

Weissman MM, Rounsaville BJ, Chevron ES: Training psychotherapists to participate in psychotherapy outcome studies: identifying and dealing with the research requirement. Am J Psychiatry 139:1442–1446, 1982

Depression:
Recent Research and
Clinical Advances

Myrna M. Weissman, Ph.D.
Gerald L. Klerman, M.D.

Interpersonal psychotherapy (IPT) was initially developed as a brief treatment for acute depression. Most of the new applications of IPT developed over the past decade involve variants of mood disorder other than acute major depression—for example, recurrent depression, dysthymia, depression comorbid with other conditions, or depression in special populations such as adolescents and the elderly. An adaptation of IPT for bipolar disorder is in preparation.

As new applications for IPT were being developed, there was an acceleration in our understanding of the epidemiology of mood disorders, including bipolar disorder, major depression, and dysthymia. There is clearer understanding of the rates and risk factors of these disorders, of

Preparation of this chapter was supported in part by Grants MH-43525, MH-28274, and MH-43077 from the National Institute of Mental Health and the John D. and Catherine T. MacArthur Foundation. Permission to reproduce the following has been obtained: a portion from M. M. Weissman "Epidemiology Overview," in *Psychiatry Update: American Psychiatric Association Annual Review, Vol. 6.* Edited by Hales RE, Frances AI. 574-588, 1987; portions of G. L. Klerman, M. M. Weissman, "Increasing Rates of Depression," *JAMA* 261:2229–2235, 1989; tabular material from S. Moldin, T. Reich, J. Rice, "Current Perspectives on the Genetics of Unipolar Depression," *Behavior Genetics* 21:211–242, 1991. Permission has also been granted to reproduce major portions of M.M. Weissman, G.L. Klerman "Depression: Current Understanding and Changing Trends," in the *Annual Review of Public Health*, Vol. 13, 1992.

comorbidity and social morbidity, and of the changing patterns, nationally and cross-nationally. Notions about the age at onset of these disorders have changed considerably (Christie et al. 1988). It is now recognized that depression can occur prepubertally and often begins in adolescence, and that family history (i.e., the presence of a mood disorder in a first-degree biological relative) is one of the most important risk factors. Considerable data, based on controlled clinical trials, are now available on the efficacy of a broad range of pharmacological and psychotherapeutic treatments, acute and maintenance, for the various types of mood disorders.

In this chapter we review the advances over the past decade in understanding the epidemiology, familial nature, pharmacological treatment, and morbidity of mood disorders. This material is presented as background because the initial phase of IPT involves educating the patient about the disorder. This information will, of course, require updating as new findings emerge.

Diagnosis and Classification

Mood disorders refers to a group of clinical conditions whose common feature is the presentation by the patient of disturbed mood, either depression or elation. This distinction does not imply a common etiology. It is likely that the mood disorders are biologically heterogeneous comparable to the situation for mental retardation or jaundice. The major distinction in mood disorders is between bipolar and the depressive disorders and between, within the depressive disorders, major depression and dysthymia.

The concept of a mood disorder (sometimes called *affective disorder*) itself is worthy of note. This chapter could not have been written two decades ago. The conditions that are today grouped together as mood disorders were treated separately in DSM-II (American Psychiatric Association 1968) as part of either psychosis or neurosis, the two predominant psychiatric categories in the 1960s.

Over the past decade, diagnostic criteria have been specified for the major mental disorders. These criteria, which are based on type, number, frequency, and duration of symptoms as well as on exclusions, were codified in 1980 in DSM-III (American Psychiatric Association 1980). Minor revisions were made in the classification and were published in 1987 as DSM-III-R (American Psychiatric Association 1987). A further revision, DSM-IV, will appear in late 1993.

In DSM-III, the distinction between psychotic and neurotic conditions was abolished, and a number of depressive conditions, first called affective and then mood disorders in DSM-III-R, were brought together. The separation of depressions into bipolar and major depression is widely accepted because of differences in family patterns, effective treatment, and natural course.

A broad outline of the DSM-III-R classification of mood disorders is given in Table 2–1. Each disorder can be further classified by severity, whether it is in remission, or whether psychotic features are present, and each has a category ["Not Otherwise Specified (NOS)"] for patients who typically do not fit the criteria for subclassification. Each diagnosis has specified criteria, and criteria for the major categories are given below.

Bipolar Disorder

The presence of *mania* defines bipolar disorder. Mania is a distinct period when the predominant mood is either elevated, expansive, or irritable and when there are associated symptoms, including hyperactivity, pressure of speech, racing thoughts, inflated self-esteem, decreased need for sleep, distractibility, and excessive involvement in activities that have high potential for painful consequences. Mania without major depression, sometimes called "unipolar" mania, is uncommon but does occur.

Table 2–1.   DSM-III-R classification of mood disorders

Bipolar disorder	Depressive disorders
Mixed	Major depression
Manic	—single episode
Depressed	—recurrent
Cyclothymia	Dysthymia
Bipolar disorder (NOS)	—primary or secondary
	—early or late onset
	Depressive disorder (NOS)

Note. NOS = not otherwise specified.

Bipolar disorder can present as either a manic or a depressive state. *Cyclothymia* is a mild chronic form of mood swings and is of interest because of its aggregation in the biological relatives of patients with bipolar disorder. For this reason, it is considered to be part of the spectrum of bipolar disorder. However, it is often difficult to differentiate the boundaries between cyclothymia and normal moods.

Individual Depressive Disorders

Following DSM-III-R, there are a number of depressive disorders.

Major depression. The essential feature of major depression is either a dysphoric mood or a loss of interest or pleasure in all, or almost all, of usual activities and pastimes. The disturbance is prominent, relatively persistent, and associated with other symptoms, including appetite disturbance, change in weight, sleep disturbance, psychomotor agitation or retardation, decreased energy, feelings of worthlessness or guilt, difficulty concentrating or thinking, thoughts of death or suicide, and/or suicide attempts. Major depression is only diagnosed in the absence of manic symptoms (currently or in the past). There is general agreement that major depression is a heterogeneous disorder, and there is no consensus and little empirical basis for most of the subtypes used clinically such as endogenous, seasonal, or melancholic depression.

Dysthymia. The essential feature is a chronic disturbance in mood (involving either depressed mood or loss of interest or pleasure in all or almost all usual activities and pastimes) and associated symptoms, but not of sufficient severity or duration to meet the criteria for major depression. The primary distinction between dysthymia and major depression is that the former is chronic but symptomatically less severe, and it must persist for at least 2 years in order to meet the criteria. There is controversy as to whether dysthymia is an independent disorder or a variant of major depression. At least in some cases the dysthymia is probably prodromal of major depression or the residual of untreated major depression. At this point these issues have not been resolved, and in DSM-III-R dysthymia is categorized by whether it occurs as primary or secondary to another disorder and by patient age at onset, with age 21 being the division.

Depressive Symptoms (Minor Depression and Subclinical Depression)

There are a large number of patients who have depressive symptoms but do not meet the criteria for either dysthymia or major depression and do not have manic episodes. These patients often appear in primary care and medical clinics and are important from the public health point of view because of the high prevalence and disability among these patients. These depressive symptoms, which do not appear in the official DSM-III nomenclature, may be classified as an adjustment disorder if they occur within 3 months (but persisting no more than 6 months) of a major identifiable psychosocial stressor. The large number of patients with these symptoms represent a considerable social cost (Horwath et al. 1992; Johnson et al. 1992).

Epidemiology

With the exception of a few studies in Europe and Scandinavia, epidemiological approaches were infrequently applied to the study of psychiatric disorders in the community until the 1970s. The major obstacle to such studies was the lack of specification of the diagnostic criteria and the difficulty in obtaining reliable diagnoses.

The period after World War II in the United States was one of considerable activity in the epidemiology of mental impairment and health. Several classic epidemiological studies of this period were completed, including studies showing the relationship between social class and mental illness, the effects of changing traditions and values in a small town, and the effects of urban life. These studies demonstrated the importance of poverty, urban social stress, and social change in the development of impairment. The investigators used sophisticated statistical and sampling techniques but had at their disposal symptom or impairment scales that could not be used to generate rates of specific psychiatric disorders. The findings from these studies did not have a major impact on clinical psychiatry (Weissman 1987; Weissman and Klerman 1978).

Psychiatric epidemiology, clinical psychiatry, and clinical research did not begin to converge until the mid-1970s. The introduction into psychiatry of specified diagnostic criteria, along with standardized methods of assessing signs and symptoms of psychiatric disorders that were necessary to make the criteria, provided the technology for systematic diagnoses in epidemiological studies. There was considerable skepticism among epidemiological researchers as to the ability to use these methods in community studies. These methods were first applied in 1975 in a small community study of 500 subjects living in New Haven, Connecticut, and were shown to be feasible and reliable (Weissman and Myers 1978). In the late 1970s President Carter's Commission on Mental Health requested data on the magnitude of psychiatric illness in the community for planning mental health programs, which gave impetus to the next phase of studies.

In 1980 the National Institute of Mental Health (NIMH) Epidemiologic Catchment Area (ECA) study was initiated using the Diagnostic Interview Schedule (DIS), a new instrument developed specifically for large-scale epidemiological studies of psychiatric disorders (Robins et al. 1981). The purpose of the ECA study was to collect data on the rates, risk factors, and treatment patterns of the major mental illnesses in the community. The study, which is based on data from over 18,000 persons living in five communities in the United States (New Haven, Connecticut; St. Louis, Missouri; Baltimore, Maryland; Durham, North Carolina; and Los Angeles, California), forms the basis of our current understanding of the epidemiology of the major psychiatric disorders (Robins and Regier 1991).

Parallel developments were being undertaken in England (Brown and Harris 1978; Smith and Weissman 1992; Wing et al. 1978). As knowledge of the ECA study grew, similar studies using the identical methodology were undertaken in different parts of the world (see Table 2–2). In many cases, the staff in other countries were trained in the use of the DIS by Robins and her team in St. Louis, Missouri. Thus, for the first time, independent, cross-national comparisons of epidemiological rates using data obtained with similar methods are now possible. The findings from these studies for the mood disorders will be summarized.

Bipolar Disorder

The community-based lifetime prevalence rates in the United States for bipolar disorder are about 1% (ranging from 0.7% to 1.6%). The rates are lower (0.4%–0.6%) in Edmonton, Canada; Puerto Rico; and Seoul, Korea. Only an annual rate has been reported in Florence, Italy, and this rate

(1.3%) is similar to the United States lifetime rates. The similarity in lifetime United States and annual Florence rates may be due to the use of physicians as interviewers in Florence or to the fact that bipolar disorder is a chronic illness. The similarities rather than the differences in cross-national rates are notable, with the exception of Taiwan (about 0.1% and 0.16%). However, the rates for most psychiatric disorders, and particularly the mood disorders, are lower in Taiwan and, based on the limited unpublished data available, Shanghai (W. Lui, personal communication, 1990). Without data from Chinese living outside of the Republic of China (Taiwan) or the People's Republic of China, it is not possible to determine if this finding is unique to the Chinese.

Table 2–2.   Lifetime prevalence rates (%) for bipolar disorder, major depression, and dysthymia based on community surveys using the Diagnostic Interview Schedule and DSM-III diagnoses in adults ages 18 and over

	Time	N	Bipolar	Lifetime prevalence rates (%)a	
				Major depression	Dysthymia
ECA (United States)	1980–1983	18,572	1.2	4.4	3.0
New Haven	1980	5,034	1.6	5.8	3.2
Baltimore	1981	3,481	1.2	2.9	2.1
St. Louis	1981	3,004	1.6	4.4	3.8
Durham	1982	3,921	0.7	3.5	2.3
Los Angeles	1983	3,132	1.1	5.6	4.2
Edmonton	1983	3,258	0.6	8.6	3.7
Puerto Rico	1984	1,551	0.5	4.6	4.7
Florence[b]	1985	1,000	1.3	6.2	2.6
Seoul	1984	5,100	0.4	3.4	2.2
Taiwan	1982	11,004	—		
Urban		5,005	0.16	0.9	0.9
Small towns		3004	0.07	1.7	1.5
Rural area		2,995	0.10	1.0	0.9
New Zealand	1986	1,498	—	12.6	—

Note. ECA = Epidemiologic Catchment Area.
[a]Rates rounded off to one decimal in most cases.
[b]Only annual prevalence rate reported.

The rates of bipolar disorder are similar in men and women. There is a trend for increased risk in urban areas. The patient's mean age at onset is in the late teens and early 20s, with many onsets occurring in adolescence. There is some suggestion of temporal changes of the rates of bipolar disorder, with an increase of rates and an earlier age at onset in the cohorts born since 1940 (Gershon et al. 1987; Lasch et al. 1990). Family history, although not assessed in the community surveys, remains one of the most important risk factors for bipolar disorder (see below).

Marital problems and depression have often been found to be closely associated, although the specific type of depression has usually not been specified. The rates of bipolar disorder are highest for persons who are cohabitating but not married; who have a history of divorce regardless of their current marital status; or who have never married. The rates are lowest in married or widowed persons without a history of divorce. However, assumptions about any causal relationship require caution. A breakup of a marriage may be a response by the well spouse to the stress of living with a depressed person, or it may be brought about by the affected person's attributing his or her distress to failings in the spouse (Henderson et al. 1979).

Major Depression

Major depression is considerably more prevalent than bipolar disorder and, unlike bipolar disorder, is more prevalent in women than in men. There is also more variability in the rates by site. The lifetime rates vary between 2.9% to 5.8% in the United States sites, including Puerto Rico (Table 2–2). The higher rate in New Haven is undoubtedly due to the use of slightly broader criteria for major depression that specify a duration of 1 week rather than 2 weeks. The rates are highest in Edmonton, Canada and New Zealand. Again, Taiwan has low rates, ranging from 0.9% to 1.7%.

Korea, unlike Taiwan, is a more westernized country, and the lifetime prevalence rate of major depression (3.4%) is comparable to the lower end of the ECA five-site range. It is of note, too, that most non–United States studies sampled more homogeneous communities than did the ECA five-site study, which by design had diverse ethnic, racial, and socioeconomic samples. Puerto Rico's data on major depression resembled the ECA results, with a lifetime prevalence of 4.6%.

A number of risk factors in major depression have emerged from community studies. Female sex continues to be the clearest and most consistent risk factor in most sites as well as in family studies (Klerman and Weissman 1989). Positive family history of major depression, although not assessed in community studies, is a risk factor as well and will be discussed later in this chapter. The ECA found few black-white differences in rates of major depression once social class and education were controlled. However, as noted before, the Chinese appear to have substantially lower rates of major depression than do United States whites or blacks as reflected in the rate in Taiwan as well as in unpublished rates from an epidemiological study conducted in Shanghai, China. Unfortunately, there are no data from Japan.

The rates for major depression are higher in urban areas than in rural areas (Blazer et al. 1986), but there is not a strong effect for social class. As with bipolar disorder, a history of divorce or separation had a profound effect on increasing rates of major depression. More specifically, continuously married and never-married people had the lowest rate and divorced people had the highest.

Dysthymia

Dysthymia is slightly less prevalent over a lifetime than major depression. The exceptions are Puerto Rico and Taiwan, where lifetime risk for major depression and dysthymia are about equal within each country. Dysthymia in the United States, including Puerto Rico, ranges between 2.1% and 4.7%. The rate of dysthymia is considered lower in Taiwan (0.9% to 1.5%). In all countries studied, the rate in females is about twice as high as that in males.

The variations found with race, marital status, and urban/rural areas in dysthymia are similar to those found for major depression. However, for dysthymia, unlike major depression, there is a significant inverse relationship with income, especially in young persons. The rates increase or level off with age until after age 65. With major depression or bipolar disorder, the rate begins to decrease around age 45. The similarity in rates and risk factors, and the high comorbidity between major depression and dysthymia (termed *double depression*), have raised questions about whether these are distinct disorders. This issue is still unresolved.

Changing Rates of Depression

There is reasonably consistent evidence for a change in the rates of major depression, with higher rates in more recent birth cohorts and an earlier age at onset (Klerman and Weissman 1989; see Figure 2–1). This observation was first made in the 1960s and 1970s based on the following findings: 1) admission at hospitals for affective illness had increased between 1950 and 1970 as compared with the previous three decades; 2) the average age at onset for major depression in clinical samples was considerably younger than had been reported before World War II; 3) childhood depression was seen in increasing frequency in pediatric and psychiatric settings; 4) an increase in suicide attempts and deaths among adolescents was noted; and 5) the rates of major depression based on community studies in the elderly population were low (Klerman et al. 1985). However, investigations of temporal changes in the rates of depression and other psychiatric disorders prior to the mid-1980s were hampered because of a lack of large systematic studies using standardized diagnostic criteria. Thus, it was not possible to tell whether the differences observed in rates were real or rather due to changing methodology, treatments, or concepts.

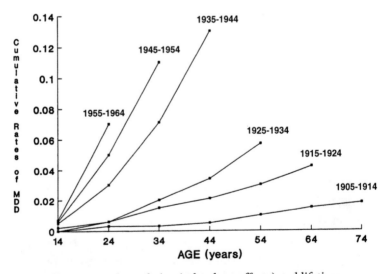

Figure 2–1.   The temporal trends (period-cohort effects) and lifetime prevalence of major depression, from the NIMH Epidemiologic Catchment Area study at five sites. Includes both sexes, white only.

The ECA study in the United States, as well as several large family studies of relatives of depressed patients using diagnostic methods comparable to those of the ECA, suggested the following (Hagnell et al. 1982; Karno et al. 1987; Klerman and Weissman 1989; Lavori et al. 1987; Wickramaratne et al. 1989):

1. Temporal changes in the rates of major depression, including an increase in the rates of the cohorts born after 1940
2. A decrease in the age at onset along with an increase in rates in the teenage and early adult years (see Figure 2–1)
3. An increase in rates for the cohorts born between 1960 and 1975, with an increase in the rates of depression for all ages but particularly younger age groups in that period
4. A persistent gender effect, with the risk of major depression consistently two or three times higher in women than in men
5. A persistent family effect, with the risk of major depression about two to three times higher in the first-degree relatives of depressed patients compared with control subjects
6. A suggestion of the narrowing of the differential risk to men and women because of a greater increase in the risk of major depression among young men

These trends were noted in epidemiological studies, as previously described, in the United States, Germany, Canada, and New Zealand, but they were not found to the same extent in studies conducted in Korea or Puerto Rico.

Various efforts have been undertaken to explain the findings and to determine whether they could be artifacts due to selective mortality and/or institutionalization, selective migration, changing diagnostic criteria, threshold changes in reporting among mental health professionals and/or society at large, reporting bias of interviewers, and recall problems among the elderly population (Klerman and Weissman 1989).

In disorders with familial aggregation, exclusive genetic interpretations are ruled out by observations of temporal changes because genes are unlikely to change in a relatively short time. The environmental risk factors for depression that have also been suggested include changes in the ratio of males to females; increased amount of urbanization; greater geographic mobility, which results in loss of attachments; increasing social anomie; changes in family structure; alteration in the role of women, especially the increased number of women in the labor force; and shifts in occupational patterns.

Thus far, the increase in the rate over time and the increase by birth cohort have been best established for major depression. However, two independent studies have shown that the same increase may be occurring for bipolar disorder (Gershon et al. 1987; Lasch et al. 1990).

Future Directions in Epidemiological Studies of Psychiatric Disorders

The DSM-III-R system has not been universally used outside the United States. A new diagnostic method, Schedules for Clinical Assessment in Neuropsychiatry (SCAN), is being field-tested in 20 centers in 11 countries (Wing et al. 1990). The aim is to develop a comprehensive procedure for clinical examination that is also capable of generating many of the categories of the ICD-10 (World Health Organization 1992), as well as the DSM-III-R and DSM-IV. The Composite International Diagnostic Interview (CIDI), based on the DSM-III-R and ICD-9 (World Health Organization 1979), has also been developed (Robins et al. 1988). The two instruments are complementary in that the CIDI is designed for use in large community surveys that necessitate the employment of lay interviewers, whereas the SCAN can only be used in its full form by clinically trained professionals. The availability of two diagnostic methods that bridge the major classification systems will facilitate future cross-national comparative studies.

Lastly, it should be noted that none of the epidemiological studies mentioned included children even though it is quite clear that mood disorders as well as many of the major mental illnesses often first occur in adolescence and, to a lesser extent, in childhood. Currently, there is field-testing of diagnostic methods applicable to epidemiological studies of children ongoing at Columbia University, Yale University, Emory University, and the University of Puerto Rico in preparation for a multisite epidemiological study of children that will be comparable to the ECA study for adults. By the year 2000 we can expect that information on the epidemiology of childhood psychiatric disorders will be available.

Genetics

Evidence for the role of genetic factors in bipolar disorder and, to a lesser extent, major depression has accumulated over the past two decades based on twin, adoption, and family studies. The interest in the genetics of bipolar disorder has been stimulated recently by the findings of linkage between bipolar disorder and markers on chromosome 11 and the X chromosome (Blehar et al. 1988). The failure to replicate these findings has been a disappointment and highlights the scientific problems in applying the new genetic approaches to complex disorders.

In 1990, the NIMH launched a multisite collaborative program to study the genetics of bipolar disorder as well as schizophrenia and Alzheimer's disease. The NIMH's goal is to establish a national resource of immortalized cell lines and psychiatric histories in reliably diagnosed pedigrees and to collect sufficiently large samples to detect any linkage. The focus in the first year has been in the standardizing of the assessment procedures across sites.

Bipolar Disorder

The selection of bipolar disorder for this first NIMH Collaborative Genetics initiative derives from the reasonably strong evidence from twin, adoption, and family studies for the genetic transmission of bipolar disorder. The mode of transmission, the spectrum of bipolar disorder, and the relationship between bipolar disorder and major depression are unclear (Gershon et al. 1987; Tsuang et al. 1980; Weissman et al. 1982). With increasing chromosome markers to map the entire genome, perhaps more definitive information will become available on linkage using restriction fragment length polymorphisms.

The findings of linkage could well call for additional family and epidemiological work to identify other factors, both genetic and nongenetic, that may modify the expression of a disorder. It has been noted that the concordance in monozygotic twins for bipolar disorder is much below 100%, so other factors may be operating. The finding of possible temporal changes in the rates of bipolar disorder implies that there are environmental factors in the expression of the disorder.

Major Depression

The phenotypic heterogeneity of unipolar major depression presents a problem when recombinant DNA approaches are used, and the search in family and clinical studies has been for a subtype(s) of major depression that might be homogeneous and possibly genetic. Twin data generally support the role of genetic factors in some of the unipolar depressions, particularly psychotic depression (Torgersen 1986). These findings do not, however, extend to all subtypes of major depression and seem less likely with dysthymia. However, the twin studies completed using modern diagnostic criteria have been based on very small samples, so conclusions about concordance cannot be drawn. A large twin study by Kendler at the University of Virginia is underway and may clarify these issues.

Over the past decade there have been several well-designed family

Table 2–3. Morbid risk of depression in first-degree relatives of unipolar depressive probands

Reference[a]	Percent (N) at risk	
Winokur et al. 1982	11.2	(305)
Gershon et al. 1982	16.6	(133)
Baron et al. 1982	17.7	(143.5)
Weissman et al. 1984	18.4	(287)
Bland et al. 1986	8.6	(763)[b]
Stancer et al. 1987	24.4	(282)
Rice et al. 1987[a]	28.6	(1,176)
Giles et al. 1988[a]	34.9	(43)
McGuffin et al. 1988		
Outpatient treatment only	24.6	(199.5)
Inpatient and outpatient treatment	11.8	(187)
Kupfer et al. 1989		
Recurrent depressive probands	20.7	(725)

[a] See Modlin et al. 1991 for references.
[b] Unadjusted number and morbid risk.
Source. Reprinted from S. O. Moldin, T. Reich, J. Rice: "Current Perspectives on the Genetics of Unipolar Depression." *Behavior Genetics* 21:211–242, 1991. Copyright 1991, Plenum Publishing Corporation. Used with permission.

studies which indicate quite clearly that major depression is highly familial (see Table 2–3) (Moldin et al. 1991). The lifetime rate of major depression in first-degree relatives ranges from 8.6% to 34.9%, which is usually about two- to threefold higher than in relatives of matched comparison groups and somewhat higher than in the general population. The study that found the lowest rate of major depression in relatives also had the oldest patients with later ages at onset (Bland et al. 1988). No substantial increase of bipolar disorder has been found in the relatives of patients with major depression.

There is a long history of searching for specific homogeneous subtypes of major depression. Some of the subtypes suggested as possibly being homogeneous and more biological, such as endogenous or melancholic depression, have not been shown to have a higher familial aggregation than the nonendogenous, nonmelancholic subtypes. However, an increased familial aggregation and a specificity of transmission of early age at onset (less than 20 years of age) of major depression have been demonstrated (Weissman et al. 1984).

For major depression, adoption studies have been inconclusive. A recent adoption study from Stockholm did not find a higher rate of depression in the biological parent of adopted-away depressed offspring (von Knorring et al. 1983). The lack of an association may be due to the study's reliance on hospital records. Moreover, these data are at variance with other adoption studies of major depression (Wender et al. 1986).

Dysthymia

There are several family studies of dysthymia underway, and information will be forthcoming in the next few years. The family studies of patients with major depression find that dysthymia aggregates in first-degree relatives, suggesting that dysthymia is on the spectrum of major depression.

Depression in Children

Whether or not a precise genetic etiology of the mood disorders is determined, the findings on familial aggregation have public health implications for children. Until recently, the conventional wisdom was that children were not capable of becoming depressed. In fact, before 1972, there were no textbooks of psychiatry that mentioned depression in children. With the increased use of systematic diagnostic assessments of children over the past decade, it has become clear that depression does occur in prepubertal children and is common in adolescence. Moreover, the offspring of depressed parents are at increased risk for depression as well as a variety of other types of social, school, and health problems.

There have been several research efforts underway to understand the clinical characteristics, familial aggregation, treatment, and course of depression in children. Although most of the studies have been on the children of parents with major depression (Beardslee et al. 1985; Hammen et al. 1990; Keller et al. 1986; Orvaschel et al. 1988; Weissman et al. 1987), there have been some studies of the children of bipolar parents (e.g., Anderson and Weissman, in press).

In general, the findings show that major depression in a parent increases the risk for psychiatric disorders in his or her children, particularly major depression and anxiety disorders. In addition, the children of depressed parents are more impaired in school and with peers, and have higher rates of developmental and medical problems compared with children of nondepressed parents.

Although the children of parents without psychiatric disorder also develop major depression, their rate is significantly lower and the age at onset may be later, most commonly in the mid-teens and rarely prepubertally. In the one study that found specificity of transmission of age at onset of major depression between parent and child, all the prepubertal depression was found in the offspring of parents with major depression occurring before age 20 (Weissman et al. 1987). A 2-year follow-up study of the same cohort suggested that depressions that occur in the children of nondepressed parents tend to be more transient and milder (Fendrich et al. 1991).

Based on a limited number of studies, the children of bipolar parents appear to be at increased risk for psychiatric disorders and possibly cyclothymia. Because bipolar disorder is less common than major depression, large samples of children may be required before an an effect is shown. However, if the proband is defined as the adolescent with bipolar illness, and the rates of illness are assessed in the adolescent's first-degree relatives (i.e., siblings and parents), then an increased risk for both major depression and bipolar illness in the relatives is found (Puig-Antich et al. 1989;

Strober et al. 1988). It is unclear if bipolar disorder occurs prepubertally and, if so, what are the early signs.

A related question regarding depressed children has to do with the continuity between childhood and adult depression. To date, not one longitudinal study has sampled groups of children who are depressed, using modern diagnostic criteria, and followed them into adulthood. The study that comes closest to having the ideal design (Harrington et al. 1990) used a "catch-up longitudinal design" to assess adult psychiatric status and social adjustment of 52 depressed children and adolescents who were compared with 52 individually matched control subjects. Harrington et al.'s major findings were that the depressed children were at an increased risk for mood disorders in adult life and had elevated risk of psychiatric hospitalization and treatment. These children were no more likely than the control group to have nondepressive adult psychiatric disorders. These findings strongly suggested that there was substantial specificity and continuity in mood disturbance between childhood and adult life.

Information from long-term follow-up of depressed children to determine the continuity between childhood and adult disorders may clarify two puzzling findings: namely, that depressed children do not have the same good response to the tricyclic antidepressants as is seen in adults, and that these children's sleep patterns and cortisol response during depression are somewhat different from those seen in adults, although the biological studies on depressed children are limited. Better understanding of the nature of depression in childhood and its relationship to adult depression could have implications for treatment and earlier preventive intervention.

Social Morbidity and Quality of Life

The social morbidity and impairment of functioning in work and marriage in patients with major depression have been well documented for over two decades. What has been unclear, though, is how their functioning compares with that of patients who have chronic medical conditions, or whether patients with depressive symptoms that do not meet criteria for DSM-III disorders are impaired. These latter patients represent a large number who are seen in primary care and medical clinics but who do not generally come to the attention of mental health professionals (Regier et al. 1978).

The recent Rand Medical Outcomes Study (MOS) (Stewart et al. 1989; Tarlov et al. 1989) monitored the patterns of morbidity outcome in health care in patients with major depression, dysthymia, or depressive symptoms not meeting the full criteria of either disorder. Patients with chronic medical conditions, including hypertension, diabetes, coronary artery disease, angina, arthritis, back problems, lung problems, and gastrointestinal problems, were compared as well as a sample of patients who had acute but not chronic medical problems (Wells et al. 1989). Of the 11,000 patients sampled, 466 had depressive symptoms that did not meet the criteria of a disorder, and an additional 168 met the criteria for a depressive disorder. These patients were monitored over 2 years, and an assessment was made of the number of days in bed, self-perceived current health status, and extent of body pain in the past month.

The major finding was that among the patients seen by medical clinicians, those with major depression had poorer current health status than those with depressive symptoms alone. Patients in the two depressive samples and the eight chronic medical samples were compared as to physical activities, such as sports, climbing stairs, walking, dressing, and bathing; normal social role performance at work or in the household; and social functioning with friends and relatives. Patients with depressive symptoms had significantly worse social functioning and reported significantly more days in bed than did patients with six of the eight chronic medical conditions, the main exception being coronary artery disease. Depressive symptoms and current medical conditions had additive effects with regard to measures of patient functioning and well-being. The functioning of depressed patients was comparable to, and at times worse than, that of patients with a number of chronic medical conditions (Klerman 1989).

In a separate study, excessive mortality from multiple causes was found in a large community sample derived from the ECA of depressive subjects over the age of 55 years (Bruce and Leaf 1989). Previous reports of mortality among depressed patients that were also based on community samples indicated an excess of death by suicide and accidents for younger depressed patients. In older age groups, suicide became less prominent, while chronic medical conditions, especially cardiovascular disease, provided the excess mortality.

Treatment

Pharmacological

Since the 1960s, there have been advances in the treatment of depression, a decrease in hospitalization, reduction in the duration of an episode, and strategies developed for prevention of relapse and recurrence. Most treatment for all mood disorders is now ambulatory. The tricyclic antidepressants have been available for over two decades, and their therapeutic value for major depression was noted in the early 1960s. It is only recently that there has been sufficient experience with the range of doses and with blood-level determinations. There is excellent evidence that the symptoms of depression can be reduced in 2 to 4 weeks with pharmacological treatment, usually a tricyclic antidepressant.

Soon after the introduction of the antidepressants, it became apparent that a high percentage of patients relapsed following short-term treatment. Thus, continuation therapy strategies were common in clinical practice and became the subject of several research studies. The goals of continuation treatments are 1) to sustain the remission brought about by short-term treatment, 2) to prevent relapse, and 3) to facilitate social and economic functioning. There is no agreement as to the optimal duration of continuation drug treatment, although commonly 6 months to 2 years of treatment has been shown to be efficacious. Beyond 1 or 2 years, treatment is considered as maintenance or prophylactic. The longest studies of drug therapy (i.e., 3 years' duration) show clearly that maintenance treatment of lithium for bipolar disorder and tricyclic antidepressants for major depression will markedly reduce relapse rates.

For a large number of patients, mood disorders fit the model of chronic illness, with periods of remission and recurrence. For many, the need for treatment beyond the acute phase increasingly is supported by follow-up and treatment studies. Over the past decade, a number of newer antidepressants have appeared with a wide variety of chemical structures and pharmacological profiles (Blackwell 1987). These drugs have been aimed at counteracting or eliminating problems with the original generation of antidepressants by reducing the anticholinergic effects (i.e., dry mouth and urinary retention), lowering cardiac toxicity and seizure thresholds, and/or reducing weight gain. One new drug, fluoxetine, a compound with highly specific action on serotonin reuptake, has received a considerable amount of publicity in the lay press. This attention is partially because it has few anticholinergic side effects and does not produce weight gain. A number of new serotonin reuptake blockers are coming on the market. Whether their antidepressant effects are remarkably different from those of the other available compounds is not fully clear.

In regard to other new areas of pharmacological treatment research, efforts are underway to test the efficacy of antidepressants in the treatment of patients with dysthymia, a disorder that has up to now been treated primarily in the domain of psychotherapy. The data on the efficacy of tricyclic antidepressants in the treatment of depressed children and adolescents are limited and inconclusive. Data on the efficacy of tricyclic antidepressants in geriatric depressed patients based on controlled clinical trials are also limited. However, the data that are available suggest that the usual antidepressant drugs in lower doses are efficacious in this population and that the side effects are problematic. These populations—dysthymic patients, depressed children and adolescents, elderly persons—clearly need further study.

The full details for treatment of bipolar disorder as well as our scientific understanding have recently been summarized in a book by Goodwin and Jamison (1990). This book in itself is an achievement of this past decade because of its reliance on and gleanings from empirical evidence.

Psychotherapy

During the past two decades, there has been noticeable improvement in the quality of psychotherapy outcome studies, as discussed in Chapter 3. Many of these new standards have been devoted to depression, and a number of psychotherapies specified for depression have been developed.

The NIMH Depression Awareness, Recognition, and Treatment Program (DART)

Emerging epidemiological findings on the prevalence and morbidity of depression, available treatments, and numerous studies of clinical practices in primary care and other general medical settings have indicated that only one-half of patients diagnosed with depressive and other psychiatric conditions are detected by general and family practitioners. In 1989, the NIMH initiated a program of secondary prevention of depression, the Depression Awareness, Recognition, and Treatment Program (DART). This program is comparable to the one initiated by the National Heart, Lung and Blood Institute to educate the public about the treatment of hypertension.

Initial efforts have focused on educating the public and professionals about the availability of effective treatments for severe disorders, particularly bipolar and recurrent unipolar depression. In the early policy discussions on the focus of the DART, relatively low priority was given to patients with milder depressions, including those with depressive symptoms seen in general medical health settings. It is still too early to know if the program will have an effect in improving detection and treatment of depression. A strong evaluation component has not been added to the program.

Conclusions

There has been considerable progress in understanding the epidemiology and familial patterns of the mood disorders and in testing new treatments. The challenge of the next decade will be 1) to bridge the gap between our understanding of treatment efficacy and the delivery of service; 2) to identify the genetic mechanism(s), particularly for bipolar disorder; and 3) to learn more about the continuity between childhood and adult depression so that appropriate interventions can occur earlier. The opportunities for secondary and tertiary prevention have increased. With increased knowledge of risk factors, particularly familial risk factors suggestive of genetic contribution for some of the mood disorders, the opportunity for primary prevention now seems less remote.

References

American Psychiatric Association: Diagnostic and Statistical Manual of Mental Disorders, 2nd Edition. Washington, DC, American Psychiatric Association, 1968
American Psychiatric Association: Diagnostic and Statistical Manual of Mental Disorders, 3rd Edition. Washington, DC, American Psychiatric Association, 1980

American Psychiatric Association: Diagnostic and Statistical Manual of Mental Disorders, 3rd Edition, Revised. Washington, DC, American Psychiatric Association, 1987

Anderson CE, Weissman MM: Family studies of affective disorders, in Depression in Children and Adolescents. Edited by Koplewicz HS, Klass E. London, Harwood Academic Publishers (in press)

Beardslee WR, Keller MB, Klerman GL: Children of parents with affective disorder. International Journal of Family Psychiatry 6:283–299, 1985

Blackwell B: Newer antidepressant drugs, in Psychopharmacology: The Third Generation of Progress. Edited by Meltzer HY. New York, Raven, 1987, pp 1041–1049

Bland RC, Newman SC, Orn H: Age of onset of psychiatric disorders. Acta Psychiatr Scand 77:43–49, 1988

Blazer DG, Crowell BA, George LK, et al: Urban-rural differences in depressive disorders: does age make a difference? in Mental Disorders in the Community: Progress and Challenge. Edited by Barrett J, Rose RM. New York, Guilford, 1986, pp 32–46

Blehar MC, Weissman MM, Gershon ES, et al: Family and genetic studies of affective disorders. Arch Gen Psychiatry 45:289–292, 1988

Brown GW, Harris TO: Social Origins of Depression: A Study of Psychiatric Disorder in Women. London, Tavistock, 1978

Bruce ML, Leaf PJ: Psychiatric disorders and 15-month mortality in a community sample of older adults. Am J Public Health 79:727–730, 1989

Christie KA, Burke JD, Regier DA, et al: Epidemiologic evidence for early onset of mental disorders and higher risk of drug abuse in young adults. Am J Psychiatry 145:971–975, 1988

Fendrich M, Weissman MM, Warner V: Longitudinal assessment of major depression and anxiety disorders in children. J Am Acad Child Adolesc Psychiatry 30:67–74, 1991

Gershon ES, Hamovit J, Guroff JJ, et al: Birth-cohort changes in manic and depressive disorders in relatives of bipolar and schizoaffective patients. Arch Gen Psychiatry 44:314–319, 1987

Goodwin FK, Jamison KR: Manic-Depressive Illness. New York, Oxford University Press, 1990

Hagnell O, Lanke J, Rorsman B, et al: Are we entering an age of melancholy? Psychol Med 12:279–289, 1982

Hammen C, Burge D, Burney E, et al: Longitudinal study of diagnoses in children of women with unipolar and bipolar affective disorder. Arch Gen Psychiatry 47:1112–1117, 1990

Harrington R, Fudge H, Rutter M, et al: Adult outcomes of childhood and adolescent depression. Arch Gen Psychiatry 47:465–473, 1990

Henderson S, Duncan-Jones P, Byrne DG, et al: Psychiatric disorder in Canberra: a standardized study of prevalence. Acta Psychiatr Scand 60:355–374, 1979

Horwath E, Johnson J, Klerman GL, et al: Depressive symptoms as relative and attributable risk factors for first onset major depression. Arch Gen Psychiatry 49:817–823, 1992

Johnson J, Weissman MM, Klerman GL: Service utilization and social morbidity associated with depressive symptoms in the community. JAMA 267:1478–1483, 1992

Karno M, Hough RL, Burnam MA, et al: Lifetime prevalence of specific psychiatric disorders among Mexican Americans and non-Hispanic whites in Los Angeles. Arch Gen Psychiatry 44:695–701, 1987

Keller MB, Beardslee WR, Dorer DJ, et al: Impact of severity and chronicity of parental affective illness on adaptive functioning and psychopathology in their children. Arch Gen Psychiatry 43:930–937, 1986

Klerman GL: Depressive disorders: further evidence for increased medical morbidity and impairment of social functioning. Arch Gen Psychiatry 46:856–860, 1989

Klerman GL, Weissman MM: Increasing rates of depression. JAMA 261:2229–2235, 1989

Klerman GL, Lavori PW, Rice J, et al: Birth-cohort trends in rates of major depressive disorder among relatives of patients with affective disorder. Arch Gen Psychiatry 42:689–693, 1985

Lasch K, Weissman MM, Wickramaratne PJ, et al: Birth cohort changes in the rates of mania. Psychiatry Res 33:31–37, 1990

Lavori PW, Klerman GL, Keller MB, et al: Age-period–cohort analysis of secular trends in onset of major depression: findings in siblings of patients with major affective disorder. J Psychiatr Res 21:23–36, 1987

Moldin SO, Reich T, Rice J: Current perspectives on the genetics of unipolar depression. Behav Genet 21:211–242, 1991

Orvaschel H, Walsh-Allis G, Ye W: Psychopathology in children of parents with recurrent depression. J Abnorm Child Psychol 16:17–28, 1988

Puig-Antich J, Goetz D, Davies M, et al: A controlled family history study of prepubertal major depressive disorder. Arch Gen Psychiatry 46:406–418, 1989

Regier DA, Goldberg ID, Taube CA: The de facto U.S. mental health services system. Arch Gen Psychiatry 35:685–693, 1978

Robins LN, Regier DA (eds): Psychiatric Disorders in America: The Epidemiologic Catchment Area Study. New York, Free Press, 1991

Robins LN, Helzer JE, Croughan J, et al: National Institute of Mental Health Diagnostic Interview Schedule: its history, characteristics, and validity. Arch Gen Psychiatry 38:381–389, 1981

Robins LN, Wing J, Wittchen H-U, et al: The Composite International Diagnostic Interview: an epidemiologic instrument suitable for use in conjunction with different diagnostic systems and in different cultures. Arch Gen Psychiatry 45:1069–1077, 1988

Smith AL, Weissman MM: The epidemiology of affective disorders, in Handbook of Affective Disorders, 2nd Edition. Edited by Paykel ES. Edinburgh, Churchill Livingstone, 1992, pp 111–129

Stewart AL, Greenfield S, Hays RD, et al: Functional status and well-being of patients with chronic conditions: results from the Medical Outcomes Study. JAMA 262:907–913, 1989

Strober M, Morrell W, Burroughs J, et al: A family study of bipolar disorder in adolescence: early onset of symptom linked to increased familial loading and lithium resistance. J Affective Disord 15:255–268, 1988

Tarlov AR, Ware JE Jr, Greenfield S, et al: The Medical Outcomes Study: an application of methods for monitoring the results of medical care. JAMA 262:925–930, 1989

Torgersen S: Genetic factors in moderately severe and mild affective disorders. Arch Gen Psychiatry 43:222–226, 1986

Tsuang MT, Winokur G, Crowe RR: Morbidity risks of schizophrenia and affective disorders among first-degree relatives of patients with schizophrenia, mania, depression and surgical conditions. Br J Psychiatry 137:497–504, 1980

von Knorring AL, Cloninger CR, Bohman M, et al: An adoption study of depressive disorders and substance abuse. Arch Gen Psychiatry 40:943–950, 1983

Weissman MM: Epidemiology overview, in Psychiatry Update: American Psychiatric Association Annual Review, Vol 6. Edited by Hales RE, Frances AJ. Washington, DC, American Psychiatric Press, 1987, pp 574–588

Weissman MM, Klerman GL: Epidemiology of mental disorders. Arch Gen Psychiatry 35:705–712, 1978

Weissman MM, Myers JK: Affective disorders in a U.S. urban community. Arch Gen Psychiatry 35:1304–1311, 1978

Weissman MM, Kidd KK, Prusoff BA: Variability in rates of affective disorders in relatives of depressed and normal probands. Arch Gen Psychiatry 39:1397–1403, 1982

Weissman MM, Wickramaratne P, Merikangas KR, et al: Onset of major depression in early adulthood: increased familial loading and specificity. Arch Gen Psychiatry 41:1136–1143, 1984

Weissman MM, Gammon GD, John K, et al: Children of depressed parents: increased psychopathology and early onset of major depression. Arch Gen Psychiatry 44:847–853, 1987

Wells KB, Stewart A, Hays RD, et al: The functioning and well-being of depressed patients: results from the Medical Outcomes Study. JAMA 262:914–919, 1989

Wender PH, Kety SS, Rosenthal D, et al: Psychiatric disorders in the biological and adoptive families of adopted individuals with affective disorders. Arch Gen Psychiatry 43:923–929, 1986

Wickramaratne PJ, Weissman MM, Leaf PJ, et al: Age, period, and cohort effects on the risk of major depression: results from five United States communities. J Clin Epidemiol 42:333–343, 1989

Wing JK, Mann SA, Leff JP, et al: The concept of "case" in psychiatric population surveys. Psychol Med 8:203–217, 1978

Wing JK, Babor T, Brugha T, et al: SCAN: Schedules for Clinical Assessment in Neuropsychiatry. Arch Gen Psychiatry 47:589–592, 1990

World Health Organization: International Classification of Diseases, 9th Revision (ICD-9). Geneva, World Health Organization, 1979

World Health Organization: International Statistical Classification of Diseases and Related Health Problems, 10th Revision (ICD-10). Geneva, World Health Organization, 1992

The Place of Psychotherapy in the Treatment of Depression

Gerald L. Klerman, M.D.
Myrna M. Weissman, Ph.D.

As described in the preceding chapters, there have been considerable advances in our knowledge about the nature of depression, including its clinical, epidemiological, and genetic aspects, as well as in the development of alternative treatments. During the same period as these advances in our knowledge of depression have proceeded, there have been concurrent advances in psychotherapy outcome research in general and in the developments of new psychotherapies specifically designed for treatment of depression. In this chapter we review these developments and assess the current place of psychotherapy in the treatment of depression. The rapid development of many new psychopharmacological agents with established efficacy for treatment of depression has strongly influenced research and clinical practice. This material will provide a background for subsequent chapters discussing interpersonal psychotherapy (IPT) and its recent applications.

Background to Psychotherapy Research

While psychological modes of healing have been practiced by almost all cultures throughout human history, psychotherapy, as a professional activity, is a relatively new development, beginning about 100 years ago. Techniques such as suggestion, reassurance, magical intonations, appeals to supernatural forces, exorcism of demonic possession, and others have been employed by healers through the centuries; only recently have these techniques been made rational, scientific, and professionalized.

In the past 100 years, a wide variety of psychotherapies have developed, and the practice of psychotherapy has flourished in the United States and parts of South America and Western Europe. Since the end of World War II, there has been rapid expansion in the types of psychotherapy. In 1978, Parloff et al. identified over 200 different types of psychotherapy used in clinical practice, and by now, in the 1990s, these numbers have grown.

There has simultaneously been growth in the types and numbers of professionals who have been trained for the application of psychotherapy. A number of professional groups provide training in psychotherapy for their members. Psychiatry, psychology, and social work constitute the disciplines with the largest number of psychotherapists. Moreover, there are also alcohol and drug abuse counselors and marriage and family therapists. Members of the clergy, priests, ministers, and rabbis are often trained in pastoral counseling.

In addition to diversity of training background and professional affiliation, psychotherapists perform their services in diverse settings. While the majority of psychotherapists work in solo private practice on a fee-for-service basis, there are large numbers who are employed in mental health centers, psychiatric hospitals, psychiatric clinics, social agencies, and schools and universities. Increasingly, counseling is also becoming available in industry through the employee assistance programs (EAPs), which were originally set up for identification and referral of workers with problems related to alcoholism but have since expanded their purview to include drug abuse, depression, family problems, and emotional stress. A major impetus to this expansion has been the increasing coverage of psychotherapeutic services via health insurance and other third-party payment systems.

Parallel to these developments in psychotherapy, there have been increasing numbers and types of psychopharmacological agents offering relief from symptoms of anxiety, distress, tension, and depression. There is a large degree of overlap between the symptoms influenced by psychopharmacological agents and those treated by psychotherapists. This overlap has often led to controversy over the relative role, utility, and efficacy of psychological and biological treatments and competition and rivalry between professional groups.

These developments in psychopharmacology and psychotherapy are reflective of the increasingly psychological orientation of American society as a whole. With increased urbanization, education, and the expansion of middle-class life-style, the desire and demand for psychotherapeutic and mental health services have increased. The utilization of mental health services has rapidly increased, gradually closing what had been a very large gap after World War II between the need for treatment and services, and the availability of professionals and facilities.

Establishing the Efficacy of Psychotherapy

For decades there have been debates about the usefulness and efficacy of psychotherapy. We date the onset of the current era in psychotherapy efficacy research to the publication in 1952 of the controversial and polemical article by Eysenck (1952). In his article, Eysenck reviewed the available studies as to the efficacy of psychotherapy, mostly based on psychodynamic psychotherapy or Rogerian client-oriented techniques. The author was very critical of the quality of the research design and methodology and concluded that the available evidence did not support conclusions of efficacy of available psychotherapies, particularly psychodynamic psychotherapy and client-oriented psychology. In addition, Eysenck heralded the appearance of new forms of psychotherapy based on principles of behavior theory and predicted that these treatments would be more efficacious than standard treatments.

Eysenck's article was experienced by psychotherapists, particularly psychodynamically oriented psychotherapists, as an attack on their field. They responded with a vigorous defense of the available evidence. A number of additional review articles appeared citing studies that Eysenck had not included and offering different interpretations of the findings than had been put forth by Eysenck (Bergin 1963; Bergin and Strupp 1972; Erwin 1980; Luborsky 1954).

More important than the lively debates and exchange of articles and letters about psychotherapy have been the improvements in design and methodology of studies to test the efficacy of this modality. A major force in these improvements has come from the National Institute of Mental

Health (NIMH), through which intramural and extramural research staffs, notably those of Drs. Parloff and Elkin, are working in collaboration with the Psychotherapy Research Review Committee, headed by D. W. Fiske (Elkin et al. 1985; Fiske et al. 1970).

The Fiske committee published a set of guidelines for the design and methodology of psychotherapy outcome studies (Fiske et al. 1970). These guidelines increasingly became the basis for review of grant applications by NIMH grant review committees and contributed greatly to the establishment of new standards. The emphasis on outcome studies is itself worthy of note. For many decades, the psychotherapy research field had been caught up in a debate between those who advocated process research and those who advocated outcome research. The majority of clinicians and researchers seemed to favor process research, hopeful of finding new techniques to enhance the efficacy of interventions during the psychotherapeutic session. Many investigators were skeptical of the appropriateness of efficacy studies at all, both in terms of their theoretical basis and of what were perceived to be immense practical obstacles to their being carried out. There was concern about the size of samples required to show differences between treatments, the lack of available methodology for assessing outcomes (particularly those related to personality functioning), and the lack of techniques for specifying the psychotherapy process itself. Another product of this endeavor was the publication of a compendium of outcome measures, recommended for use in psychotherapy efficacy studies (Waskow 1975; Waskow and Parloff 1975).

Specific Versus Nonspecific Factors

Notable in the controversy about efficacy studies on psychotherapy was the debate over specific versus nonspecific factors in psychotherapy outcome. An influential group of critics of psychotherapy research, led by Jerome Frank (1969, 1974; Frank and Frank 1991), emphasized the importance of nonspecific factors, particularly the relationship between the psychotherapist and the patient (usually referred to as "client"). These individuals did not question that psychotherapy is effective. They argued that the major determinants of the efficacy of psychotherapy did not lie in any specific set of techniques derived from the body of specific theory or empirical research, but rather that the success of psychotherapy was dependent upon the quality of the relationship between psychotherapist and patient. On the one hand, the client (i.e., patient) comes into psychotherapy expectant and desirous of change, demoralized but still hopeful and, for the most part, cooperative. If he or she is met by a warm, empathic human being, a relationship of trust and sharing rapidly develops. Thus, it is argued, the specific techniques—be they behavioral, dynamic, or interpersonal—matter little in determining the outcome of the psychotherapeutic process.

Current Standards for Psychotherapy Outcome Research

In spite of these controversies and objections, a small but stalwart band of psychotherapy researchers initiated a series of outcome studies through the 1960s and 1970s (Karasu 1982; Luborsky et al. 1975; see Weissman et al. 1987 and Weissman 1979 for reviews). Based on these researchers' experience, increasing agreement emerged as to the requirements for adequately designed and executed research projects. These requirements included the following:

1. The randomized clinical trial design has been accepted as the most valid source of evidence for the efficacy of psychotherapy. The randomized trial had been originally developed for the evaluation of drugs, but its techniques have diffused into nonpharmacological interventions, such as surgery, radiation therapy, electroconvulsive therapy (ECT), vaccinations (e.g., the polio vaccine), and, finally, psychological treatments, including psychotherapy.

2. The target conditions for psychotherapy have been increasingly specified. In this process, more use has been made of operationalized diagnostic criteria, such as the Research Diagnostic Criteria (RDC; Spitzer et al. 1978) or, more recently, the DSM-III (American Psychiatric Association 1980) and DSM-III-R (American Psychiatric Association 1987) criteria. Whereas in the past, psychotherapy was often advocated for vaguely defined "neuroses" and "personality difficulties," these conditions have undergone increasing differentiation, and the criteria for their diagnosis have been further specified by reliable and valid diagnostic algorithms. As these changes in methodology have been applied to a selection of patients for psychotherapy studies, the hetero-

geneity of patient samples has decreased considerably and the clinical relevance of psychotherapy outcome has increased as psychotherapy studies have been targeted for specific clinical groups, such as schizophrenia being treated in the hospital, schizophrenia being treated in aftercare, anxiety disorders, phobias, obsessive-compulsive states, eating disorders such as anorexia and bulimia, and depression.

3. Structured interviews for obtaining information necessary for judgments of inclusion and exclusion criteria have been developed. Most psychotherapy protocols identify a target population for inclusion (i.e., schizophrenic patients, phobic patients, depressed patients) but also describe exclusion criteria (e.g., suicidality, alcoholism, drug abuse). While, for the most part, psychotherapy trials have relied on clinical judgment for these diagnostic assessments, there is increasing use of structured interviews, such as the Schedule for Affective Disorders and Schizophrenia (SADS; Endicott and Spitzer 1978) and the Diagnostic Interview Schedule (DIS; Robins et al. 1981), or, more recently, the Structured Clinical Interview for DSM-III-R (SCID; Spitzer et al. 1992). In English and Europeans centers, the Present State Examination (PSE), developed by Wing and associates (1974), has been utilized.

4. The use of new statistics, such as Kappa, to estimate reliability of categorical judgments has now become standard. For reliability of continuous variables, interclass coefficients have long been used.

5. Estimates of statistical power have often resulted in the awareness that large sample sizes are needed to determine the efficacy of a treatment—larger samples than can be provided by any single institution. Having long been used in psychopharmacological studies, the multicenter trial has slowly become utilized in psychotherapy outcome studies (Elkin et al. 1985; Klerman et al. 1974; Weissman et al. 1981).

6. An innovative development has been the improvement of treatment specification through the use of treatment manuals, which standardize the treatment and facilitate the training of therapists. These manuals, as well as standardized criteria of therapist competence, have improved techniques for training therapists for participation in clinical trials of psychotherapies (Chevron and Rounsaville 1983; Rounsaville et al. 1988).

7. Techniques and procedures have been developed for the training of psychotherapists in specified treatments. This process has required the

prior establishment of manuals, and monitoring techniques have been used to ensure that the treatment as delivered adheres to the manual.

8. In the evaluation of outcome, multiple observers are now standard. In addition to patient self-report and therapists' observations, it has become standard to have an independent evaluator who assesses the patient at periodic intervals without knowledge of the specific treatment that the patient is receiving. These assessments by independent observers are almost always based on standardized rating scales, such as the Hamilton Rating Scale for Depression (Ham-D; Hamilton 1960), the reliability and validity of which have been established independently.

9. In the evaluation of outcome, multiple domains of symptoms and functioning have become standard. The first priority, of course, is the assessment of psychopathology either by clinician evaluation, such as with the Ham-D, or by patient self-report using paper-and-pencil tests such as the Beck Depression Inventory (BDI; Beck et al. 1961) or the Zung Depression Rating Scale (Zung 1965). In addition to measures of psychopathology, it has become increasingly evident that assessments of social functioning and quality of life are useful. Most assessment batteries used today in psychotherapy outcome research involve multidimensional outcomes. This approach has the potential disadvantage of increasing the time spent by the patient in assessment sessions, and there may be inadvertent psychotherapeutic benefits through these extensive and time-demanding procedures that confound assessment of outcome of control treatments in clinical trials.

10. Most recent psychotherapy studies have specified the duration of treatment, usually between 12 and 20 weeks. Recently, studies of longer duration have appeared.

11. Naturalistic follow-up studies have been utilized to describe the clinical course of the patients subsequent to the experimental treatment phase. In these follow-ups, there is particular interest in the treatments received, both psychological and psychopharmacological, after the patient leaves the clinical trial.

12. Complex multivariate statistical techniques have increasingly been used for the analysis of the data.

It is acknowledged that the techniques described above have led to increased complexity and research costs of psychotherapy trials. These developments, however, have contributed to increasing data on the efficacy of psychotherapy for specific disorders.

The Relationship of Psychotherapy Research to Clinical Practice

There is still a wide gulf between psychotherapy research and the clinical practice of psychotherapy. Psychotherapy researchers often complain that their findings are not given attention by practitioners and that, in general, research findings seem to have little influence on clinical practice. On the other hand, clinical practitioners complain that the topics initiated for psychotherapy research seem trivial and tangential to the major issues of clinical practice. Most clinicians using psychotherapy have strong convictions about the desirability and feasibility of the particular form of treatment in which they have been trained and with which they are identified. There is evidence, however, that psychotherapy practice gradually becomes more eclectic, with admixtures of behavioral and interpersonal techniques added to the standard corpus of psychodynamic techniques.

A major stimulus for recent change in psychotherapists' practice derives from the development of psychopharmacological agents and the challenge that these agents pose to psychotherapy. As new psychopharmacological agents have been developed and their efficacy demonstrated through controlled clinical trials, a reevaluation of the role of psychotherapy in many disorders has been required. Clinical states that previously were the province of psychotherapy, such as phobias, anxiety disorders, obsessions and compulsions, and personality disorders, have become the targets of newly developed psychopharmacological agents. The patient and clinician are now confronted with the choice of which specific type of treatment to utilize, and within the broad array of psychopharmacological and psychological treatments, there has been increased differentiation and diversification.

This situation with respect to the relationship between psychotherapy research and clinical practice is a deviation from the ideal of rational therapeutics, a concept that applies in other branches of medical treatment. In other branches of medicine, findings from research studies are rapidly diffused within the clinical community and influence clinical behavior, particularly with regard to diagnostic practices, prescription of medications, or utilization of nonpharmacological procedures. Likewise, findings from psychotherapy research studies, particularly outcome studies, should ideally influence clinical practice and result in changes in the behavior of psychotherapists with respect to selection of type of psychotherapy, duration of treatment, frequency of sessions, use of combined drugs and psychotherapy, involvement of the family, and other aspects of clinical practice. Conversely, problems encountered in clinical practice would become the subject for new investigation and research. This ideal relationship relies heavily on the so-called "medical model" and the intensifying relationship of biological science to clinical medicine. Whether a similar relationship will crystallize between psychological and behavioral science and clinical psychotherapy is still uncertain.

The Humanistic Critique

There are critics of the use of clinical trials to evaluate psychotherapy, both among clinical practitioners and among researchers. The extreme critics argue that the approach itself is based on invalid assumptions. They challenge the basic concept of mental illness as a discrete disorder, instead emphasizing the continuity between normal states of personality functioning and clinical dysfunction. Humanistic values and concerns are widespread and deeply felt within the practitioner community. Humanistic critics argue that the uniqueness of individual patients and their complexity and diversity make randomization of treatment inappropriate. The uniqueness of each patient is regarded both as a scientific proposition and as a tenet of the humanistic credo.

Moreover, it is argued that the outcome measures chosen to assess the efficacy of treatment—usually symptom scales and measures of social functioning—do not do justice to the complexity of the human personality. The goals of psychotherapy, it is argued, are not so much to treat specific disorders, but to help patients resolve their conflicts and facilitate the achievement of their personal goals and aspirations. In the humanistic model, psychotherapy is not regarded as a treatment for a clinical condition—the medical model—but as a humanistic endeavor, individually suited to the patient and therapist.

New Developments in the Psychotherapy of Depression

As described in the preceding section of this chapter, over the last 10 years there has been considerable improvement in the quality and quantity of information on the efficacy of psychotherapy treatment in comparison and in combination with pharmacotherapy of adults with major depression. Several short-term psychotherapies developed specifically for depression, particularly cognitive therapy, IPT, and some psychotherapies based on behavior approaches, have been specified in manuals. These manuals standardize the treatment and are used in the training of therapists conducting the treatment in the clinical trials (Klerman 1991). Similar information on the efficacy of psychotherapy is not available for persons with bipolar disorder or dysthymia, or for adolescents with major depression, although several clinical trials are now in the planning phase. In 1987 there were 18 clinical trials testing the efficacy of these psychotherapies in homogeneous samples of patients with major depression (Weissman et al. 1987). By 1991 there were probably close to 30 trials completed or in process.

Justification for the Use of Psychotherapy in the Treatment of Depression

In recent decades, drugs have become the standard treatment for major depression, at least in the research literature, if not in clinical practice. At the same time, we believe that there is an important place for psychotherapy.

Psychotherapy is widely used, and there is extensive clinical experience that preceded the advent of drugs that should not be discarded. The use of psychotherapy for the treatment of depression rests upon two premises. First, the symptom picture and psychological state of the depressed patient should be clarified. This picture includes many psychological themes such as memories of the past, fears for the future, and concerns over self-esteem, as well as the expression of a variety of affect states, mostly dysphoric, including depression itself, guilt and shame, anger and irritability (perhaps to the extent of rage and hatred), anxiety, tension, and feelings of an inability to cope associated with helplessness, hopelessness, and worthlessness. Suicidal thoughts and preoccupations are also part of the clinical picture. Second, as recent studies have indicated, focused forms of psychotherapy, particularly those treatments for mild to moderate forms of ambulatory depression, have been found to be efficacious.

In some clinical circles and residency training programs, an expectation has developed that all patients that meet DSM-III criteria for major depression should receive antidepressant medication. We do not interpret the available evidence as justifying that practice, particularly for mild to moderate cases. The results of recent studies, particularly the NIMH Treatment of Depression Collaborative Research Program (Elkin et al. 1989), indicate equivalent efficacy for drugs and psychotherapy. It is true that the onset of action of medication is often more rapid (i.e., within 2 days to 4 weeks), but by the end of 6 to 8 weeks, an equivalent degree of efficacy is usually achieved.

Some psychotherapists claim that psychotherapy of the acute episode of depression will have enduring effects and prevent recurrence and relapse. This claim is based on the presumption that psychotherapy is a learning process and that the experience of psychotherapy during the acute episode will be generalized and will result in changes in coping style and adaptive resources that, later, may prevent the recurrence of depressive episodes. While this is a widely held view, we are not convinced that the available evidence yet justifies that view. However, the evidence from the Pittsburgh study reported by Frank et al. (1990) suggests that for recurrent depressions, even once monthly, maintenance IPT had modest efficacy in preventing relapse. In this debate it is important to distinguish enduring effects of acute treatment (12–20 weeks) from continuation and maintenance treatment as used in the Pittsburgh study. Moreover, patients come to the treatment situation with expectations and their own values as to how they would hope to have their depression treated. Many patients value psychotherapy because they believe it keeps responsibility and control with them and enhances their autonomy and mastery.

We stated in the preface to this volume that we believe that patients' treatment needs are best met by the availability of a variety of treatments—both psychological and psychopharmacological. Assuming that the efficacy evidence warrants the decision, patients should have a choice among efficacious treatments.

Moreover, there are some special considerations concerning women, children, and adolescents. Epidemiological studies show clearly that the age at onset and highest prevalence of major depression is in women in their reproductive years. Thus, evidence that a nonpharmacological treatment can reduce symptoms of depression and diminish relapse through the period of pregnancy and nursing is of considerable potential importance in public health.

For children and adolescents, the situation is equally as pressing. The few clinical trials of antidepressants with depressed children and adolescents have not been positive, and the dangers of suicide by overdose and the problems of cardiotoxicity in children are well known. A similar case can be made for elderly persons. Although there is ample evidence for the efficacy of antidepressants at reduced dosage for elderly patients, the side effects and medical contraindications of these agents often preclude their use in this age group.

Despite the evidence for the efficacy of drugs, some depressed patients, for any number of other reasons, cannot or do not want to take them, and psychotherapy offers another alternative. Finally, whatever the etiology of a psychiatric disorder, these disorders have consequences in the patient's social, family, and work functioning and also may be exacerbated by problems in these areas. Consequently, psychotherapy can play an important rehabilitative role.

New Strategies for the Psychotherapy of Depression

Skepticism about the place of psychotherapy as a treatment for specific psychiatric disorders in many research and academic centers recently has been tempered by specification of the treatments in manuals and by new data on efficacy. One of the notable developments over the past two decades has been the increasing number of controlled clinical trials testing the efficacy of psychotherapy for specific disorders using methods comparable to those used in the testing of pharmacotherapy (see Weissman et al. 1987 for summary). Therapists' characteristics that influence outcome and improve patient specification have been delineated and usually involve patient selection according to standardized diagnostic criteria such as the RDC or DSM-III-R.

For depressive disorders, in particular, the evidence for the efficacy of psychotherapy based on controlled clinical trials has been growing, although the evidence is not as conclusive as that for drug therapy. A number of new psychotherapies to be used specifically for the treatment of depression have been developed (for reviews, see Weissman 1978, 1979; Weissman et al. 1987). Some studies have included comparisons with medication or the combination of medication and psychotherapy. These new psychotherapies have been the subject of extensive and critical review (see Glass et al. 1980; Hirschfeld and Shea 1989; Manning and Frances 1990; Rush 1982; Shea et al. 1988; Strupp and Binder 1984).

Psychoanalysis and Psychodynamic Psychotherapy

For a major part of the 20th century, especially through World War II and during the 1960s and 1970s, psychoanalytic ideas dominated the psychological study and interpretation of depression, and psychoanalysis and psychodynamic psychotherapy were the major modalities used in psychotherapy. All psychodynamic psychotherapies rest on the assumption that the origin of depression lies in early childhood experience and stress the importance of loss or disappointment and the existence of impaired characterological functioning preceding the onset of the acute episode, with emphasis on narcissism, dependency, repressed expression of frustration and anger, and excess guilt and an overactive conscience (Gaylin 1968). These personality traits render the individual vulnerable to blows to self-esteem, usually from interpersonal losses and disappointments, which serve as the precipitant for the acute symptomatic episode. Psychoanalytic psychotherapy does not usually identify symptom reduction as a primary goal. Rather, the goal of psychoanalytic psychotherapies is to effect personality change, particularly at the unconscious level, and improvement in symptoms and social functioning will follow accordingly. The emphasis in the treatment sessions is on the exploration of conscious and unconscious material; reconstruction of childhood developmental experiences, with particular emphasis on intrafamilial transactions with parents and siblings; and the extensive use of the transference.

A number of modifications of psychoanalysis have been applied to depressed patients, although not necessarily as an explicit goal. The early efforts at short-term therapy come from the work of Ferenczi in Hungary and Alexander in the United States in the late 1930s and 1940s. A major source of innovation was the English group at the Tavistock Clinic, initially guided by Balint and continued by Malan (1979). Other contributors to short-term dynamic psychotherapy include Davenloo in Montreal (1980), Sifneos and Mann in Boston (Sifneos 1979), Strupp and associates at Vanderbilt University in Tennessee (Strupp and Binder 1984), and Luborsky and associates in Philadelphia (Luborsky 1984).

Although these approaches are widely discussed and the subject of frequent symposia and workshops, there are no published controlled trials targeted at clinical depression. The one exception is Luborsky et al. in Philadelphia, who applied their technique, called "supportive-expressive dynamic psychotherapy," to a controlled trial of psychotherapy in Veterans Administration hospital patients who had the diagnosis of opiate dependence and were receiving methadone and peer counseling by ex-addicts. Using randomization, subsamples received either cognitive-behavior therapy or supportive and expressive therapy. The published results indicate greater improvement in the group receiving the psychotherapies, particularly in the presence of depression.

Behavioral Approaches

A number of behavioral approaches have been developed, particularly in the United States and United Kingdom. Many of these approaches have their theoretical source in the works and ideas of Skinner, but they also incorporate theory and principles from classic Pavlovian conditioning.

The first behavioral formulation of depression was described by Ferster (1973), who hypothesized that depression involves a loss of positive reinforcement. Lewinsohn et al. have modified and extended this formulation to emphasize the role of social learning, arguing that depressed patients lack the normal repertoire of social skills to elicit positive reinforcement from their social environment. Lewinsohn et al. (1984) have made this formulation the basis for their social learning therapy, called "Coping With Depression," which is conducted in an educational mode as part of a 16-week group format, organized as a didactic course, involving homework, self-monitoring, and exposure to positive events.

Other behavioral approaches have been developed by Rehm and by Bellack et al. (1980), based on social skills training. All of the behavioral approaches emphasize patients' self-monitoring on a daily basis between sessions, scheduling of activities, enhancement of assertiveness, and other skills.

Cognitive-Behavior Therapy

The most popular new technique of short-term psychotherapy is cognitive-behavior therapy (CBT). This approach, developed by Beck et al. (1979), combines a comprehensive theory of the psychogenesis of depression with highly specific therapeutic interventions described in detail in the published manual. Beck's basic thesis is that the psychopathology of depressed patients involves what he calls the "cognitive triad": negative self-image, which involves viewing oneself as defective, inadequate, deprived, worthless, and undesirable; a tendency to see the external world as negative, demanding, and defeating; and an expectation of failure and punishment and continued hardship, deprivation, and failure in the future. In CBT the interventions are focused on these cognitive distortions, and specific therapeutic interventions are described in the manual and in training.

In practice, CBT includes a number of behavioral techniques, including role playing, monitoring of mood, and task assignment (i.e., "homework"). A number of controlled clinical trials of CBT have been reported, and the general conclusion is that it shows efficacy for the treatment of ambulatory depression. In addition, there are claims that the short-term efficacy is sustained and that patients with successful short-term results will have a prevention of recurrences. Combination with medication is usually recommended by cognitive therapists (Simons et al. 1986). CBT was one of the psychotherapies selected for evaluation in the NIMH Treatment of Depression Collaborative Research Program.

Group and Marital Therapies

A number of variations of group therapy and of marital and family therapy have been described for depression. Docherty (1989) has identified cognitive group therapy as the best evaluated among the group therapies for depression, and he cites five studies that report group cognitive therapy to be superior to some control condition (i.e., usually waiting list).

Psychotherapy of Specific Types of Depression

As noted previously, almost all of the studies of short-term psychotherapy of depression developed in the past two decades have been evaluated in ambulatory patients with DSM-II diagnosis of psychoneurotic depressive reaction or DSM-III diagnosis of major depression. The rationale for this approach has been that, among the various forms of depression, the outpatient, nonpsychotic, and nonbipolar forms of depression would be most likely to be responsive to psychotherapy as a primary treatment intervention.

At this juncture, it would be valuable to briefly review the various DSM-III categories of depression to determine the current evidence for the possible value of psychotherapy.

Bipolar Disorder—Manic Phase

With very rare exceptions, most psychiatrists and psychotherapists would not attempt to treat a manic episode with psychotherapy alone, but would rely on medication, often in the hospital setting. Attention to the structure of the psychosocial milieu and the interpersonal transactions between manic patients and the staff has been described, but individual forms of psychotherapy alone without medication are seldom employed and probably are not to be recommended.

On the other hand, as the acute episode has resolved and the patient enters a long-term continuation and maintenance therapy, usually with lithium, psychotherapy has an important adjunctive or rehabilitative role. Like psychoeducational techniques and family methods, psychotherapy also enhances the efficacy of medication, as described in detail by Goodwin and Jamison (1990). These authors also emphasize the value of local patient self-support groups. In this respect it is of note that the National Depressive and Manic Depressive Association has recently gained national attention, based in large part on a coalition of local self-support groups.

Glick, Clarkin, and associates (1985) have reported results of a controlled trial of inpatient family therapy, indicating that, of the various diagnostic groups involved in the study, bipolar patients, particularly females, responded best to a psychoeducational family intervention.

Bipolar Disorder—Depressed Phase

Far more common in clinical practice than manic episodes are episodes of depression in patients with a previous history of manic episodes who thus meet the criteria for bipolar disorder. While the symptomatology of these patients as they present themselves for treatment is very similar in many respects to acute episodes of unipolar major depression, the propensity of these patients to switch into mania is an important therapeutic issue. There are many who believe that tricyclics are particularly prone to induce this switch, and that tricyclics or antidepressants should not be used alone in the treatment of acute episodes of depression and bipolar patients, but that lithium, and perhaps monoamine oxidase inhibitors, should be combined. The controlled trials on this issue are still not conclusive.

For these patients, psychotherapy in combination with the medication plays an important adjunctive and rehabilitative role, and the guidelines put forth by Goodwin and Jamison are particularly of value.

Cyclothymia

There are no controlled studies of the efficacy of psychotherapy with cyclothymic patients. In clinical practice, these patients are treated with psychotherapy alone or in combination with lithium. However, no systematic studies, controlled or uncontrolled, are available.

Major Depression and Its Subtypes

There are a number of subtypes of major depression for which psychotherapy alone is not recommended as the primary treatment. However, it must be noted that this recommendation is based on clinical experience and not on the results of systematic studies. For psychotic depression, in particular, the primary mode of treatment is medication and/or electroconvulsive therapy (ECT). Psychotherapy (individual, group, and family) may have a valuable adjunctive role, particularly in the aftercare of hospitalized patients and maintenance therapy.

Melancholic, or Endogenous, Depression

The proper treatment for the melancholic, or endogenous, subtype of depression is controversial. The development of the concept of melancholic depression is closely allied to the introduction of tricyclic antidepressants. Many experienced psychopharmacologists interpret the available evidence as indicating that tricyclic antidepressants are specifically indicated for melancholic patients and that psychotherapy is of limited value, except when used in combination with medication. Partial support for this is based on analysis of a subset of the New Haven–Boston Collaborative Study of the Treatment of Acute Depression (Klerman et al. 1982), in which a small subsample of endogenous depression patients did better on amitriptyline than with psychotherapy alone. In contrast, Elkin et al. (1985) reported that in the NIMH Treatment of Depression Collaborative Research Program, RDC endogenous features were not found to be a strong predictor of response to imipramine. These authors reported that RDC endogenous patients who were treated with IPT also did well, and they questioned the specificity of this particular depressive subtype for tricyclic medication.

Adjustment Disorder With Mood Disturbance

Although not usually considered an affective or mood disorder, significant numbers of patients experience episodes with strong depressive features in acute response to stressors. The overlap between this diagnosis and post-traumatic stress disorder has not been clearly established. Although there are no controlled studies, patients with these symptoms often receive psychotropic drugs, often a benzodiazepine, antianxiety agent, or perhaps a tricyclic. Various forms of psychotherapy and counseling are widely employed by clinicians with these patients, although there are few controlled studies. Klerman et al. (1987) reported the efficacy of a brief psychosocial intervention for patients with distress seen in a primary care, general medical facility. There was some evidence for the efficacy of a brief, modified form of IPT, called "interpersonal counseling," that was administered by psychiatric nurses under supervision (for a detailed description, see Chapter 11).

Conclusions

Many treatments are suitable for depression. The depressed patient's interests are best served by the availability and scientific testing of different psychological and pharmacological treatments to be used alone or in combination. Ultimately, clinical testing and experience will determine which is the best treatment for a particular form of depression.

References

American Psychiatric Association: Diagnostic and Statistical Manual of Mental Disorders, 3rd Edition. Washington, DC, American Psychiatric Association, 1980

American Psychiatric Association: Diagnostic and Statistical Manual of Mental Disorders, 3rd Edition, Revised. Washington, DC, American Psychiatric Association, 1987

Beck AT, Ward C, Mendelson M, et al: An inventory for measuring depression. Arch Gen Psychiatry 42:667–675, 1961

Beck AT, Rush AJ, Shaw BF, et al: Cognitive Theory of Depression. New York, Guilford, 1979

Bellack AS, Hersen M, Himmelhoch JS: Social skills training for depression: a treatment manual (abstract). Catalog of Selective Documents in Psychology 10:2156, 1980

Bergin AE: The effects of psychotherapy: negative results revisited. Journal of Clinical and Counseling Psychology 10:244–250, 1963

Bergin AE, Strupp HH: Experimental and Quasi-Experimental Designs for Research. Chicago, IL, Aldine-Atherton, 1972

Chevron ES, Rounsaville BJ: Evaluating the clinical skills of psychotherapists: a comparison of techniques. Arch Gen Psychiatry 40:1129–1132, 1983

Davenloo H: Short-Term Dynamic Psychotherapy, Vol 1. New York, Jason Aronson, 1980

Docherty JP: Group psychotherapy of depression, in Comprehensive Textbook of Psychiatry/V, 5th Edition, Vol 1. Edited by Kaplan HI, Sadock BJ. Baltimore, MD, Williams & Wilkins, 1989, pp 944–951

Elkin I, Parloff MB, Hadley SW, et al: NIMH Treatment of Depression Collaborative Research Program. Arch Gen Psychiatry 42:305–316, 1985

Elkin I, Shea MT, Watkins JT, et al: National Institute of Mental Health Treatment of Depression Collaborative Research Program: general effectiveness of treatment. Arch Gen Psychiatry 46:971–983, 1989

Endicott J, Spitzer RL: A diagnostic interview: the Schedule for Affective Disorders and Schizophrenia. Arch Gen Psychiatry 35:837–844, 1978

Erwin E: Psychoanalytic therapy: the Eysenck agreement. Am Psychol 35:435–443, 1980

Eysenck HJ: The effects of psychotherapy: an evaluation. Journal of Consulting Psychology 16:319–324, 1952

Ferster CB: A functional analysis of depression. Am Psychol 10:857, 1973

Fiske DW, Hunt HF, Luborsky L, et al: Planning of research on effectiveness of psychotherapy. Arch Gen Psychiatry 22:22–32, 1970

Frank E, Kupfer DF, Perel JM, et al: Three-year outcomes for maintenance therapies in recurrent depression. Arch Gen Psychiatry 47:1093–1099, 1990

Frank JD: Common features account for effectiveness. International Journal of Psychiatry 7:122–127, 1969

Frank JD: Common features of psychotherapies and their patients. Psychother Psychosom 24:368–371, 1974

Frank JD, Frank JB: Persuasion and Healing. Baltimore, MD, Johns Hopkins University Press, 1991

Gaylin W (ed): The Meaning of Despair. New York, Jason Aronson, 1968

Glass GV, Smith ML, Miller N: The Benefits of Psychotherapy. Baltimore, MD, Johns Hopkins Press, 1980

Glick ID, Clarkin JF, Spencer JH, et al: A controlled evaluation of inpatient family intervention. Arch Gen Psychiatry 42:882–886, 1985

Goodwin FK, Jamison KR: Manic-Depressive Illness. New York, Oxford University Press, 1990

Hamilton M: A rating scale for depression. J Neurol Neurosurg Psychiatry 25:56–62, 1960

Hirschfeld RMA, Shea MT: Mood disorders: psychosocial treatments, in Comprehensive Textbook of Psychiatry/V, 5th Edition, Vol 1. Edited by Kaplan HI, Sadock BJ. Baltimore, MD, Williams & Wilkins, 1989, pp 933–944

Karasu TB (ed): Psychotherapy Research: Methodological and Efficacy Issues. Washington, DC, American Psychiatric Association, 1982

Klerman GL: The efficacy of psychotherapy: scientific and public policy issues. Presidential address at the annual meeting of the Association for Clinical and Psychosocial Research, New Orleans, LA, May 1991

Klerman GL, DiMascio A, Weissman MM, et al: Treatment of depression by drugs and psychotherapy. Am J Psychiatry 131:186–191, 1974

Klerman GL, Weissman MM, Prusoff BA: RDC endogenous depression as a predictor of response to antidepressant drugs and psychotherapy, in Typical and Atypical Antidepressants. Edited by Costa E, Racagni G. New York, Raven, 1982, pp 165–174

Klerman GL, Budman S, Berwick D, et al: Efficacy of a brief psychosocial intervention for symptoms of stress and distress among patients in primary care. Med Care 25:1078–1088, 1987

Lewinsohn PM, Antonuccio DO, Steinmetz JL, et al: The Coping With Depression Course: A Psychoeducational Intervention for Unipolar Depression. Eugene, OR, Castalia, 1984

Luborsky L: A note on Eysenck's article "The Effects of Psychotherapy: An Evaluation." Br J Psychol 45:129–131, 1954

Luborsky L: Principles of Psychoanalytic Psychotherapy: A Manual for Supportive-Expressive Treatment. New York, Basic Books, 1984

Luborsky L, Singer B, Luborsky L: Comparative studies of psychotherapies: is it true that "Everyone has won and all must have prizes?" Arch Gen Psychiatry 32:995–1008, 1975

Malan DH: Individual Psychotherapy and the Science of Psychodynamics. London, Butterworth, 1979

Manning D, Frances A (eds): Combined Pharmacotherapy and Psychotherapy for Depression. Washington, DC, American Psychiatric Press, 1990

Parloff MB, Waskow IE, Wolfe BE: Research on therapist variables in relation to process and outcome, in Handbook of Psychotherapy and Behavior Change, 2nd Edition. Edited by Garfield SL, Bergin AE. New York, Wiley, 1978, pp 233–282

Robins LN, Helzer JE, Croughan J, et al: National Institute of Mental Health Diagnostic Interview Schedule. Arch Gen Psychiatry 38:381–389, 1981

Rounsaville BJ, O'Malley S, Foley S, et al: Role of manual-guided training in the conduct and efficacy of interpersonal psychotherapy for depression. J Consult Clin Psychol 56:681–688, 1988

Rush AJ: Short-Term Psychotherapies for Depression. New York, Guilford, 1982

Shea MT, Elkin I, Hirschfeld RMA: Psychotherapeutic treatment of depression, in American Psychiatric Press Review of Psychiatry, Vol 7. Edited by Frances AJ, Hales RE. Washington, DC, American Psychiatric Press, 1988, pp 235–255

Sifneos PE: Short-Term Dynamic Psychotherapy: Evaluation and Technique. New York, Plenum, 1979

Simons AD, Murphy GE, Levine FL, et al: Cognitive therapy and pharmacotherapy for depression: sustained improvement over one year. Arch Gen Psychiatry 43:43–48, 1986

Spitzer RL, Endicott J, Robins E: Research Diagnostic Criteria: rationale and reliability. Arch Gen Psychiatry 35:773–782, 1978

Spitzer RL, Williams JBW, Gibbon M, et al: Structured Clinical Interview for DSM-III-R: User's Guide. Washington, DC, American Psychiatric Press, 1992

Strupp HH, Binder JL: Psychotherapy in a New Key: A Guide to Time-Limited Dynamic Psychotherapy. New York, Basic Books, 1984

Waskow IE: Selection of a core battery, in Psychotherapy Change Measures: Report of the Clinical Research Branch (DHEW Publ No [ADM]-74-120). Edited by Waskow IE, Parloff MB. Bethesda, MD, National Institute of Mental Health, 1975, pp 3–30

Waskow IE, Parloff MB (eds): Psychotherapy Change Measures: Report of the Clinical Research Branch (DHEW Publ No [ADM]-74-120). Bethesda, MD, National Institute of Mental Health, 1975

Weissman MM: Psychotherapy and its relevance to the pharmacotherapy of affective disorders: from ideology to evidence, in Psychopharmacology: A Generation of Progress. Edited by Lipton MA, DiMascio A, Killam KF. New York, Raven, 1978, pp 1313–1321

Weissman MM: The psychological treatment of depression. Arch Gen Psychiatry 36:1261–1269, 1979

Weissman MM, Prusoff BA, Klerman GL: Drugs and psychotherapy in acute depression. Arch Gen Psychiatry 38:115–116, 1981

Weissman MM, Jarrett RB, Rush JA: Psychotherapy and its relevance to the pharmacotherapy of major depression: a decade later (1976–1985), in Psychopharmacology: The Third Generation of Progress. Edited Meltzer HY. New York, Raven, 1987, pp 1059–1069

Wing J, Cooper J, Sartorius N: The Description and Classification of Psychiatric Symptoms: An Instructional Manual for the PSE and CATEGO System. London, Cambridge University Press, 1974

Zung WWK: A self-rating depression scale. Arch Gen Psychiatry 12:63–70, 1965

Interpersonal Psychotherapy and Its Adaptations for Depression

Maintenance Interpersonal Psychotherapy for Recurrent Depression

Ellen Frank, Ph.D.
David J. Kupfer, M.D.
Cleon Cornes, M.D.
Susan M. Morris, L.S.W.

After so many times, it seems like depression not only rules your life, it *is* your life. You keep telling yourself that "this, too, will pass" and it does eventually. Then the depression comes back again and again. After a while, it just seems like nothing can ever help, and that you'll never get control of your life.

A 53-year-old woman with a history
of five episodes of unipolar depression

A single episode of unipolar depression can be a devastating experience. Recurrent unipolar depression has the potential to be a chronically disabling condition. The identification of the

Portions of this chapter have been adapted from the following publications: E. Frank: "Interpersonal Psychotherapy as a Maintenance Therapy for Patients With Recurrent Depression." *Psychotherapy* 28:259–266, 1991; E. Frank, D. J. Kupfer, J. M. Perel, et al.: "Three-Year Outcomes for Maintenance Therapies in Recurrent Depression." *Archives of General Psychiatry* 47:1093–1099, 1990; E. Frank, D. J. Kupfer, E. F. Wagner, et al.: "Efficacy of Interpersonal Psychotherapy as a Maintenance Treatment for Recurrent Depression: Contributing Factors." *Archives of General Psychiatry* 48:1053–1059, 1991; D. J. Kupfer, E. Frank, V. J. Grochocinski, et al: "Delta Sleep Ratio: A Biological Correlate of Early Recurrence in Unipolar Affective Disorder." *Archives of General Psychiatry* 47:1100–1105, 1990 recurrent patient has become less problematic in recent years with the advent of more precise and sophisticated diagnostic criteria; however, successful prophylactic treatment of recurrent depression has remained an elusive goal.

Early treatment studies did not yield encouraging findings as to the prognosis for these patients. From 1978 to 1982, the Depression Prevention Clinic at Western Psychiatric Institute and Clinic in Pittsburgh, Pennsylvania, served as one of five centers in the National Institute of Mental Health (NIMH) Collaborative Study Group (NIMH-PRB) comparing lithium, imipramine, and a lithium/imipramine combination as maintenance treatment for recurrent unipolar disorder as well as bipolar disorder. This study, the findings of which were published by Prien et al. in 1984, involved 150 patients with recurrent depression treated in a 2-year maintenance trial. Of the 88 patients with unipolar depression whose index episode was considered severe, the most effective treatment—active imipramine—had only a 48% success rate in preventing new episodes over a 2-year period. Another study published in 1984 by Glen et al. reported a 3-year maintenance trial of 131 patients with unipolar depression. The maintenance-phase success rate for patients in this study was under 35% for patients in the active medication groups.

Clearly, there was room for improvement in maintenance treatment strategies for recurrent depression. While pharmacotherapy had certainly proven efficacious in the acute treatment of major depression, a majority of individuals with recurrent illness were not being helped by medication-only treatment approaches. In 1985, the National Institute of Mental Health/National Institutes of Health Consensus Development Panel on Recurrent Mood Disorders emphasized the evidence of the chronic and recurrent nature of mood disorders and the need for long-term maintenance treatment planning. This prompted consideration of combining one of the depression-specific psychotherapeutic approaches with maintenance pharmacotherapy.

Researchers have employed interpersonal psychotherapy (IPT) in both short-term and long-term treatment trials of depression. In the original study of this treatment approach, Klerman and colleagues (1974) examined the effects of 8 months of psychotherapy in women whose depression had remitted following 6 to 8 weeks of amitriptyline therapy. At the conclusion of the continuation treatment, patients receiving no treatment (the low-contact condition) demonstrated a relapse rate of 36%, compared with 12% in the amitriptyline group, 16.7% on the IPT-alone group, and 12.5% in the combination group. This study provided an estimate of the efficacy of IPT on relapse rates and social adjustment and for a long time was the only controlled trial reported in the literature that examined the prophylactic effectiveness of psychotherapy. A second study, by DiMascio et al. (1979), and the recently completed NIMH Treatment of Depression Collaborative Research Program (Elkin et al. 1989) demonstrated that IPT was an effective short-term treatment for depression. In the three-site NIMH research program, more than half (57% to 59%) of the patients completing 16 weeks of treatment were symptom-free. When more severely depressed patients were examined, IPT was the only treatment that approached imipramine in efficacy.

A primary reason for considering IPT as a long-term prophylactic treatment was the evidence that, even in the face of complete symptomatic remission, patients with a history of recurrent depression continue to show marked impairment in social adjustment. Data from the Pittsburgh site of the NIMH-PRB pointed to the continuing presence of work and social impairment even in the maintenance phase of depression treatment (D. J. Kupfer and E. Buzzinotti, unpublished data, 1992).

The self-rated version of the Social Adjustment Scale (SAS; Weissman and Bothwell 1976) was used during the several phases of the NIMH study. In order to verify the clinical impression of continued social impairment despite absence of clinical symptoms, SAS data were analyzed at three points in time in 40 unipolar patients treated at the Pittsburgh site who had entered the maintenance phase of the study. Using the presence of at least moderate impairment in a minimum of two or more of six role areas, we found that all patients entering the study met this criterion. At the *beginning* of the maintenance period (approximately 6 months after onset of treatment), 75% of the patients, in spite of considerable clinical improvement, continued to demonstrate moderate impairment in two or more role areas. The most striking finding was that 6 *months into maintenance treatment,* 69% of the patients continued to demonstrate at least moderate impairment in two or more role areas, and 59% showed this level of impairment in three or more role areas. In both assessments in the maintenance period, patients were considered symptom-free from a clinical standpoint. Yet they reported difficulties in social functioning that were different from those encountered by the normal control subjects studied by Weissman and Paykel (1974).

It was our hypothesis that such impairments contribute in important ways to a patient's vulnerability to recurrence. A treatment that focuses exclusively on the interpersonal context of the patient's life might offer the opportunity to intervene in such a way that one aspect of the patient's vulnerability would be reduced or eliminated.

Maintenance interpersonal psychotherapy (IPT-M) is the form of maintenance treatment that grows logically from such a hypothesis. IPT-M is based upon the premise that, along with the biological vulnerabilities and personality traits that may contribute to the pathogenesis of depression, recurrent depression always occurs within a psychosocial and interpersonal context. IPT-M was designed to maintain recovery and reduce vulnerability to future episodes by focusing on the interpersonal context of depression. Unlike IPT, which as an acute treatment emphasizes the psychosocial context associated with the episode itself, IPT-M emphasizes the psychosocial context of the remitted state in which the patient appropriately has taken on more responsibilities and has increased social contacts. By helping the patient develop more effective strategies for coping with social and interpersonal problems, IPT-M attempts to function as "preventive medicine" in this new context, thus enabling the patient to reduce the stresses that are associated with the remitted state and therefore reduce the risk of recurrence.

Maintenance interpersonal psychotherapy was modified from IPT specifically for use in the Maintenance Therapies in Recurrent Depression protocol conducted in the Department of Psychiatry, University of Pittsburgh School of Medicine, Western Psychiatric Institute and Clinic. This was a 3-year outcome study of IPT alone and in combination with medication. Initial treatment consisted of combined imipramine (150 to 300 mg) and IPT in weekly sessions for 12 weeks, followed by four biweekly sessions and then monthly sessions until the patient stabilized. Once a stable remission had been sustained for 20 weeks, during which time patients continued to be treated with imipramine and IPT, the 128 subjects who had achieved recovery were randomly assigned to one of five treatment groups: 1) IPT-M alone; 2) IPT-M with active imipramine; 3) IPT-M with placebo; 4) medication clinic visits with active imipramine; or 5) medication clinic visits with placebo. The maintenance form of IPT was developed for this phase and consisted of monthly sessions focused on one or more of the IPT interpersonal problem areas. Patients were seen monthly for 3 years or until they experienced a full recurrence of symptoms and met criteria for a new episode of major depression.

One of the principal questions that this study was designed to address was whether IPT, offered either alone or in combination with pharmaco-therapy, would help to prevent new episodes of depressive illness in pa-tients with a history of recurrences. The description of IPT-M that follows is based on the treatment experiences of eight IPT-M therapists who treated 16 pilot IPT-M cases and more than 75 maintenance treatment protocol cases.

Development of Maintenance Interpersonal Psychotherapy

The adaptation of IPT to a maintenance format began with the develop-ment of an IPT-M pilot treatment manual. This pilot manual was based primarily on the IPT manual written by Klerman, Weissman, and their colleagues, later published in *Interpersonal Psychotherapy for Depression* (Klerman et al. 1984).

Only clinicians who had been trained by Dr. Bruce Rounsaville or Ms. Eve Chevron of the Yale University Depression Research Unit, and who had been certified as competent acute IPT therapists by Drs. Klerman and Weissman, were chosen for the pilot-testing phase of IPT-M. Additional therapists were subsequently trained by Cleon Cornes, M.D., who was originally trained in IPT for participation in the NIMH Treatment of Depression Collaborative Research Program and had been designated as a certified IPT trainer by Drs. Klerman and Weissman. Each therapist in-volved in the pilot-testing phase was required to read the pilot manual and to attend several group meetings conducted by the first author, where general issues of both maintenance treatment and the adaptation of IPT to maintenance treatment were discussed. After participating in this initial preparation, each therapist was asked to treat a minimum of two pilot IPT-M cases for a period of 18 months. This entailed treating fully remitted patients with recurrent unipolar depression who had previously been treated with a combination of imipramine and weekly IPT. These patients, all of whom continued on their acute treatment medication regimen throughout the maintenance treatment, were seen for 18 maintenance sessions of 45 to 50 minutes' duration.

During the pilot-testing period, therapists met on a weekly basis in a group supervision format with Dr. Cornes. All of the pilot IPT-M sessions were videotaped to provide discussion material for the group supervision sessions. The focus of the group supervision sessions was on adherence to the basic tenets of IPT, as well as exploration of the dynamics specific to therapeutic intervention with patients in remission.

Initial pilot sessions were also audiotaped in order to allow independent raters to monitor the content of IPT-M sessions using a psychotherapy rating scale developed especially for this project. It was thus possible to monitor and standardize the treatment offered by IPT-M therapists to a criterion equivalent to those sessions that had been judged acceptable IPT sessions by the Yale University supervisors. Major requirements for the pilot testing of a psychotherapy in a refined controlled-trial methodology were thus met in the development of IPT-M. The treatments were standardized and monitored, both openly in the group supervision sessions and independently by objective raters, to ensure treatment integrity. Treatment sessions were of comparable length (45 to 50 minutes), and all patients received the same number and frequency of sessions. Therapists were uniformly trained and competent in the specific therapy and were deemed appropriate for the patient population based on their experience in treating depressive outpatients and with delivering acute IPT treatment.

Description of Maintenance Interpersonal Psychotherapy

Maintenance interpersonal psychotherapy differs from the acute treatment from which it is derived in terms of its goals and its timing, as well as the number and sometimes the kind of problem areas addressed. Our therapeutic approach with IPT-M takes these differences into account, thus allowing for a more expansive treatment scope than had been possible in IPT and for a pattern of less frequent therapeutic contacts.

Goals of Treatment

Because IPT-M begins with patients who are fully remitted, its goal is to maintain the patient in the euthymic state rather than bring about the remission of an acute episode. In order to accomplish this, the IPT-M therapist is vigilant for early signs of interpersonal problems similar to those identified as having contributed to the patient's most recent depressive episode or to previous episodes of depression. The therapist works with the patient to enhance those strengths that were present prior to the patient's illness and/or those that began to emerge as the most recent depressive episode remitted. The patient is also encouraged to be alert to the appearance of the somatic and cognitive changes that were characteristic of prior depressive episodes. When symptoms are reported to the IPT-M therapist, both therapist and patient plan strategies to circumvent the emergence of a new episode. These strategies focus primarily on interpersonal techniques for improving the patient's mood and functioning.

Timing of Treatment

Timing of sessions in IPT-M is also different from that in acute IPT treatment. IPT-M was scheduled on a once-a-month basis in the Maintenance Therapies in Recurrent Depression protocol. This was considered ideal timing for IPT-M because the population for whom it is intended are asymptomatic, the projected length of treatment is several years, and the goal of treatment is to prevent new episodes rather than treat a current episode of depression.

There were two types of responses observed in our patients to the once-a-month scheduling of IPT-M. Some patients experienced decreased contact as a loss and had a difficult time moving from the weekly acute IPT sessions, through the transition period of biweekly sessions required in the study protocol, to the final schedule of monthly maintenance sessions. Several patients approached their first maintenance sessions with a defeatist attitude and complained that they could see no benefit to be gained from meeting so infrequently. Other patients were directly or indirectly hostile and expressed anger either at the therapist or at the research protocol for reducing the frequency of sessions. The patient's disappointment or hostility sometimes led to the adoption of a "reporting" stance in the first few monthly sessions. When this occurred, the therapist would raise this as a therapeutic issue. Such patients tended to resolve their initial discomfort with the timing of IPT-M sessions within one to two sessions. It should be noted that the majority of patients actually had no difficulty with the transition, probably because the monthly schedule seems appropriate to most patients in early remission: frequent enough to provide a secure base but not so frequent as to interfere with their view of themselves as well.

Problem Areas in IPT-M

Unlike IPT, which helps the patient develop more productive strategies for coping with social and interpersonal problems associated with the onset of depressive symptoms and with those that develop as an immediate conse-quence of depression, IPT-M emphasizes those problems that persist dur-ing remission or that develop as a consequence of remission. In acute IPT, generally only one or, at most, two major problem areas can be addressed. In IPT-M, which was designed as a multiyear course of therapy, it is virtually impossible and actually countertherapeutic to restrict the treat-ment to a single problem area. Throughout the course of IPT treatment, often a number of interpersonal themes emerge that cannot become the major focus of treatment. The therapist makes note of these additional themes and reserves them for possible exploration in IPT-M. In the major-ity of cases, the focus in IPT-M is on a combination of the traditional problem areas of role transitions, role disputes, and interpersonal deficits. Grief reactions are rarely a focus in IPT-M unless a death occurs during the course of maintenance treatment. As in acute IPT, emphasis in IPT-M is placed on elicitation of feelings and nonjudgmental exploration of the affective quality of relationships, using familiar therapeutic techniques such as reassurance, clarification, reality testing of perceptions and perfor-mances, modification of interpersonal communication, and pursuit of rewarding adaptive interpersonal behaviors.

Role Transitions

As indicated above, the focus in IPT-M usually consists of a combination of the four basic problem areas. Individuals experiencing role transitions are helped to view their new role in the most positive, least restrictive manner. Patients are encouraged to see their new role as an opportunity for growth, and they are helped to regain their self-esteem and sense of mastery in relation to the demands of the new role. They are guided to a realistic appraisal of what may have been lost in the transition, and are encouraged to develop a social support system and a repertoire of social skills that can be called upon in the new role.

We have found that a majority of IPT-M patients need to address the role transition they make from depressed individual to well individual. While for some this is a relatively easy transition, for others the experience of remaining consistently well for a long period of time can be disconcerting both to the patient and to the patient's significant others. This is especially true for patients who have suffered years of recurrent depressive episodes. Long-term commitments that the patient had felt uncomfortable making when ill become possible once the patient is in remission. Family members and co-workers may also begin to demand more than the patient feels confident that he or she can provide. Adapting to the exciting but often frightening possibilities and responsibilities that go along with being fully recovered can require considerable therapeutic work.

As we have noted elsewhere (Frank et al. 1987a), about one-half of the patients reaching the maintenance phase of the Maintenance Therapies in Recurrent Depression protocol had essentially normal personality profiles when assessed in a remitted state. Personality assessments were done both by self-report, using the Hirschfeld-Klerman Personality Battery (Hirschfeld et al. 1987), and by clinician rating, using the personality assessment form developed for the NIMH Treatment of Depression Collaborative Research Program (Elkin et al. 1985). The other half of the patient group who entered maintenance treatment displayed clinically significant personality pathology, especially avoidant and dependent features.

When beginning maintenance treatment, individuals who were free of personality pathology tended to view themselves and were viewed by their significant others as "well persons" who occasionally experienced episodes of dysfunction. These patients rarely experienced difficulty as they moved into the maintenance phase of the study. However, patients with chronic personality pathology were more likely to find the "well" role unfamiliar. As with any role transition, the newly found energy and assertiveness associated with remissions often created a temporary disequilibrium in these patients' interpersonal realm. This transition out of the "sick role" frequently became at least a temporary focus of IPT-M for some patients, as in the following case:

Ms. N. is a 29-year-old obese single white female who was experiencing her fourth episode of depression when she entered the protocol. She is the youngest daughter of six children born into a strict Italian Catholic family. Her mother had died several years earlier. The patient reported that she had been very close to her mother and was devastated by her death. For most of her life Ms. N. had lived in the family home. She had moved away on one occasion but could not handle the situation financially and returned home after a few months. At the time she entered treatment, the patient was living with her father, a younger brother, and her paternal grandfather. She was not working and had primary caretaking responsibilities for her grandfather, who was demented, incontinent, and bedridden.

The focus in acute IPT was on interpersonal disputes. Ms. N. and her father were frequently at odds, especially since she was dependent upon him for income. Ms. N. was able to gain insight into the fact that caring for her grandfather was really quite a burden to her; however, any mention to her father about an out-of-home placement for the grandfather was met with anger and disapproval. Ms. N. and the therapist spent time reviewing her communication style, which was generally whiny and non-assertive, and worked on approaching her father about the grandfather's care from a more adult standpoint. Although her father remained adamant that her grandfather should remain at home, Ms. N. was able to begin to set limits for herself regarding his care as she worked on issues of self-esteem and assertiveness. She was also able to recognize her desire to have her father be more supportive and loving as her mother had been, and to acknowledge the dissonance between this expectation and reality. She worked to lessen her own reactivity to her father's demands and concentrate on her own needs.

During the course of maintenance treatment, the therapeutic focus shifted to role transitions. Because of the persistent nature of her depressive episodes, Ms. N. had never been able to sustain consistent employment or become involved in a committed relationship. She had always wanted to marry and have children, much as her mother and older sisters had done. As her current episode remitted, the patient began looking to move beyond her dependent homemaker role and seek employment and increase her social contacts. She found work as a waitress, which helped her to become less financially dependent on her father for the first time in years. She was able to lose weight and improve her appearance, and found herself being approached by men. She began dating and became involved with a man who had a 10-year-old son. She ultimately became engaged to this man and spent much of the remaining maintenance phase discussing the ramifications of the many changes she had experienced since entering treatment.

Interpersonal Disputes

Because patients in IPT-M are seen over such a long period of time, it is only natural that some interpersonal disputes would develop and become the focus of treatment. These may occur within the context of marriage, family, work, or social settings. IPT techniques can readily be applied when these disputes occur. The therapist helps the patient to identify the nature of the dispute, guides the patient in making choices about a plan of action, and encourages the patient to modify maladaptive communication patterns whenever possible. If such modification is impossible or undesirable, the patient is encouraged to reassess expectations for the relationship.

Experience with IPT-M has shown that one or two relationships in the patient's life seem to emerge as those that are occasional or chronic sources of difficulty. The nature of IPT-M allows the therapist and patient to work together over an extended period of time in order to identify characteristic destructive patterns of interaction early in their development, to disrupt those dysfunctional patterns before they become ingrained, and to try out new patterns of interaction. The following case illustrates these points:

Ms. Y. is a 47-year-old married white female who had experienced yearly episodes of depression since age 18. During the winter months, Ms. Y. became depressed and isolative. She tended to tailor her life around these depressive episodes and overfunctioned when well. Ms. Y. was the oldest of six children and had become responsible for her siblings at an early age because of her parents' ongoing marital difficulties. She matured quickly and essentially functioned as an adult at an early age. Ms. Y. married soon after high school. Her own marriage was characterized by conflicts related to her husband's alcohol abuse.

Ms. Y. was a full-time homemaker; her husband worked in a local steel mill. The couple had four children: two daughters, ages 32 and 27, and two sons, ages 25 and 16. The oldest son also abused alcohol. Ms. Y. tended to take on much of the responsibility of running the household and thus fostered dependence in her husband and sons.

The focus in acute IPT was on role transitions. As Ms. Y. began feeling less depressed, she recognized her pattern of being overly responsible for others and not attending to her own needs. Her oldest son announced his engagement during this phase of treatment, and Ms. Y. utilized this opportunity to detach and begin taking less responsibility for her own grown children. She was able to take pride in the fact that she was not taking on more responsibility than she needed to for her son's wedding.

She also began focusing on the role transition from being a parent to not being needed as much in that role. She successfully processed the many conflicted feelings she had about this change and began focusing on other ways to fill her time. To her surprise, her family reacted well to these changes, which helped to add to her increasing confidence and self- esteem.

In maintenance treatment, issues of interpersonal disputes with her husband began to take precedence. As the patient negotiated the move from being a full-time parent, she found herself reassessing the marital relationship. She was able to recognize that her depression had often been reactive to her husband's off-again, on-again drinking habits, and to acknowledge the necessity of detaching and not taking responsibility for his drinking. The patient actively sought outlets for her energies, including increasing social contacts. The therapist remained supportive of the patient during this period. Her husband was ultimately able to admit his drinking problem and joined Alcoholics Anonymous, although he continued to have difficulty in maintaining sobriety. Ms. Y. was able to continue decreasing her own reactivity to her husband's behavior.

The interpersonal disputes between the couple intensified midway through the maintenance phase when Ms. Y.'s youngest daughter disclosed that she had been sexually abused as a child by her father. Although upset by this revelation, the patient did not become depressed. She was able to focus on the impact of her daughter's disclosure on herself and on the family's relationships. This involved processing the guilt, sadness, and anger that she felt. Ms. Y. also used earlier IPT work on not getting overinvolved by setting healthy boundaries for herself related to the relationship between her husband and their daughter, instead of rushing to "fix" things. She remained supportive of her daughter and, in fact, participated in her daughter's incest support group. She was able to remain detached when her husband increased his drinking, and she continued to remain active in her outside activities in addition to joining Alanon.

Ms. Y. successfully negotiated the transition from being a full-time parent during early IPT, utilizing the increased self-confidence this gave her to work on her marital disputes during the maintenance phase. Her husband's past and present behavior posed serious challenges to her recovery, but the patient was able to detach successfully and attend to her own needs. She was proud of these accomplishments and was hopeful for the future because of her success in treatment.

Interpersonal Deficits

Interpersonal deficits are a focus of treatment in the maintenance phase of IPT for those patients whose deficits do not ameliorate with the resolution of the depressive episode. The IPT-M therapist works to reduce the patient's social isolation and enhance the quality of any existing relationships. In IPT-M, as in the Stage-2 work described with IPT patients showing interpersonal deficits (see Klerman et al. 1984), emphasis is placed on helping the patient apply what is learned in treatment to outside situations. When there are no current meaningful relationships, the focus of treatment is on past relationships, the relationship with the therapist, and the beginnings of new relationships. Each attempt at a new relationship, whether successful or not, is looked at in terms of correctable deficits in the patient's communication skills and interpersonal style.

As we have noted above, many of the patients in the Maintenance Therapies in Recurrent Depression protocol fell into the avoidant/dependent personality spectrum (Frank et al. 1987a). Patients with these traits need encouragement to change their social interactions and attend more to their interpersonal needs. Some of these patients need to form more independent, self-reliant styles so as to feel less at the mercy of others in their interpersonal relationships. The long course of IPT-M provides a secure base from which patients can explore new interpersonal styles and seek support and reinforcement in the therapy, as in the following case:

Mr. D. is a 38-year-old single white male who was in his fourth episode of depression when he sought treatment at our clinic. Mr. D. lived alone in the country and worked independently as a draftsman. He was the youngest of three children. Both parents were deceased, as was one sibling. He was not close to his surviving sister, and he had no close friends. Mr. D. had never had any significant relationships in his life. He generally presented as a very avoidant, lonely man. Mr. D. was obese, had low self-esteem, and was nonassertive. His primary complaints centered around his dissatisfaction with his work and his social isolation.

The focus of acute IPT was interpersonal deficits. Because Mr. D. had no outside relationships, the therapist-patient relationship assumed primary importance. The patient was able to review his past relationships with his parents, who were described as isolative, taciturn people who put little stock in friendships. Mr. D., who had never been encouraged to socialize, felt he had little to offer others. He was able to identify a typical pattern of moving toward people, becoming fearful of rejection, and then withdrawing into his house.

As Mr. D.'s depression lifted, his functioning at work improved. He was able to devote more energy to nurturing the creative parts of himself.

He enrolled in a photography class and exhibited considerable talent in this medium. The positive nature of this experience encouraged the patient to continue making changes. He was able to lose 70 pounds, which added to his self-esteem. He joined a public-speaking class and tried seeking out new friends. The therapist remained supportive and encouraging as Mr. D. began taking these steps to decrease his isolation.

In the maintenance phase of treatment, therapeutic work continued to revolve around the theme of interpersonal deficits. Mr. D. was able to explore his fears about entering into new relationships and recognize the extent of his own low self concept. It was during the maintenance phase that Mr. D. identified himself as homosexual. This was a source of considerable anxiety and shame for the patient, and marked the first time that he had ever disclosed his sexual orientation. The therapist expressed nonjudgmental acceptance, which greatly helped to decrease Mr. D.'s anxiety.

Throughout the course of IPT-M, Mr. D. continued to focus on his fears of rejection and low self-esteem as they related to the process of "coming out" and becoming comfortable in the gay community. He was able to join a support group at a local gay and lesbian counseling center, and he began dating for the first time in his life. The therapist helped Mr. D. decrease his anxiety in this regard by role-playing various scenarios and providing feedback when he reported new interactions.

Although Mr. D. continued to experience some difficulties in relating to others, he was able to use therapy to develop a broader repertoire of social skills and increase his self-confidence. He also was able to acknowledge that the maintenance therapy had supported and encouraged a great deal of positive growth, and he derived satisfaction and pride from the fact that he had successfully maintained a positive relationship with his therapist throughout the 3 years of treatment.

Grief Reactions

Grief reactions are not usually a focus in IPT-M unless a death occurs during the course of the maintenance treatment. Should this happen, the treatment strategies utilized parallel those employed in IPT, with one exception: the therapist normalizes the symptoms the patient is experiencing by clarifying distinctions between a normal grief reaction and a depressive episode.

At times, a loss during the course of maintenance treatment may trigger unresolved feelings about an earlier death. In that event, the IPT-M therapist employs the strategies suggested by Klerman et al. (1984) for treatment of unresolved grief reactions:

Ms. P. was a 39-year-old married white female who at the time she entered treatment lived with her husband, three teenage sons, and a daughter. She had a history of multiple depressive episodes beginning at age 16 and had been hospitalized once for depression. Ms. P. had married at age 18 and moved out of state with her husband. Their first child was born 2 years later. The family had numerous financial problems, and the patient went to work at a canning factory, where she began an affair with her supervisor, a man 20 years her senior. Prior to the current depressive episode, the patient had been treated for endometriosis and had had a hysterectomy, and was laid off from her factory job of 15 years. This also resulted in the termination of the extramarital affair with her supervisor.

Acute IPT treatment focused primarily on the distant relationship between the patient and her husband and her residual guilt regarding the extramarital affair. Because Ms. P. was unable to find work, the therapist also helped her to deal with the unresolved role transition from working mother to full-time homemaker. Her oldest son left home to join the military during this time, and the patient was able to adapt to this change, which also reinforced the need for the patient and her husband to face their marital problems as their children grew older. This remained a focus as the patient proceeded into maintenance treatment.

Approximately 1 year into therapy, Ms. P.'s youngest child, her 12-year-old daughter, was killed in an auto accident. Psychotherapy focus shifted to the grief reaction of the patient. For the next several months, the patient was able to use therapy to mourn for her child and to process the impact that this tragedy had on family relationships. She was able to discuss the sorrow and guilt she had about not being able to bear more children, an issue that she had not been able to discuss with her husband until it was "diffused" by bringing it up in therapy.

With the help of the therapist, Ms. P. was able to distinguish her quite natural grief reaction from a recurrence of depression. Her mood remained stable throughout the course of the protocol, and by the study's end she was continuing to feel well and had become involved with a new business she had bought with her husband. This new business venture was seen in a positive light and gave the patient and her husband a reason to work together. It also gave Ms. P. a focus and direction in life, which she felt had been missing since she had lost her job and which had been further challenged by her daughter's death.

Cautions for the IPT-M Therapist

Our experience using IPT-M has indicated certain cautions for the IPT-M therapist. These include 1) being alert for patients having difficulty switching from more frequent acute treatment sessions to monthly maintenance treatment, 2) being aware of one's own concerns as a therapist about the maintenance format, 3) being judicious about the use of interpretation, and 4) being vigilant regarding possible recurrences of depression.

As noted previously, some patients experience the decreased therapeutic contacts in IPT-M as a loss and have difficulty moving to the monthly session format. The IPT-M therapist is advised to recognize the possibility that the patient may have some difficulty managing the transition. Initially, some patients tend to return to the therapeutic focus of earlier acute treatment experiences. The therapist can reinforce these efforts, as in the following case, by noting that it is to the patient's credit that he or she is independently continuing to address an issue raised many months earlier:

> Ms. A. is a 39-year-old married white female who had suffered yearly episodes of depression since her early 20s but had never previously sought treatment. During the acute phase of IPT, she focused on her interpersonal disputes with her husband, whom she described as "a nice guy" but very dependent on her and possibly also depressed. Ms. A. felt unable to confide in her spouse about her problems and concerns. She had few outside supports and thus greatly valued the therapeutic relationship. The patient used therapy to work on issues of assertiveness and self-esteem, and she was able to begin negotiating a more independent relationship with her husband.
>
> Because of Ms. A.'s high regard for the therapeutic relationship and the progress she had made during the initial IPT sessions, the transition to the continuation phase of treatment was difficult for the patient. She perceived the decreased frequency of treatment contacts as "slowing down," and voiced concerns about losing the therapeutic relationship, which she saw as a primary source of support. Ms. A. also responded with a minor increase in symptoms, presenting with some overeating, mood lability, and general distress and anxiety. Although her overall functioning was not impaired, she and her husband began arguing more. An extra treatment session was added when Ms. A. complained of increased symptoms. The therapist worked to reassure the patient that she was not experiencing a recurrence of depression. The positive gains that she had made during acute IPT were reviewed and reinforced, and the therapist praised Ms. A.'s desire to continue working on her treatment issues. During this time, the patient's husband entered individual therapy himself. This helped to stabilize the couple's relationship and reestablish the interpersonal focus of Ms. A.'s own therapy as she moved into maintenance treatment.

Equally important to consider are concerns that the IPT-M therapist may have about maintenance treatment. Therapists in the Maintenance Therapies in Recurrent Depression protocol had some initial questions about whether a true therapeutic relationship could be maintained when patients were seen so infrequently; they also were concerned that sessions might deteriorate to mere diaries of the events of the previous month.

While one consistent problem focus is neither possible nor sensible in IPT-M, patients and therapists can and do maintain a consistent therapeutic relationship on a monthly basis. IPT-M is offered to patients who are already familiar with and who have experienced the conceptual framework of IPT. It is the nature of this treatment that various problem areas emerge and recede when patients are seen once a month over a multiyear maintenance treatment period. Patients and therapists are, nevertheless, able to retain a consistent approach to these various problem areas because of their long-standing relationship. In fact, there exists a subgroup of patients who make major therapeutic breakthroughs as a result of moving from weekly to monthly contacts. These individuals seem to benefit from the longer distance between sessions and are able to bring richer material to the monthly sessions as a result of having had more time between appointments to observe and process the interpersonal context of their lives and to experiment with new behaviors.

While it is possible for patients to address major interpersonal problems on a once-a-month basis, therapeutic interpretations of material presented must be made judiciously. The overzealous IPT-M therapist runs the risk of making an overstimulating interpretation that might leave the patient vulnerable between sessions, wondering what the therapist might have meant or even questioning the value of the treatment. This could result in a negative transference reaction or acting-out behavior when the therapist has only a limited capacity to deal with such problems on the basis of one session per month.

Given the insidious nature of recurrent depression, it is crucial that therapists be aware of early warning signs of emerging episodes. The patient should be encouraged to monitor somatic and/or cognitive symptoms that had been indicative of prior depressive episodes, and to report any such changes to the therapist. Such vigilance can aide in the planning of treatment strategies to prevent the recurrence of a new episode, as in the following case:

Ms. F. is a 55-year-old married white female with a history of three fully documented episodes of depression. She reported that several times during her late adolescence and early adult life she had experienced dysphoria and disruption in neurovegetative functioning to the extent that she may have actually suffered other depressive episodes.

Ms. F. had been married for more than 30 years to a man who was an elementary school teacher. Mr. F.'s position brought him into contact with many other women, including both colleagues and parents. This had always been a difficult situation for Ms. F., for she suspected that many of these women were attracted to her husband, who by all accounts was a charming and pleasant man. Her discomfort was exacerbated by the fact that the current president of the school board was an unmarried woman who had intruded herself enormously both on her husband's professional life and on their married and family life. The couple had had many disagreements about the situation and had been unable to resolve the problem to Ms. F.'s satisfaction.

As Ms. F.'s depression improved, her complaints about her husband significantly lessened. She ceased to feel suspicious about his fidelity and was able to use therapy to help improve her communication with him. Husband and wife were able to work together so that they could come to some agreement on how to handle the situation with the school board president.

Throughout the course of maintenance treatment, the therapist noted that whenever Ms. F. was feeling even slightly more depressed, she became preoccupied with thoughts about the extent to which her husband might be romantically involved with other women. When she was not depressed, she was never bothered by ideas about her husband's fidelity. The therapist was able to use the long-term therapeutic relationship to gently point this out to the patient. Several times during the course of the maintenance treatment, the patient came in reporting that her thoughts had again turned to relationships between her husband and his female colleagues. Rather than viewing these thoughts as representing an issue that needed to be brought up with her husband, Ms. F. and her therapist were able to identify them as the possible start of a new episode. Together, they decided upon a course of action that would be most likely to keep her from going into another episode of depression. This included Ms. F.'s devoting more time to her own needs and focusing less on the needs and desires of others.

This strategy had the effect of improving Ms. F.'s mood several times during the course of maintenance treatment. On each occasion, by the time she returned for her next monthly visit, she reported that she was no longer concerned about her husband's female colleagues, and she was essentially free of depressive symptoms.

Efficacy of Maintenance Interpersonal Psychotherapy

One of the most important factors in assessing the prophylactic efficacy of a treatment modality is whether that treatment modifies the course of the disorder. IPT-M was developed specifically for use in the Maintenance Therapies in Recurrent Depression protocol. The study was designed to explore the relative effectiveness of five maintenance treatment strategies in preventing or delaying a recurrence of depressive illness in a group of high-risk patients (Frank et al. 1990). Entrance criteria were particularly stringent, requiring subjects between ages 21 and 65 years to be seen initially in their third or more episode of unipolar depression. In the acute stage of treatment, patients were treated with IPT for 12 weeks according to the methods described by Klerman et al. (1984), and were maintained on 150 to 300 mg of imipramine. Blood plasma levels of imipramine/desipramine were continuously monitored, and dosages were adjusted if patients complained of intolerable side effects.

Once patients had stabilized (as indicated by a Hamilton Rating Scale for Depression [Hamilton 1960] score of 7 or less and a Raskin score [Raskin et al. 1969] of 5 or less), they entered into the 20-week continuation phase of treatment. After the first 12 IPT sessions, patients began to see their psychotherapists with decreasing frequency in preparation for the monthly schedule of the maintenance phase. Patients were seen biweekly for the next 8 weeks, then monthly until they had sustained remission of symptoms for a period of 20 weeks. No changes were made in any patient's medication regimen during this phase. Patients were then randomly assigned to one of the five maintenance treatment conditions: 1) IPT-M alone; 2) IPT-M with active imipramine therapy continued at the acute treatment dosage; 3) IPT-M with placebo; 4) medication clinic visits with active imipramine therapy; and 5) medication clinic visits with placebo.

At the last continuation treatment session, patients were informed whether they would continue in monthly psychotherapy or switch to monthly medication clinic visits, and whether they would continue to receive medication tablets. However, both patients and members of their treatment teams remained blind as to whether they were receiving active medication or placebo. Patients were seen monthly for 3 years in the maintenance phase, or until they experienced a recurrence of depressive illness.

Of the 230 patients entered in the study, 128 ultimately entered into the maintenance therapy phase. In the maintenance treatment phase, 26 patients were assigned to IPT-M alone; 25 to IPT-M and active imipramine; 26 to IPT-M with placebo; 28 to medication clinic and active imipramine; and 23 to medication clinic with placebo. Random assignment to these groups ensured that they were equivalent with respect to demographic, baseline clinical, and short-term and continuation treatment characteristics.

Of the 128 patients who entered the maintenance phase, only 22 (17%) failed to complete the protocol: 3 eventually developed medical problems that were incompatible with continued imipramine treatment, 1 moved out of the country, 15 elected to drop out of the study or were terminated for noncompliance with the protocol, and 3 were discontinued for various other reasons.

The mean survival time for the total group of 128 patients was 75.7 ± 61.8 weeks, with a median of 54.4 weeks. The mean survival times for each of the five treatment conditions are provided in Table 4–1. Groups receiving active imipramine had the longest mean survival time. Because 50% of the patients did not have a recurrence, no median can be reported for these groups. Using Cox's proportional hazards model, imipramine at a maintenance dosage of approximately 200 mg was thus proven to be highly effective in delaying recurrence ($P < .0001$).

Equally important are the findings regarding IPT-M. Groups receiving IPT-M either alone or with placebo survived nearly twice as long as did the group of patients receiving medication clinic and placebo. The overall survival analysis showed a significant effect ($P < .05$) for psychotherapy in extending survival time, and when the two groups receiving active medication were omitted from the analysis, the effect for IPT-M was shown to be slightly greater ($P < .04$). However, comparison of the group receiving IPT-M with active imipramine with the group medication clinic with imipramine failed to demonstrate a statistically significant advantage of combined treatment ($P = .81$). Although no statistically significant advantage was found to support the hypothesis that IPT-M would enhance the effect of maintenance pharmacotherapy, our experience with IPT-M itself suggests that this is a viable therapeutic modality with high acceptance by both patients and therapists. It may be that our strategy of continuing the acute treatment dose of medication rather than reducing patients to a so-called maintenance dose produced a ceiling effect in terms of survival time, precluding the possibility of observing an additive effect for IPT-M.

Potential Predictors of the Efficacy of Maintenance Interpersonal Psychotherapy

There are a number of factors that can contribute to the efficacy of a treatment. Variables that seem to influence the efficacy of IPT-M include both the psychobiological profile of the patient and factors in the patient/therapist dyad.

Biological Correlates

Several investigative groups pursuing treatment research have incorporated biological measures, particularly sleep electroencephalographic and neuroendocrine studies, in their outcome research (Jarrett et al. 1990; Kupfer et al. 1990; Rush et al. 1989). The most common and predictable sleep abnormalities of depression include sleep continuity disturbance, shortened rapid eye movement (REM) latency, a change in the temporal distribution of REM sleep, and diminished slow wave or delta sleep. De-

Table 4–1. Survival time in five maintenance treatment conditions for 3 years

Group	Mean survival time (weeks)	Median survival time (weeks)
Medication clinic and active imipramine	124 ± 13	—[a]
IPT-M and active imipramine	131 ± 10	—[a]
Medication clinic and placebo	45 ± 11	21
IPT-M alone	82 ± 13	54
IPT-M and placebo	75 ± 12	61

[a]Because 50% of the patients did not have a recurrence, no median can be reported for these groups.
Source. Adapted from Frank et al. 1990.

pressed individuals tend to progress into REM sleep more rapidly, have increased REMs in the first half of the night, and demonstrate a gradual diminution of delta sleep throughout the night, with lower delta-wave intensity during the first rather than the second non-REM period. Non-depressed individuals typically demonstrate a linear decrease in delta sleep throughout the night.

Our research team examined the ratio between the average delta wave counts in the first and second non-REM periods of patients in the Maintenance Therapies in Recurrent Depression protocol. We found that this delta-sleep ratio can serve as a predictor of both short-term and long-term (prophylactic) treatment outcome (Kupfer et al. 1990). Analysis of data on the 74 patients who were assigned to the three treatment cells that involved no active medication demonstrated that a lower delta-sleep ratio could predict survival time following discontinuation of drug therapy. The delta-sleep ratio appears to provide a marker of vulnerability to early recurrence following discontinuation of pharmacotherapy. Thus, it may be possible to use this ratio to identify those recurrent unipolar patients most likely to remain well when provided IPT-M alone on a monthly basis. Even though the average clinician may not have ready access to a sleep laboratory, in the case of the patient for whom nonpharmacological maintenance is clearly indicated on other grounds, the inconvenience and expense associated with obtaining electroencephalographic sleep studies may be well worth it.

Treatment Specificity

Another important trend in psychotherapy research is the exploration of the effect of treatment specificity in relation to outcome. To determine whether the prophylactic effect of monthly sessions of IPT was a function of specific features of the psychotherapeutic intervention, the contribution of the quality of IPT sessions to survival time was examined (Frank et al. 1991). The specificity of IPT-M was monitored through use of the Therapy Rating Scale, modeled after the scale developed by DeRubeis et al. (1982) for use in the NIMH Treatment of Depression Collaborative Research Program study (Elkin et al. 1989). The Therapy Rating Scale was designed to assess the extent to which therapy sessions were characterized by interpersonal interventions, somatic interventions (i.e., interventions appropriate to the medication clinic approach), or contamination interventions (i.e., cognitive-behavioral or psychoanalytic interventions). Each IPT-M therapy session was audiotaped, and a 7-minute segment beginning 5 minutes after the start of the session was later rated by trained undergraduate raters. The raters were blind to subjects' treatment conditions and to the number of months since the latter's assignment to the maintenance phase.

Among patients not receiving active medication, patients who received less specific IPT demonstrated a median survival time of 18.1 weeks, whereas patients who received more specific IPT demonstrated a median survival time of 101.7 weeks. The impact of treatment specificity was not moderated by baseline clinical severity, by severity at the time of random assignment, or by differences among clinicians. Rather, specificity appeared to be a stable feature of individual patient/therapist dyads.

This effect was found not to reflect the influence of one or two particularly talented therapists, but seemed instead to be a function of the ability of specific patient/therapist dyads to focus on interpersonal concerns. Each therapist studied had some patients with whom such intensive focus was possible and others with whom it was not. Individual clinicians were found to have different ratings with different patients, suggesting that the patient-therapist relationship is, indeed, bidirectional (Docherty 1989).

Populations for Whom Maintenance Interpersonal Psychotherapy Is Indicated

Maintenance interpersonal psychotherapy appears to be especially indicated for a number of special populations, including women, individuals with complicating medical conditions and drug intolerance, and elderly persons.

Women and IPT-M

The development of preventative maintenance strategies is especially relevant for women, given the female-to-male ratio of close to 2:1 in those patients seeking treatment for unipolar depression (Weissman and Klerman 1985; Weissman et al. 1984), and the even higher ratio of females to males presenting for treatment. It is noteworthy that 78% of patients in our Maintenance Therapies in Recurrent Depression protocol were female. Although no significant treatment-by-gender effects were noted in the overall survival analysis, when only those patients receiving IPT-M alone were examined, there is some evidence that IPT-M may have had greater prophylactic capacity for the females than for the males (median survival = 75.9 versus 10.3 weeks, P = .069).

A number of issues can complicate the clinical presentation and course of depression in women. Among the factors that deserve special attention and make IPT-M a particularly attractive treatment strategy are the unique importance of social environment and social relations, the desire to become pregnant and to nurse an infant, menstrual cycle effects on symptomatology, and complications in symptomatology and interpersonal functioning that occur subsequent to rape victimization, incest, or battering.

Many theories emphasize social factors as possible contributors to gender differences in rates of depression. While a range of genetic, hormonal, and personality theories have been proposed regarding women's vulnerability to depression, the literature on women in therapy has placed emphasis on potential differences in women's interpersonal environments. Interpersonal psychotherapy may be especially helpful for women because it focuses on relationships that are core to a woman's identity and self-esteem. For depressed women, the ability to regain and maintain good quality relational functioning may be a particularly important aspect of empowerment and recovery from depression, and of more importance to the maintenance of remission than are other potential foci of therapy.

Maintenance interpersonal psychotherapy also appears to be a viable treatment option for women in their child-bearing years. Although it was once assumed that pregnancy was associated with lower rates of psychiatric disorders, our own work documents the high incidence (46%) of pregnancy-related affective disorders in women with recurrent depression (Frank et al. 1987b). The desire to become pregnant, the pregnancy itself, and the desire to nurse may preclude the use of antidepressants, making IPT-M a particularly attractive treatment option.

A clear majority of women experience noticeable changes in mood in the late luteal phase of their menstrual cycles, with approximately 5% experiencing symptoms that severely affect their functioning (Rivera-Tovar and Frank 1990). In treating depressed women, clinicians need to be sensitive to monthly fluctuations in mood and consider whether increases in symptoms represent relapse or recurrence, or a more temporary symptom magnification related to the menstrual cycle. A maintenance approach to psychotherapy increases the ability to monitor such mood fluctuations and to initiate special therapeutic work aimed at helping women anticipate and cope with these changes.

Women in the United States are exposed to victimization, including incest, marital violence, and rape, at rates much higher than those for men. There is now substantial evidence that rape-related (Frank et al. 1988) and battering-related (O'Leary et al. 1989) depressive symptoms are responsive to psychotherapeutic intervention. Recovered depressed women with a history of victimization may be especially vulnerable to relapse or recurrence in the absence of a psychotherapeutic approach to maintenance that can support the fragile self-esteem observed in these women.

The Need for Alternatives to Psychopharmacological Interventions

The use of antidepressants may be problematic in individuals who suffer from a range of medical conditions, including autoimmune disorders (e.g., lupus, thyroid disease), cardiovascular disorders, or medical conditions for which the patients are taking medication. Substantial numbers of patients may need to discontinue antidepressant medication when it interacts with other medical conditions or treatments. Family planning needs may also necessitate discontinuation. Although electroconvulsive therapy (ECT) represents an acute treatment alternative, concerns also exist regarding patient refusal and medical contraindications. Furthermore, it is not clear that maintenance ECT is an effective prophylactic, and it is certainly not a convenient one. Thus, although considerable data exist suggesting that somatic treatments protect against relapse and recurrence, many patients may have side effects or risks that counterbalance these benefits. Even for individuals who are appropriate candidates for somatic treatments, IPT at an acute and maintenance level may provide distinct advantages beyond symptomatic remission. These include an increased effectiveness in interpersonal relationships and a deeper comprehension of personal vulnerabilities to depression that can lead to lower incidence rate of recurrence.

Patients also often find medication side effects to be intolerable. Over long-term treatment, side effects that seemed tolerable during the initial treatment may be reexamined by patients who are free of depressive symptoms. One of the most frequently cited side effects of tricyclic antidepressants is undesired weight gain. In the Maintenance Therapies in Recurrent Depression protocol, 13.3% of subjects experienced a weight gain of greater than 10% during the acute and continuation phases. The problem of weight gain may be particularly relevant for women, given the prominence of weight concerns among American females. Seemingly minor side effects such as this one may have important significance over longer periods of time. The use of maintenance psychotherapy in the form of IPT-M represents a viable alternative for the group of patients who cannot tolerate or refuse to take antidepressant medications over long-term periods.

Elderly Patients and IPT-M

Many features of IPT-M are particularly attractive as a treatment for depressed elderly persons. Elderly persons often suffer from a number of concurrent medical conditions and are more likely either to not tolerate the side effects of antidepressant medications or to resist consideration of additional pharmacotherapy. Furthermore, the specific problem areas addressed in both IPT and IPT-M are particularly relevant to the lives of older individuals. We are currently engaged in a long-term trial of the efficacy of IPT as a maintenance strategy in elderly patients with a diagnosis of recurrent depression. A description of the modifications we have made in IPT for use with elderly patients appears in Chapter 7 of this volume.

Acknowledgments

The development of maintenance interpersonal psychotherapy was supported in part by National Institute of Mental Health Grants MH-29618 and MH-30915. We acknowledge our indebtedness to the dedicated clinicians whose work is described in this chapter: Elaine Buzzinotti, M.S.; Jack Cahalane, M.S.W.; Steve Carter, Ph.D.; Lynne Eninger, M.S.W.; Debra Frankel, M.S.W.; Carol Hughes, M.S.W.; and Carole Webster, M.S.W. We also wish to thank Gerald L. Klerman, M.D.; Myrna Weissman, Ph.D.; Bruce Rounsaville, M.D.; and Eve S. Chevron, M.S. for their consultation in the development of IPT-M and for the training of the original group of therapists.

References

DeRubeis RJ, Hollon SD, Evans MD, et al: Can psychotherapies for depression be discriminated? A systematic investigation of cognitive therapy and interpersonal therapy. J Consult Clin Psychol 50:744–756, 1982

DiMascio A, Weissman MM, Prusoff BA, et al: Differential symptom reduction by drugs and psychotherapy in acute depression. Arch Gen Psychiatry 36:1450–1456, 1979

Docherty JP: The individual psychotherapies: efficacy, syndrome-based treatments and the therapeutic alliance, in Outpatient Psychiatry: Diagnosis and Treatment, 2nd Edition. Edited by Lazare A. Baltimore, MD, Williams & Wilkins, 1989, pp 624–644

Elkin I, Parloff MB, Hadley SW, et al: National Institute of Mental Health Treatment of Depression Collaborative Research Program: background and research plan. Arch Gen Psychiatry 42:304–316, 1985

Elkin I, Shea T, Watkins JT, et al: National Institute of Mental Health Treatment of Depression Collaborative Research Program: general effectiveness of treatments. Arch Gen Psychiatry 46:971–982, 1989

Frank E: Interpersonal psychotherapy as a maintenance therapy for patients with recurrent depression. Psychotherapy 28:259–266, 1991

Frank E, Kupfer DJ, Jacob M, et al: Personality features and response to acute treatment in recurrent depression. Journal of Personality Disorders 1:14–26, 1987a

Frank E, Kupfer DJ, Jacob M, et al: Pregnancy-related affective episodes among women with recurrent depression. Am J Psychiatry 144:288–293, 1987b

Frank E, Anderson B, Stewart BD, et al: Efficacy of cognitive behavior therapy and systematic desensitization in the treatment of rape trauma. Behavior Therapy 19:403–420, 1988

Frank E, Kupfer DJ, Perel JM, et al: Three-year outcomes for maintenance therapies in recurrent depression. Arch Gen Psychiatry 47:1093–1099, 1990

Frank E, Kupfer DJ, Wagner EF, et al: Efficacy of interpersonal psychotherapy as a maintenance treatment for recurrent depression: contributing factors. Arch Gen Psychiatry 48:1053–1059, 1991

Glen AIM, Johnson AL, Shepherd M: Continuation therapy with lithium and amitriptyline in unipolar depressive illness: a randomized, double-blind, controlled trial. Psychol Med 14:37–50, 1984

Hamilton M: A rating scale for depression. J Neurol Neurosurg Psychiatry 23:56–62, 1960

Hirschfeld RMA, Klerman GL, Clayton PJ, et al: Assessing personality: effects of depressive state on trait measurement. Am J Psychiatry 144:288–293, 1987

Jarrett RB, Rush AJ, Khatami M, et al: Does the pretreatment polysomnogram predict response to cognitive therapy in depressed outpatients? Psychiatry Res 33:285–299, 1990

Klerman GL, DiMascio A, Weissman M, et al: Treatment of depression by drugs and psychotherapy. Am J Psychiatry 131:186–191, 1974

Klerman GL, Weissman MM, Rounsaville BJ, et al: Interpersonal Psychotherapy for Depression. New York, Basic Books, 1984

Kupfer DJ, Frank E, Grochocinski VJ, et al: Delta sleep ratio: a biological correlate of early recurrence in unipolar affective disorder. Arch Gen Psychiatry 47:1100–1105, 1990

O'Leary KD, Barling V, Arias I, et al: Prevalence and stability of physical aggression between spouses: a longitudinal analysis. J Consult Clin Psychol 57:263–268, 1989

Prien RF, Kupfer DJ, Mansky PA, et al: Drug therapy in the prevention of recurrences in unipolar and bipolar affective disorders: a report of the National Institute of Mental Health Collaborative Study Group comparing lithium carbonate, imipramine, and a lithium carbonate–imipramine combination. Arch Gen Psychiatry 41:1096–1104, 1984

Raskin A, Schulterbrandt J, Reatig N, et al: Replication of factors of psychopathology in interview, ward behavior, and self-report ratings of hospitalized depressives. J Nerv Ment Dis 148:87–98, 1969

Rivera-Tovar A, Frank E: Late luteal phase dysphoric disorder in young women. Am J Psychiatry 147:1634–1636, 1990

Rush AJ, Giles DE, Jarrett RB, et al: Reduced REM latency predicts response to tricyclic medication in depressed outpatients. Biol Psychiatry 26:61–72, 1989

Weissman MM, Bothwell S: The assessment of social adjustment by patient self-report. Arch Gen Psychiatry 33:1111–1115, 1976

Weissman MM, Klerman GL: Sex differences in the epidemiology of depression. Arch Gen Psychiatry 34:98–111, 1985

Weissman MM, Paykel E: The Depressed Woman: The Study of Social Relationships. Chicago, IL, University of Chicago Press, 1974

Weissman MM, Leaf PJ, Holzer CE, et al: The epidemiology of depression: an update on sex differences in rates. J Affective Disord 7:179–188, 1984

Conjoint Interpersonal Psychotherapy for Depressed Patients With Marital Disputes

Myrna M. Weissman, Ph.D.
Gerald L. Klerman, M.D.

Conjoint interpersonal psychotherapy for depressed patients with marital disputes (IPT-CM) is an adaptation of interpersonal psychotherapy (IPT) designed for the treatment of depression occurring in the context of marital disputes. IPT-CM, like IPT, is a brief, weekly treatment. It differs from IPT in that a conjoint treatment format involving the spouse is used, and it focuses on only one of the four problem areas associated with depression for which IPT was developed: interpersonal marital disputes.

A manual describing the specific strategies, techniques, scripts, and case examples is available in draft form and may require modification for further use in research and practice (Rounsaville et al. 1986). In this chapter we summarize key aspects of the manual and describe the results of a small clinical trial (Foley et al. 1989).

The IPT-CM treatment extends individual IPT techniques for use with the identified depressed patient and her or his spouse. It also incorporates aspects of currently available marital therapies, particularly those that emphasize dysfunctional communication, and focuses on bringing about improvement in a small number of target problem areas.

Background

The basic approach of IPT to clinical depression has been described in detail (Klerman et al. 1984; also see Chapter 1). We build upon that previous material in describing the specific role of marital discord and disputes in depression and the rationale for conjoint therapy.

Epidemiological Studies and Life Events Research

Numerous epidemiological and clinical studies assessing the role of life events have documented that marital discord and marital disputes are highly associated with clinical depression (Bloom et al. 1978; Briscoe and Smith 1973; Brown and Harris 1978; Coyne 1976).

The most recent epidemiological data, derived from the National Institute of Mental Health (NIMH) Epidemiologic Catchment Area (ECA) study (Robins and Regier 1991), indicate that statements of dissatisfaction with current marital relations are highly associated with major depression (Leaf et al. 1986; Weissman 1987). These findings are consistent in community studies using self-rating scales of depressive symptoms (Olin and Fennell 1989).

Similarly, life events research indicates that when depressed patients in treatment are asked to identify the life events occurring in the recent past, marital discord figures prominently among the patients' attributions of the events preceding the onset of the current episode of clinical depression. More recent studies on marital satisfaction, stress, and coping in depressed patients continue to show the serious impact of depression on marital relations (Gotlib and Whiffen 1989a, 1989b), although some studies question the direction of the effect (Fincham et al. 1989; Jacobson et al. 1989; Schmaling and Jacobson 1990).

In treating depressed patients with interpersonal disputes, it became apparent to us that a significant proportion of the interpersonal role disputes involved the marriage partner. For example, in a study examining life stress in relationship to the onset of depression (Paykel et al. 1969), the most commonly reported life stress in the 6 months prior to the onset of clinical depression was an increase in arguments with the spouse. Furthermore, in our early study of 150 depressed patients treated in a maintenance trial for over 9 months with tricyclic antidepressants alone, individual IPT alone, or the combination, over 40% of the patients, all females, reported marital conflict as the stress associated with the onset of their depression (Rounsaville et al. 1978, 1979, 1980).

Recent Social Changes

It is likely that marital disputes in relation to depression have increased over recent decades in modern urban industrialized societies. With an increased emphasis on individual fulfillment, relaxation of previous sexual restrictions, availability of contraceptive devices, and changed attitudes toward abortion, marriage, and child-rearing, an increasing number of couples are experiencing difficulties in resolving their expectations of marriage. Disputes arise over such issues as the woman's participation in the work force, sexual activities and their frequency, management of finances, allocation of household tasks (e.g., shopping, cooking, housekeeping, decorating), and the division of labor in child-rearing. In this historical context of recent social change, where altering sex roles and changing patterns of marriage and family life are the norm, depression appears to be occurring more frequently, particularly among younger age groups (Klerman and Weissman 1989).

Marital Discord and Depression

Depression preceding the marital problems. Extensive research on the cognitive difficulties associated with depression as discussed by Beck et al. (1979) indicates that patients, when depressed, have a limited capacity to consider a positive outcome to current difficulties. Similarly, research on learned helplessness when extended to the marital situation indicates why many married individuals, when confronted alone with difficult problems, are unable to initiate moves that would allow them first to master, and then later to potentially resolve, marital disputes.

Marital discord as "cause" of depression. Theoretically, we have proposed that depression is more likely to occur as a mood or a syndrome when an individual feels helpless, hopeless, and unable to influence the behavior of a significant other. The disappointment and frustration incurred by these helpless feelings mobilize the fear that there will be a disruption of the patient's relationship with the significant other and, thus, that there will be a disruption of the attachment bond. In this context, the marriage relationship is seen as a special and intense form of the attachment bond; the relationship of the attachment bond to depression has been described in great detail by Bowlby (1969).

Limitations of Individual Psychotherapy in Marital Disorder

Conducting individual psychotherapy with depressed patients with interpersonal marital disputes has shown that working only with the identified patients may be limited. The absence of the spouse prevents direct renegotiation of disputed role expectations. Information gathered in a session comes from only one party to the dispute, a party whose perception and interpretation of the events are potentially biased by involvement in the dispute and the wish to appear blameless and without culpability. Portrayal of the self as the innocent victim is a common theme in individual psychotherapy of mental disputes.

Added to these theoretical and empirical observations was the suggestion by Gurman and Kniskern (1978) that individual, as compared with couples, treatment of patients with marital problems would be more likely to precipitate a divorce.

Characteristics

Like IPT, IPT-CM is defined by the following characteristics:

1. Placing emphasis on depression [At least one party to the dispute, usually the wife, must have a clinically diagnosed depression. IPT-CM accepts the concept of depression as a clinical disorder and differs from many other forms of family or marital therapy, which deemphasize Axis I clinical disorders in the patient or spouse.]
2. Setting of time-limited goals, with an emphasis on improving depressive symptoms and marital relationships and a deemphasis on changing the personality of the individuals

3. Developing a structured and comparatively operationalized treatment plan
4. The psychotherapist's taking an active and directive therapeutic stance
5. Fostering an early positive relationship and an alliance with the couple
6. Avoiding analysis of the patient/therapist relationship (transference) as the major focus of the treatment
7. Encouraging change in the interpersonal relationship between the couple outside of the session

The concepts and techniques used in IPT-CM could be applied to other forms of disputes outside the marital situation as well as to disputes involving nonmarried couples, both heterosexual and homosexual, who are not involved in a legally contractual marriage. However, for the purpose of initiating research, the initial formulations and clinical trial focused on those disputes that take place between two heterosexuals who are legally married.

Clinical Goals

The goals of IPT-CM are to facilitate a remission of the acute depressive episode and to promote resolution of the role dispute via renegotiation of role relations between the marriage partners. IPT-CM may not be applicable in cases in which one or both partners have an ongoing extramarital affair or in which both partners are not willing to participate even with the goal of bringing about a less disruptive separation. In addition, if the spouse of the identified patient has a psychotic mental disorder such as current mania or schizophrenia, it is unlikely that the strategies would be applicable, especially in the absence of medication (Prusoff et al. 1980).

The Process

The basic methods of IPT-CM are the same as in IPT except that the spouse is involved in each session. After the initial evaluation, as in IPT, managing the patient's depressive symptoms is the primary goal. Because the entrance into conjoint marital IPT for depression is through the prior identification of a clinically depressed spouse, the treatment has two complementary sets of goals: a) the individual goals of the depressed patients, the most important of which is a reduction of depressive symptoms; and b) the joint goals of the couple so as to improve their marital functioning.

The Initial Phase: Assessment, Diagnosis, and Therapeutic Contract

Assignment of the current depressive episode should involve primary inquiry of the identified patient. However, the nondepressed spouse should be present during at least one session of the assessment process. Because many depressed patients are reluctant to share this information with those who are close to them, the spouse may learn about the degree and severity of the patient's depression, something which the patient may previously have been reluctant to discuss.

Eliciting the nondepressed spouse's version of the depression may take place either intermittently while the therapist is directing questions to the patient, or sequentially following the completion of questioning that is directed primarily to the patient. Inquiry is also made about how the spouse has attempted to handle the patient's depression.

Evaluating the Clinical Status of the Spouse

Because the first goal of therapy is the treatment of the identified patient's depression, the spouse may feel left out of this phase of the treatment or, alternatively, may feel blamed for the depression. To guard against this, the therapist should attempt to include the spouse in every task described below. For example, in taking the history of the identified patient's depression, the therapist should gather a parallel history of the current depressive episode from the spouse's viewpoint.

An evaluation of the clinical status of the spouse is undertaken. The same clinical review as used with the patient can be used. Studies that have evaluated psychopathology in the families of depressed probands have shown that many of the spouses of depressed patients meet specified diagnostic criteria for some psychiatric disorder, most often major depression. Determination of the spouse's psychiatric diagnosis can be of value for two reasons. First, it may become evident that the spouse of the identified patient is in need of an additional treatment intervention such as medication. Second, knowledge of significant psychopathology in the spouse will help the therapist set treatment goals that take this liability into consideration. For example, the spouse's ability to change or to be supportive of the identified patient who is attempting to recover from depression may be severely limited if the spouse is disabled by psychopathology.

The depressed patient typically presents for treatment alone and may not be expecting the therapist to recommend couples treatment, even if the patient is readily aware that marital disputes contribute to the current depressive episode. The patient may profess a willingness to enter couples treatment but state that the spouse will not come in. In this case, the therapist should at least initially pursue the possibility that the patient is reluctant to engage in couples treatment and should explore these apprehensions with the identified patient. The therapist may then try to motivate the patient for couples treatment by explaining the particular benefits of it or by appealing to the patient's sense of what is entitled to her or him as help from a spouse. For example, the therapist may act surprised and ask, "You mean your [husband/wife] wouldn't care enough about your welfare to help you out in getting over this depression?"

Finally, the therapist should offer to talk to the spouse directly about the advisability of couples treatment. In many cases where the identified patient describes the spouse as unwilling to enter treatment, the spouse is remarkably responsive to a direct call from the therapist.

Assessment of Marital Disputes in Relation to Depression

The evaluation of the marital disputes follows closely the sections of IPT that address role disputes. The initial complaints about the marriage are determined. An effort is made to define the areas in which the partners differ in their understanding and performance of marital roles. Areas in which marital role disputes often arise include responsibilities and power, finances, family (extended and nuclear), social and work activities outside the family, sexual and intimate roles, and communication. These areas are outlined in the IPT-CM manual (see Rounsaville et al. 1986).

Following the IPT manual, the stage of the marital dispute is determined as one of the following: 1) *renegotiation,* in which the patient and the significant other are openly aware of differences and are actively trying, even if unsuccessfully, to bring about change; 2) *impasse,* in which the discussion between the patient and the spouse has stopped and smoldering, low-level resentment has taken over; or 3) *dissolution,* in which the relationship is irretrievably interrupted, and the goal is to help the parties separate.

The history of the marital relationship should be reconstructed. This in itself can be a therapeutic maneuver, because it may remind the couple of happier times, ways in which they have solved problems in the past, and the continuity of the bond they have formed with each other. It is often valuable to have each partner hear the other's version of the marital history in order to clarify areas in which disputes and disagreements take place. In the context of the clinical setting, the marital history may be obtained through structured written questionnaires, many of which are available (Frank and Kupfer 1974; Frank et al. 1976; Locke and Wallace 1976; Spanier 1976; Weissman and Bothwell 1976). It is important that these be filled out by each partner individually and be reviewed together. The marital history includes information on what was going on in each partner's life at the time they first met, how they met, why they were attracted to each other, what their expectations were of marriage, how they describe their dating and courtship, and how they describe their sexual relationships, changes in roles, children, finances, disputes, and separations. At the end of the session, the couple is provided with a rationale and time frame of the treatment.

The initial inventory reviews the relationship between the depression and marital disputes—whether the patient's depression is seen as a cause of a dispute, or the dispute is a cause of the depression—and different strategies are outlined for each. An interpersonal inventory is also obtained from each partner, focusing on the history of the marital relationship from its beginning and on each partner's relationship to her or his family of origin.

The most direct way of emphasizing the therapist's neutral role is simply to point out when each spouse attempts to ally with the therapist and explicitly state that the therapist's role is not to take sides but to help the partners negotiate with one another.

Because of the acute symptoms, the depressed partner may seem more worthy of sympathy and more in need of assistance. The nondepressed spouse, on the other hand, may be seen as the victimizer who has caused the depression. To prevent this from taking place, the central strategy is for the therapist to address comments to the couple in a way that includes both partners' participation in the problem.

The Middle Phase: Renegotiating the Marital Contract

During the middle phase, the major goal is the renegotiation of the marital roles. Although the patient and the therapist may agree on marital disputes as the problem, they do not necessarily know precisely what has made the problems or how to solve them. The structure and coherence of the treatment are provided by tying new material about the marriage to the central themes and targeted problem areas noted in the early sessions. As in IPT, the options for role change are discussed as well as alternative expectations for marital roles. Improvement of communication and role renegotiation constitute a major theme. Specific scripts to be used during treatment for exploring options and alternatives are included in the manual.

A typical middle session begins with the therapist asking, "How have you two been getting along recently?" or "What has happened between you since we last met?" or "What have you been working on?"

The Therapist's Role in the Middle Sessions

The IPT-CM manual illustrates characteristics of ideal therapeutic sessions and guidelines for the therapist to foster productivity of sessions. These guidelines, which are not unique, include the following:

Phrase comments positively. The therapist can create a safe working atmosphere by phrasing comments, confrontations, and clarifications in relatively positive terms. Patients feel vulnerable and highly sensitive to criticism and blaming, particularly by the therapist with the spouse present. If either or both partners are preoccupied with concerns about being found to be the culprit by the therapist, then their participation will be guarded and they may drop from treatment.

There are several ways for the therapist to avoid being critical while still generating change. First, the therapist can validate the patient's behaviors. Many patients blame themselves excessively for behaviors that result from anger, such as deliberately hurting or inducing guilt in their partner. Extramarital affairs may be a source of great pain, compounded by guilt and recriminations. The therapist's handling of such issues should be matter-of-fact and serious, but should point out that these behaviors are common and simply indicate that the ways in which the couple have tried to solve marital problems have not worked up to this time.

The therapist can avoid blaming either partner by attributing problems not to selfish or malicious intentions or personality problems but to lack of agreement as to role expectations that the couple have had in their interactions. For example, ceaseless, unproductive arguments are not necessarily the result of stubbornness, bad faith, or irreconcilable differences, but may be caused by a failure to conduct discussions by more productive rules. Such a line of reasoning assures the couple that neither partner is specifically at fault because both partners have been following these rules and are equally responsible for changing.

The therapist, by refusing to accept the partners' negative labels for themselves, their marriage, or their actions, may elicit a complete sequential explication of events or feelings. For instance, the couple may describe the past week as "a disaster" without indicating any specific details. By forcing the couple to give a more complete account of "disastrous events" (e.g., the first open argument in years), the therapist may make the events seem understandable or even a sign of progress.

Remain nonjudgmental and communicate warmth and positive regard. This, of course, does not mean that the therapist accepts all aspects of the couple, but, rather, conveys the message that the partners' problems can be resolved and do not necessarily represent permanent features of the individuals or their relationship. In keeping with this stance, the therapist is optimistic and supportive, using such techniques as reassurance and direct advice giving when the patient is feeling most symptomatic and helpless.

Keep negative affect within bounds. The therapist should foster the expression of affect but keep it within bounds. The therapist interrupts and sets limits to uncontrolled displays of angry feelings and, at the same time, keeps discussion focused on topics of importance to the couple, while avoiding an abstract, technical, or intellectualized discussion.

Focus content on targeted problems. The therapist is responsible for keeping psychotherapy sessions focused on topics relevant to the targeted treatment goals. Goals are not left unformulated, and sessions do not pass without reference to them or to the specific subgoals that are derived from the central treatment goals. At the beginning of middle sessions, the therapist should ask the couple, "What would you like to work on today?" or "What is on your agenda?" rather than, "How are you doing?" or "How are things going?" "How did that happen?" is replaced by "How did you make that happen?"

Firmly set limits when one or both spouses interrupt or monopolize. The most direct and practical way of handling excessive interrupting or monopolizing is to set a rule against it or to simply intervene by saying something like, "Let her finish—you'll have your turn." "I can't hear when both of you are talking at once." The therapist may also take this opportunity to coach the couple in rules for communicating or arguing fairly.

Avoid alliance with one partner. When the therapist makes interventions that seem to attack a particular spouse or discovers an exclusive sympathy for one spouse's position and blame for the other spouse, the therapist may request to leave the session for a short period, review videotapes of this and other sessions, talk the case over with a supervisor or colleague, or take down and review process notes on the session. Each spouse will attempt to ally the therapist with himself or herself, but steps to prevent this from happening should be taken. For example, the therapist may emphasize the participation of both partners in problems, or he or she may speak of problems in terms of dysfunctional rules of the marital system, and so forth.

    Other issues that are described in the manual include dealing with partners who engage in incessant arguments both in and out of therapy; couples who repeatedly get sidetracked in discussions or present with a series of crises; the patient who discusses suicide, requires medication, or is silent; and so forth.

Renegotiation of the Marital Role Contract

A distinction related to how the therapist manages each session is the degree to which the couple encourage communicating with each other or through the therapist. With couples who are highly argumentative and angry, it is often pointless to simply let them engage in lengthy arguments. In such cases the therapist may choose to insist initially that the spouses' talk be done through him or her, with the patients speaking only when he or she questions them.

With less fractious couples, communication between the spouses is encouraged. This is particularly the case for disengaged, reticent couples who say too little to each other. There are other instances in which the therapist may request that the spouses talk directly to each other: "Could you tell [your spouse] directly now what you wish?" This should take place when the therapist wishes to heighten the impact of a partner's statements, or when a spouse is complaining about the other, stating a wish about what he or she would like the other to do, or making a statement that conveys affection or understanding of the spouse. When the couple is talking about communication problems, here the couple should be encouraged to demonstrate this difficulty in the session to allow further exploration of the problem. The therapist should also be alert to instances in which one spouse is "mind reading" or speaking for the other. When this takes place, the therapist may instruct the partner to ask the other what he or she thinks or feels about the issue. It is frequently helpful to encourage the partners to speak directly with each other when they are trying to resolve a particular agreed-upon dispute: "Why don't you ask [your spouse] right now what [he or she] thinks, feels, [etc.]?"

While helping the couple to identify and explore options for achieving a more satisfactory division of marital roles, it sometimes becomes apparent that one or both partners have developed role expectations based on their family of origin that are not adaptive in the current relationship. In order for the therapist to help the couple realize that there are alternatives, it is often necessary to point out that they have been acting currently as if no alternatives exist.

It may be useful to review how each spouse's family of origin has provided a model for the way the current relationship is seen. This model can be dysfunctional for several reasons. It may have worked in the family of origin, but not as well as alternative models that were also available would have. Or, it may have worked in the family of origin but is not appropriate to new problems or to the different cast of characters in the couple's life. Finally, it may not have even worked in the family of origin.

The major thrust of the intermediate phase of IPT-CM is to renegotiate roles and to put the new contract into practice. Questions such as "How do you wish your spouse to change?" may facilitate the process.

The Termination Phase

The termination phase is handled as it is in IPT. Termination and the couples' feelings about it are discussed explicitly and accomplishments are reviewed. In the last few sessions, the therapist may bolster the couple's sense of being able to handle future problems by reviewing with them areas in which they anticipate future difficulties and guiding them through an exploration of how various contingencies can be handled.

Because many couples have some discomfort with termination, a decision not to terminate should not be based solely on the patient's discomfort. If the couple do not wish to terminate, they should be instructed that they can come back but that they should wait at least 4 weeks before doing so. The exception to this are couples in which the identified patient is severely symptomatic and has shown little or no improvement in the course of therapy. Alternative treatment (i.e., drugs and/or individual psychotherapy) should be considered for either spouse alone or for the couple, depending on the specific needs in each case.

Comparison With Other
Marital Therapies

Emphasis on Depression as a Clinical Disorder

Both individual IPT and IPT-CM focus on depression as a clinical disorder. IPT-CM, like IPT, follows the general clinical point of view embodied in the DSM-III (American Psychiatric Association 1980) and DSM-III-R (American Psychiatric Association 1987), and differs from other forms of psychotherapy that deemphasize symptoms and clinical disorders. Symptoms are not regarded as epiphenomena or as an expression of an underlying personality conflict as in psychodynamic psychotherapy, or, as in many family therapies, as a failure in the family system.

A consequence of accepting the concept of clinical disorder is the willingness to conduct a diagnostic assessment and to make clinical diagnoses based on Axis I of the DSM or other comparable diagnostic criteria. By doing so, the identified patient is placed in the sick role and is encouraged to identify herself or himself as having a medically relevant disorder. Medication for the depression is used when appropriate, as determined by presenting the signs and symptoms and the medical condition of the depressed patient. For these reasons, IPT and IPT-CM are seen as health interventions that are most suitably provided by clinics and practitioners associated with medical centers, hospitals, community mental health centers, and so forth, although not necessarily by physicians.

During the initial phase of IPT-CM, considerable attention is given to eliciting the symptoms of depression, reconstructing the history of the current depressive episode in the ill spouse, and ascertaining if the patient's clinical picture meets the criteria for major depression.

Comparison With Psychodynamic Approaches

In both the individual and the conjoint marital form of IPT, the focus is on "here and now" interactions between the patient and significant others. In the case of IPT-CM, the focus more specifically is on the current marital relationship. The purely psychodynamic psychotherapist focuses on unconscious motivation and conflicts and upon mental representations of reality, whether conscious or unconscious. In these efforts, the psychodynamic psychotherapist is less concerned with interpersonal relations than with object relations, namely the mental representations of the reality of interpersonal relations.

It is the premise of psychodynamic psychotherapy that the behavior of individuals in interpersonal relations is determined not only by the actual reality of those relationships but by the special meaning, both conscious and unconscious, that the patient brings to these situations. These meanings are expressed in mental representations of object relations based on both current and past experiences. The exact relationship between past and current experiences, and the mental representations and personality functions, are not entirely clear from current psychoanalytic theory. The psychodynamic psychotherapist listens for wishes, memories, and conflicts, while the IPT-CM therapist listens for role disputes, unfulfilled or unexpressed expectations, and the manifestations of these in actual current transactions.

Comparison With Family
Strategic Approaches

A number of schools of family therapy are subsumed under the rubric of a strategic approach. These approaches place the pathology not within the individual and their thoughts or feelings, but in the structure of the system itself and the rules of the system that may govern behaviors. The goal of treatment is to change the rules by which the system operates. To accomplish this, the couple are given tasks that will cause the current system to break down outside of the therapy sessions. If the tasks are followed, the couple presumably are no longer able to function within the old rules because the rules themselves are undercut. Thus, the couple should start to behave differently, often with no idea of why they are doing so.

The role of the therapist is similar to that of a physician. Prescriptions are given, and these prescriptions frequently take the form of paradoxical interventions (i.e., interventions that seem to run counter to the stated intention of the treatment). Another technique used in the strategic approach is "reframing," which means translating current behavior into a positive statement, no matter how negative the behavior is. Most of the work of therapy is seen as taking place outside of sessions.

The IPT-CM approach and strategic therapies differ in basic concepts as well as specific techniques. IPT-CM attempts to understand the couple's problems as they relate to role disputes. Paradoxical interventions are avoided, and reframing is conceived of more as a way of developing a therapeutic alliance than of changing the couple's behavior. Tasks both within and outside the session are designed to renegotiate roles and are agreed upon as reasonable by all parties before being assigned. The emphasis in IPT-CM is on giving the couple a better understanding of their problems. The therapist explains interventions and elicits cooperation rather than prescribes tasks. Techniques such as manipulating the space in the treatment session, actualization, marking boundaries, and manipulating mood (Minuchin 1974) are avoided.

Comparison With Other
Family Systems Approaches

There are a variety of family system approaches that are highly diverse in techniques and emphasis (Steinglass 1978). Bowen (1976) emphasizes the families of origin and extended family relationships. Minuchin (1974) studies the couple's interactions in the sessions and emphasizes boundaries and alliances between family members. Other therapists emphasize communication to the exclusion of other types of interactions between family members (Watzlawick et al. 1974). What these approaches share is their common reliance on general systems theory, which focuses on dynamic processes between persons rather than on the dynamics within the persons themselves.

Comparison With Behavioral Approaches

Behavioral approaches to marital therapy involve identifying positively reinforcing aspects of marital functioning and helping the couple to increase such functioning, while simultaneously identifying negatively reinforcing behaviors and attempting to extinguish the latter (see O'Leary and Turkewitz 1978; Weiss 1978). In inducing behavior change, there is frequently an explicit contract in which the partners agree to try new positive behaviors and curtail negative ones. Behavior change is seen as taking place because of learning that results from systematically reinforced practice. Larger problems are broken into behavioral components and are then approached in a stepwise fashion. Behavioral approaches are often highly eclectic and recognize subsystems within the marriage, focusing on communication, affection, child care, and so forth. The key unifying feature of such approaches is their common base on learning therapy, which emphasizes stimulus and reinforcement contingencies rather than psychodynamic processes or dynamics of a marital or family system.

Although IPT-CM may assist the couple in increasing rewarding interactions and decreasing unrewarding ones, this is not the primary focus of the approach, which is based on changes in role expectations. In IPT-CM, as in behavioral approaches, a treatment contract is made and exercises are assigned to be accomplished between sessions. However, the contract is less tied to reinforcement contingencies, and the homework is less aimed at systematic practice of changed behavior than at helping the couple to develop a richer understanding of the problems in their marriage. It is assumed that once the couple have an understanding of their role disputes and have learned more effective ways of negotiating their problems, they will put this knowledge to use in transactions between therapeutic sessions.

Efficacy

The use of conjoint marital psychotherapy has apparent prima facie validity. It "makes sense" given the IPT conceptualization of role disputes. However rational the conjoint approach may appear, it requires empirical evaluation as does any other treatment.

Clinical Trials of Marital Therapy With Depression

In addition to the one pilot study of IPT-CM, which will be discussed later in this chapter, several published clinical trials exist that have compared individual with conjoint marital therapy for depressed patients with marital problems.

Jacobson et al. (1991) have reported findings from a study in which 60 married depressed women were assigned to either conjoint behavioral marital therapy alone, individual cognitive therapy alone, or combined individual cognitive and conjoint behavioral marital therapy. The results suggest that behavioral marital therapy was less effective than cognitive therapy for depression in maritally nondistressed couples, whereas for maritally distressed couples the two treatments were equally effective. Behavioral marital therapy was the only treatment to have a significant positive impact on a marital relationship in distressed couples, and cognitive therapy was the only therapy to enhance marital satisfaction of nondistressed couples. The absence of a nontreatment control group and the small sample in each cell limit conclusions.

A study by O'Leary and Beach (1990) included 36 maritally discordant couples with depressed wives, who were randomly assigned to marital therapy, cognitive therapy, or a waiting list control. The women given marital or cognitive therapy showed significant and clinically meaningful reduction in their depression. Those given marital therapy showed greater increases in marital dissatisfaction than those given cognitive therapy or no treatment, and these differences were maintained at 1-year follow-up. The findings thus suggest that marital therapy may be more effective than individual treatment for clinically significant marital discord with coexistent clinically significant depression. The findings are insufficient to make any kind of definitive statement other than to call for more research.

Testing the Efficacy of IPT-CM

There has been one pilot study of IPT-CM that has examined the feasibility and patient acceptance and provided preliminary evidence of efficacy as well as the relative efficacy of individual versus conjoint IPT in terms of symptoms, social functioning, and marital adjustment (Foley et al. 1989).

Selection of Patients

Eighteen couples participated in the study, and the marital partner who originally sought treatment for major depression was assigned the patient status. The patient sample consisted of 5 male and 13 female adults, married, nonbipolar, nonpsychotic, depressed outpatients ages 21 to 60. Consent to participate in either of the treatment conditions was obtained from both patient and spouse. For inclusion in the study, patients had to meet the Research Diagnostic Criteria (RDC; Spitzer et al. 1978) for a current episode of major depressive disorder following a diagnostic interview on the Schedule for Affective Disorders and Schizophrenia—Lifetime Version (SADS-L; Endicott and Spitzer 1978). Only patients who identified marital disputes as the major problem associated with the onset or exacerbation of their depression were admitted into the study. Prospective patients were excluded from the study if they or their spouses were found to be at serious risk for suicide based on a clinician's judgment of current active suicide potential.

Patients were randomly assigned to IPT or IPT-CM and received 16 weekly therapy sessions. In IPT-CM the spouse was required to participate in all psychotherapy sessions, whereas in IPT the spouse did not meet with the psychotherapist. The clinical status of all patients and spouses was assessed by a clinical evaluator at intake and at termination of each patient's treatment.

Treatments were conducted according to the IPT and IPT-CM manuals. Patients and spouses in both treatment conditions were asked to refrain from taking psychotropic medication during the study without prior discussion with their therapists, and therapists were discouraged from prescribing or arranging for prescriptions of any psychotropic medication. Only two prescriptions were written by a staff psychiatrist during the study: one patient in individual and one in conjoint marital therapy were prescribed sedatives for the treatment of insomnia.

IPT Psychotherapist Training for Research

Three therapists (a psychiatrist, a psychologist, and a social worker) administered individual IPT to depressed married subjects. Three other therapists (social workers) administered conjoint marital IPT. All therapists had extensive prior experience in the treatment of depressed subjects and were trained in IPT-CM using preliminary drafts of the manual. The training programs consisted of didactic sessions, instruction in the use of the IPT or IPT-CM manual, and supervision in the administration of the therapy. The quality of therapist performance was monitored by two expert raters, who reviewed videotapes of entire therapy sessions. All therapists were judged by the expert raters to be competently administering the treatment during the course of the study.

Assessments

Symptom status, social functioning, and marital adjustment of patients and spouses in both treatment conditions were evaluated at intake and at termination of the 16-week course of therapy. Depression and social functioning were assessed by a clinical evaluator who was blind to the treatment condition.

Patients' satisfaction with the treatment and self-ratings of improvement in therapy were assessed by patient self-report at termination. Symptoms of depression were recorded on the Hopkins Symptom Checklist–90 (SCL-90), a 90-item self-report symptom inventory constructed to measure psychopathology in medical and psychiatric outpatients (Lipman et al. 1979), and on a 21-item version of the Hamilton Rating Scale for Depression (Hamilton 1967). Social functioning was assessed on the Social Adjustment Scale (SAS; Weissman and Bothwell 1976).

Marital adjustment was measured on a 44-item version of the Locke-Wallace Marital Adjustment Test (Locke and Wallace 1976), a 32-item self-report scale that can be used to assess a subject's perceptions of the functioning of his or her marital relationship. The Spanier Dyadic Adjustment Scale (Spanier 1976) contains four empirically verified subscales: *dyadic satisfaction,* which measures a subject's feelings of happiness and contentment in the marriage; *dyadic cohesion,* which reflects the strength of the union between the marital partners; *dyadic consensus,* which assesses the extent of agreement or disagreement between marital partners on a wide variety of issues; and *affectional expression,* which characterizes a subject's view of affection and sexual relations in the marriage. On both scales, higher scores indicated higher levels of marital adjustment.

Characteristics of Patient and Spouse

There were no statistically significant differences in demographic or clinical characteristics between the two treatment groups. The 18 patients were predominantly Catholic (61%), white (94%), and from social class III or IV (39% and 33% percent, respectively). The mean patient age was 40, and patients had been married an average of 15 years prior to intake. Previous episodes of major depression were reported by 89% of the patients.

Seventy-eight percent of the spouses had a lifetime history of some form of psychiatric disorder; 50% of the spouses reported previous episodes of major depression, and an additional 17% had a history of minor depression. At intake, two of the spouses were in a current episode of major depression of sufficient severity to qualify for patient status in the study. The prevalence of major depression among the spouses is consistent with the reports of other investigators (Merikangas 1982; Weissman et al. 1982).

Acceptance and Feasibility of Treatment

Patients were easily recruited for participation in the study and accepted randomization into the two treatment groups. Two patients in IPT and one in IPT-CM terminated treatment prior to completion. One patient in IPT was unable to continue treatment after Session 12 because of a serious physical illness. Another in IPT terminated after Session 4 because of symptomatic deterioration. One patient in IPT-CM terminated after Session 13, also because of symptomatic deterioration.

Spouses in both treatment cells agreed to participate in the study and cooperated by completing periodic assessments. Spouses of patients randomized to IPT-CM were willing to participate in joint therapy sessions. In IPT-CM, only two therapy sessions were skipped and three sessions were rescheduled. In IPT, no therapy sessions were skipped and two sessions were rescheduled.

Patient evaluations of the quality of treatment did not differ by treatment cell. Patients in both groups expressed satisfaction with the treatment, felt that they had improved, and attributed improvement to their therapy.

Outcome Assessment of IPT-CM

Patients in both treatment groups exhibited a significant reduction in symptoms of depression and social impairment from intake to termination of therapy. There was no significant difference between treatment groups in the degree of improvement in depressive symptoms and social functioning by endpoint.

The Locke-Wallace Marital Adjustment Test scores at Session 16 were significantly higher (indicative of better marital adjustment) for patients receiving IPT-CM than for patients receiving IPT. Scores on the Spanier Dyadic Adjustment Scale also indicated greater improvement in marital functioning for patients receiving IPT-CM than for patients receiving IPT. At Session 16, patients receiving IPT-CM reported significantly higher levels of improvement in affectional expression (i.e., demonstrations of affection and improvement in sexual relations in the marriage) than did patients receiving IPT.

Although spouses exhibited some symptoms of depression and social maladjustment, those symptoms were not severe enough to allow for marked improvement over the course of the study: only two spouses were in current episodes of major depression at intake. Hence, neither the depression nor the social adjustment scores of spouses in either treatment group improved significantly during the therapy period. While the Locke-Wallace Marital Adjustment Test scores of spouses in both treatment groups improved, there was no significant difference in the degree of improvement in spouses between treatment groups.

Conclusions and Plans
for Future Research

The response rates to our efforts to recruit patients into the pilot study were high, probably due to the high prevalence of depression in the context of marital disputes. Attendance of both patients and spouses at treatment sessions was excellent. Only two patients (one in each treatment group) dropped out because of symptomatic failure. Patients in the IPT and IPT-CM treatment conditions improved equally in symptoms and in social adjustment during the course of therapy; however, a differential effect of treatment on marital functioning was found: patients receiving IPT-CM had greater improvements in marital adjustment and affectional expression than did patients receiving IPT.

The results should be interpreted with caution due to the pilot nature of the study, the small size of the pilot sample, the lack of a no-treatment control group, and the absence of a pharmacotherapy or combined pharmacotherapy-psychotherapy comparison group.

Plans for Future Research

Plans for future research on IPT-CM should take into account the following issues that emerged during the course of treatment in the pilot study. Because depression was prevalent among some spouses of the identified patients in the study, it seems important to examine systematically the psychiatric status of such spouses and to develop a strategy for managing the emergence of symptoms among them.

The IPT therapists who participated in the study found it difficult to focus on marital issues if the patients were severely depressed. The therapists felt that management of marital disputes would be more effective if the patients' symptoms of depression were initially brought under control (either with drugs or psychotherapy) and marital issues were addressed subsequently.

The results of this pilot study were promising enough to warrant further testing on a larger sample that includes a no-treatment control and a pharmacotherapy group. A clinical trial on such a sample may be expected to provide useful information on the best form of treatment for patients experiencing depression in the context of marital disputes. The IPT-CM manual, which is available in draft form, requires further testing in a series of clinical trials. It will need to be modified for future use.

References

American Psychiatric Association: Diagnostic and Statistical Manual of Mental Disorders, 3rd Edition. Washington, DC, American Psychiatric Association, 1980

American Psychiatric Association: Diagnostic and Statistical Manual of Mental Disorders, 3rd Edition, Revised. Washington, DC, American Psychiatric Association, 1987

Beck AT, Rush AJ, Shaw BF, et al: Cognitive Therapy for Depression. New York, Guilford, 1979

Bloom BL, Asher SJ, White SW: Marital disruption as a stressor: a review and analysis. Psychol Bull 85:867–894, 1978

Bowen M: Theory in the practice of psychotherapy, in Family Therapy: Theory and Practice. Edited by Guerin PJ. New York, Gardner Press, 1976, pp 12–22

Bowlby J: Attachment and Loss, Vol 1: Attachment. London, Hogarth Press, 1969

Briscoe CW, Smith JB: Depression and marital turmoil. Arch Gen Psychiatry 28:811–817, 1973

Brown GW, Harris T: Social Origins of Depression: A Study of Psychiatric Disorder in Women. New York, Free Press, 1978

Coyne JC: Depression and the response of others. J Abnorm Psychol 85:186–193, 1976

Endicott J, Spitzer RL: A diagnostic interview: The Schedule for Affective Disorders and Schizophrenia. Arch Gen Psychiatry 35:837–844, 1978

Fincham FD, Beach SRH, Bradbury TN: Marital distress, depression, and attributions: is the marital distress–attribution association an artifact of depression? J Consult Clin Psychol 57:768–771, 1989

Foley SH, Rounsaville BJ, Weissman MM, et al: Individual versus conjoint interpersonal psychotherapy for depressed patients with martial disputes. International Journal of Family Psychiatry 10:29–42, 1989

Frank E, Kupfer DJ: The KDS-15—A Marital Questionnaire. Pittsburgh, PA, Western Psychiatric Institute and Clinic, University of Pittsburgh, 1974

Frank E, Anderson C, Kupfer DJ: Profiles of couples seeking sex therapy and marital therapy. Am J Psychiatry 33:559–562, 1976

Gotlib IH, Whiffen VE: Depression and marital functioning: an examination of specificity and gender differences. J Abnorm Psychol 98:23–30, 1989a

Gotlib IH, Whiffen VE: Stress, coping, and marital satisfaction in couples with a depressed wife. Canadian Journal of Behavioural Sciences 21:401–418, 1989b

Gurman AS, Kniskern DP: Research on marital and family therapy: progress, perspective and prospect, in Handbook of Psychotherapy and Behavior Change: An Empirical Analysis, 2nd Edition. Edited by Garfield S, Bergin A. New York, Wiley, 1978, pp 817–901

Hamilton M: Development of a rating scale for primary depressive illnesses. British Journal of Social and Clinical Psychology 6:278–296, 1967

Jacobson NS, Holtzworth-Munroe A, Schmaling KB: Marital therapy and spouse involvement in the treatment of depression, agoraphobia, and alcoholism. J Consult Clin Psychol 57:5–10, 1989

Jacobson NS, Dobson K, Fruzzetti AE, et al: Marital therapy as a treatment for depression. J Consult Clin Psychol 59:547–557, 1991

Klerman GL, Weissman MM: Increasing rates of depression. JAMA 261:2229–2235, 1989

Klerman GL, Weissman MM, Rounsaville BJ, et al: Interpersonal Psychotherapy for Depression. New York, Basic Books, 1984

Leaf PJ, Weissman MM, Myers JK, et al: Psychosocial risks and correlates of major depression in one United States urban community, in Mental Disorder in the Community: Progress and Challenge. Edited by Barrett JE, Rose RM. New York, Guilford, 1986, pp 47–73

Lipman RS, Covi L, Shapiro AK: The Hopkins Symptom Check List: factors derived from the SCL-90. J Affective Disord 1:9–24, 1979

Locke HJ, Wallace KM: Short-term marital adjustment and prediction tests: their reliability and validity. Journal of Marriage and Family Living 38:15–25, 1976

Merikangas KR: Assortative mating for psychiatric disorders and psychological traits. Arch Gen Psychiatry 39:1173–1180, 1982

Minuchin S: Families and Family Therapy. Cambridge, MA, Harvard University Press, 1974

O'Leary KD, Beach SRH: Marital therapy: a viable treatment for depression and marital discord. Am J Psychiatry 147:183–186, 1990

O'Leary KD, Turkewitz H: Marital therapy from a behavioral perspective, in Marriage and Marital Therapy. Edited by Paolino TJ, McCrady BS. New York, Brunner/Mazel, 1978, pp 240–297

Olin GV, Fennell DL: The relationship between depression and marital adjustment in a general population. Family Therapy 16:11–20, 1989

Paykel ES, Myers JK, Dienelt MN, et al: Life events and depression: a controlled study. Arch Gen Psychiatry 21:753–760, 1969

Prusoff BA, Weissman MM, Klerman GL, et al: Research Diagnostic Criteria subtypes of depression: their role as predictors of differential response to psychotherapy and drug treatment. Arch Gen Psychiatry 37:796–801, 1980

Robins LN, Regier DA (eds): Psychiatric Disorders in America: The Epidemiologic Catchment Area Study. New York, Free Press, 1991

Rounsaville BJ, Weissman MM, Prusoff BA, et al: Marital disputes and treatment outcome in depressed women. Compr Psychiatry 20:483–490, 1978

Rounsaville BJ, Weissman MM, Prusoff BA, et al: Process of psychotherapy among depressed women with marital disputes. Am J Orthopsychiatry 49:505–510, 1979

Rounsaville BJ, Prusoff BA, Weissman MM: The course of marital disputes in depressed women: a 48-month follow-up study. Compr Psychiatry 21:111–118, 1980

Rounsaville BF, Weissman MM, Klerman GL, et al: Manual for Conjoint Marital Interpersonal Psychotherapy for Depressed Patient with Marital Disputes (IPT-CM). Unpublished manual from Yale University School of Medicine, New Haven, CT; Cornell Medical School, Payne Whitney Clinic, Columbia University College of Physicians and Surgeons, New York, 1986

Schmaling K, Jacobson HS: Marital interaction and depression. J Abnorm Psychol 99:229–236, 1990

Spanier GB: Measuring dyadic adjustment: new scales for assessing the quality of marriage and similar dyads. Journal of Marriage and Family Living 38:15–25, 1976

Spitzer RL, Endicott J, Robins E: Research Diagnostic Criteria: rationale and reliability. Arch Gen Psychiatry 35:773–785, 1978

Steinglass P: The conceptualization of marriage from a systems theory perspective, in Marriage and Marital Therapy. Edited by Paolino TJ, McCrady BS. New York, Brunner/Mazel, 1978, pp 298–394

Watzlawick P, Beavin JH, Jackson DD: Change! Principles of Problem Formation and Problem Resolution. New York, WW Norton, 1974

Weiss RL: The conceptualization of marriage from a behavioral perspective, in Marriage and Marital Therapy. Edited by Paolino TJ, McCrady BS. New York, Brunner/Mazel, 1978, pp 41–46

Weissman MM: Advances in psychiatric epidemiology: rates and risks for major depression. Am J Public Health 77:445–451, 1987

Weissman MM, Bothwell S: The assessment of social adjustment by patient self-report. Arch Gen Psychiatry 33:1111–1115, 1976

Weissman MM, Kidd KK, Prusoff BA: Variability in the rates of affective disorders in relatives of depressed and normal probands. Arch Gen Psychiatry 39:1397–1403, 1982

Interpersonal Psychotherapy for Adolescent Depression

Laura H. Mufson, Ph.D.
Donna Moreau, M.D.
Myrna M. Weissman, Ph.D.
Gerald L. Klerman, M.D.

Interpersonal psychotherapy (IPT) is a brief treatment specifically developed and tested for depressed adults (Klerman et al. 1984). Our purpose in this chapter is to describe a modification of IPT for use with depressed adolescents (*interpersonal psychotherapy for adolescent depression*; IPT-A). We describe IPT and its efficacy in adults and present the rationale for developing IPT-A. Preliminary experience with depressed adolescents treated with IPT-A will be presented, and case histories will be used to illustrate the application of this specific modality.

The decades since World War II have witnessed an expansion in the use of psychotherapy in the United States. Numerous forms of psychotherapy are being used by increasing numbers of professional psychotherapists. Recently, there has been considerable advancement in the development of

This work was supported by a grant to Dr. Weissman from the John D. and Catherine T. MacArthur Foundation Network I (Psychobiology of Depression and Other Affective Disorders), by a NARSAD Young Investigators Award to Dr. Mufson, and by the University of Chicago–Anne Pollock Lederer Foundation for the Study of Depression in Young Adults Award. Portions of this chapter appeared in the *Journal of the American Academy of Child and Adolescent Psychiatry* in July 1991. Case material has been altered to prevent identification.

methods and technologies for testing the efficacy of psychotherapy (Weissman et al. 1987b). These developments include testing with clinical trials, use of controls, development of outcome measures, specification of the therapies in manuals, and development of training programs for therapists participating in research (Chevron et al. 1983). A number of brief psychotherapies have been operationalized and detailed in manuals to facilitate testing of efficacy and training of research psychotherapists. These therapies have been tested for specific disorders, most often for the treatment of major depression. All of the clinical trials to date for major depression have been with adults in outpatient settings.

Depression is highly prevalent in adolescents. However, there is meager evidence for the efficacy of pharmacotherapy for this age group. Despite the widespread clinical use of various treatment modalities, there is not one published, controlled clinical trial on the efficacy of any individual psychotherapy in the treatment of adolescents diagnosed as depressed according to DSM-III (American Psychiatric Association 1980) or DSM-III-R (American Psychiatric Association 1987) criteria.

Adolescent Depression

The rationale for developing IPT-A is based in part on our current understanding of the nature of depression in adolescents and the currently available treatments, as will be described.

Epidemiology, Morbidity, and Course

In contrast to the debates several decades ago, it is now clear from clinical, epidemiological, family-genetic, and high-risk studies that major depression does occur in children and adolescents. Empirical studies have demonstrated that mood swings, cognitive distortions, and poor interpersonal and family relationships are not characteristics of normal adolescent growth and development (Offer 1969; Offer et al. 1981; Rutter et al. 1976), and longitudinal and epidemiological studies support that view. Prior to 1970, research was scant on childhood and adolescent depression, and, in particular, there were few epidemiological studies. Early studies relied more upon the reports from parents and teachers about the children and rarely asked the children themselves about their symptoms. More recently, children and adolescents have been shown to be reliable informants about their mental states (Orvaschel et al. 1981; Weissman et al. 1987a) and, in fact, report more affective symptoms than their parents or teachers report about them (Angold et al. 1987).

There is great variability in reports of prevalence rates of childhood depression because of variable diagnostic criteria, multiple populations, different methods for obtaining information (self-report versus structured interviews), and varying informants. The rates of depression also differ because of the use of varying definitions ranging from presence of depressive symptoms or depressed mood to presence of the disorder or syndrome as criteria. According to one study of adults with depressive disorders, the most frequent age at first onset, retrospectively reported, is in adolescence and young adulthood (Christie et al. 1988). Rates are considerably higher when depressive *symptoms,* rather than a disorder per se, are assessed.

Depressive symptoms are common in young children (Earls 1980; Richman et al. 1975) and elementary school–age children (Lefkowitz and Tesiny 1985; Smucker et al. 1986). Rutter et al. (1976) found that 40% of 14- and 15-year-olds in the Isle of Wight study reported substantial feelings of misery and depression. Kaplan et al. (1984), in a survey of 11- to 18-year-olds in a general high school population, found 13% to be mildly depressed, 7% to be moderately depressed, and 2% to be severely depressed. In the Ontario Child Health Study (Fleming et al. 1989), symptoms of depression were reported by 36.9% of boys and 55.6% of girls between the ages of 12 and 16 years. Kandel and Davies (1982), in a large epidemiological survey of high school students, found that 25% of the students reported depressed mood. In contrast, studies that examined the rate of DSM-III depressive disorder found lower rates. Garrison et al. (1989) found that 4.4% of seventh-, eighth-, and ninth-graders reported DSM-III-like depressive syndrome. In their epidemiological sample of 2,000 adolescents of ages 14 to 15 years, Rutter et al. (1976) found that 1.3% met criteria for a depressive disorder. Fleming and Offord's (1990) excellent review of 14 epidemiological studies of childhood and adolescent depressive disorders indicated a current prevalence rate for major depression in adolescents in the range of 0.4% to 6.4%. Major depression before puberty, however, is uncommon.

The symptom pattern of childhood depression is similar to that of adults as described in the DSM-III (Ryan et al. 1987; Strober et al. 1981). Childhood depression, like adult depression, is associated with substantial impairment in psychosocial functioning (Puig-Antich et al. 1985). For adolescents, this impairment includes substance abuse, suicide attempts, school dropout, and antisocial behavior (Kandel and Davies 1986; see Brent et al. 1990; Fleming and Offord 1990, for reviews). There also is comorbidity of depression with other psychiatric disorders and a high degree of family dysfunction (Geller et al. 1985; Kashani et al. 1988; Kovacs et al. 1988).

The most common epidemiological variables studied in relation to childhood and adolescent depression are age, sex, socioeconomic status, and family psychosocial factors (Kashani and Sherman 1988). There is a consistent increase in major depressive disorders from preadolescent to adolescent years (Offord et al. 1987; Ryan et al. 1986). Similarly, there is a consistent finding of an increase in rates of depression among adolescent girls in particular (Kashani et al. 1987; Rutter et al. 1976). Family risk factors for depression in adolescence include death of a parent, low family cohesion, and low levels of perceived affection between family members (i.e., affectionless control) (Fendrich et al. 1990; Reinherz et al. 1989; Wells et al. 1985).

There is as yet not one longitudinal study that has assessed depressed adolescents using DSM-III criteria at initial assessment and followed them into adulthood to determine the natural course of the illness and the prognostic significance of adolescent depression. However, there are re-lated studies which suggest that there is continuity between adolescent and adult depression and that adolescent depression has a substantial long-term morbidity (Garber et al. 1988; Harrington et al. 1990; Kandel and Davies 1986; Kovacs et al. 1984a, 1984b; Strober 1985; Strober and Carlson 1982). Kovacs et al. (1984a) reported on a short-term longitudinal study of depressed adolescents. They found that major depressive disorder and adjustment disorder with depressed mood remit most quickly, that the most chronic disorder is dysthymic disorder, and that the greatest rate of recurrence is for those adolescents with major depression and dysthymic disorder. The epidemiological and clinical data point out the need for increased attention to adolescent depression because of its significant prev-alence, associated morbidity, chronicity, recurrence, and tendency to per-sist into adulthood.

Current Treatments

Pharmacotherapy

The few controlled clinical trials of pharmacotherapy in depressed adolescents have not demonstrated efficacy. This may be due to methodological problems, such as small sample size, diagnostic variability, or the biological uniqueness of adolescents (see Campbell and Spencer 1988 for review). More recent studies on depressed adolescents have attempted to address early methodological deficiencies and have used structured diagnostic interviews and DSM-III criteria, but statistically significant differences in response between antidepressant medication and placebo were not found (Geller et al. 1990; Kramer and Feiguine 1981; Ryan et al. 1986; Strober et al. 1990).

The major classes of medications used for the treatment of adolescent depression include tricyclic antidepressants (i.e., nortriptyline, imipramine, desipramine), serotonergic antidepressants (i.e., fluoxetine), antianxiety agents (i.e., lorazepam, alprazolam, clonazepam), and neuroleptics. Neuroleptics are used to treat psychotic symptoms such as delusions and hallucinations and will not be reviewed here because psychosis precludes treatment with IPT. Antianxiety agents may be used in conjunction with antidepressants in the early stages of pharmacological treatment. Indications include nervousness, agitation, anxiety, severe insomnia, and concurrent panic attacks.

There were multiple published studies on the use of tricyclic antidepressants in children in the 1970s and early 1980s. Positive therapeutic efficacy ranged from 40% to 90%, with an average of 75% (Puig-Antich and Weston 1983). However, these studies, which were uncontrolled open trials, involved heterogeneous patient populations not diagnosed by semi-structured interviews, utilized low doses with variable length of treatment times (Puig-Antich and Weston 1983).

The most recent studies, comparing imipramine or amitriptyline to placebo in a double-blind design, have failed to demonstrate the superiority of antidepressants over placebo in the treatment of depressed children diagnosed by DSM-II criteria or Research Diagnostic Criteria (RDC) (Kashani et al. 1984; Puig-Antich et al. 1987). There are only four published studies testing the efficacy of tricyclic antidepressants in adolescents and one published study on the use of monoamine oxidase (MAO) inhibitors that used a semistructured interview to make a DSM-III diagnosis of major depression. There was no difference between placebo and tricyclic antidepressant, each yielding greater than 50% positive response.

Amitriptyline in doses up to 200 mg per day was used to treat depression in 20 adolescent inpatients (Kramer and Feiguine 1981). In the double-blind experimental design, no difference was found between placebo and medication. Ryan et al. (1986), in an open-label study, treated 34 hospitalized adolescents who met the RDC for major depression with imipramine in doses up to 5 mg/kg per day for a period of 6 weeks. Forty-four percent of the subjects improved on the medication. There was no association between positive therapeutic response and combined serum levels of imipramine and desipramine. Geller et al. (1990), in a double-blind placebo study of nortriptyline in 52 adolescents (12 to 17 years of age) meeting the RDC and DSM-III criteria for major depression, found that one-third of the subjects improved during the placebo washout period. Of the 31 subjects who completed the study, only one showed any clinical response. Strober et al. (1990) studied the efficacy of imipramine in an open-label trial of 35 depressed adolescent inpatients, ages 13 to 18, meeting the RDC and DSM-III criteria for major depression. Treatment lasted for 6 weeks with a target dose of 5 mg/kg. One patient did not complete the study. Of 25 nondelusional depressed patients, one-third were rated as responders. Of the 10 delusional depressed patients, only one responded favorably to the medication.

Two additional studies reported on the efficacy of tricyclics augmented with lithium for the treatment of depressed adolescents who failed to respond to tricyclic antidepressant therapy alone. In an open treatment study of 14 adolescents meeting the RDC for major depression, 43% of the subjects responded to the augmented treatment (Ryan et al. 1988a). However, Strober et al. (1990) reported on a small open trial of lithium augmentation in depressed adolescents who did not respond to tricyclics alone. The vast majority of subjects showed no improvement.

In an open clinical trial, MAO inhibitors, either alone or in combination, were used to treat 23 adolescents who met the RDC and DSM-III criteria for major depression and failed to respond to a 6-week course of tricyclic antidepressants (Ryan et al. 1988b). Poor dietary compliance was a major issue in this study, and the authors stated that the risks of complications due to dietary indiscretion outweigh possible benefits of the medication. Although research has demonstrated in children that serum levels seem to predict a therapeutic response, the same association was not found in one study with adolescents (Ryan et al. 1986). The 44% positive response rate over a 6-week period in 34 adolescents was independent of combined plasma levels of imipramine and desipramine. The treatment response was negatively affected by comorbid separation anxiety disorder and endogenous subtype of depression. In addition, a poorer response to tricyclic antidepressants was found in depressed young adults when compared with older adults. Consequently, the authors concluded that age was a more important variable in the adolescents' negative therapeutic response than the presence of a comorbid disorder or endogenous subtype.

Fluoxetine is currently under investigation for treatment of depression in adolescents. Because of its low profile of side effects, low lethality index, and a lack of propensity to cause weight gain, it seems very suitable for use in depressed adolescents.

There are several ongoing studies of pharmacological therapy for adolescent depression (Ryan 1990). Larger samples of depressed adolescents need to be included in well-designed studies that test the efficacy of pharmacotherapy and psychotherapy, each alone, and then in combination.

Psychotherapy

Clinicians treating depressed adolescents commonly use treatments found to be efficacious in the treatment of adults (Hersen and Van Hasselt 1987). Although there are no published studies meeting all criteria for clinical trials, there have been several studies that have examined the efficacy of psychotherapy for the treatment of depression in adolescents. Wilkes and Rush (1988) have suggested methods for adapting cognitive therapy for the treatment of nonpsychotic depressed adolescents. The authors have proposed a treatment model of cognitive therapy for this age group. This work is under further development, and a manual is being prepared by Frank et al. (E. Frank, A. Nowels, J. A. Rush, et al.: Cognitive therapy manual for depressed adolescents. MacArthur Foundation Mental Health Research Network I: Psychobiology of Depression and Other Affective Disorders, 1990). A behavioral psychoeducational approach for coping with depression, with modifications for adolescents, has been developed by Clarke and Lewinsohn (1989). A group format has also been completed and was used by Lewinsohn et al. (1990).

Reynolds and Coats (1986) reported findings from a clinical trial comparing cognitive-behavior therapy, relaxation training, and waiting list control for the treatment of depressive symptoms in 30 adolescents. Treatment was conducted in 10 small group meetings of 50 minutes over 5 weeks. The findings indicated the superiority of the two active treatments in the reduction of depressive symptoms when compared with waiting list control, and no difference between the two active treatments. This study, however, used depressive symptoms, not diagnosis, as the entrance criterion, so these findings are not generalizable to treatment of adolescents with major depressive disorder.

Lewinsohn et al. (1990) have conducted a clinical trial with 54 depressed adolescents comparing two different presentations of the Coping With Depression Course for adolescents with a waiting list control. The adolescents were diagnosed using a structured diagnostic interview and met the RDC for major, minor, or intermittent depression. Subjects in the active treatment groups received group therapy with or without treatment provided for their parents. The results showed that the subjects in the two active treatment groups improved significantly more on the depressive measures than did the waiting list group; however, there were no significant differences between the two active treatments. There was a trend for greater improvement in the subjects whose parents also participated in the treatment in comparison with the group whose parents did not participate. Although this study is the largest and best to date, it still leaves open the question of the efficacy of individual treatment for adolescent depression.

Robbins and associates (1989a), in a pilot treatment strategy for 38 adolescents hospitalized with major depression, conducted an open trial of a psychotherapy, which the authors described as being similar to IPT. They noted that 47% of the patients responded with a reduction of symptoms when treated with psychotherapy alone. The patients who did not respond were then treated with a combined tricyclic antidepressant and psychotherapy, and 92% responded. Dexamethasone nonsuppression and melancholic subtype were associated with failure to respond to psychotherapy alone. Robbins et al. conducted this study without modifying the IPT manual specifically for depressed adolescents; thus, the procedures of the treatment are not defined. Despite the lack of a standardized manual, Robbins et al. found promising results for an IPT-like treatment, which supports the need to further explore the use of IPT as a treatment for depressed adolescents.

Individual psychotherapy is of considerable clinical interest in the treatment of adolescents. A number of thoughtful papers by leading clinicians have described their experiences and views (Bemporad 1988; Cytrn and McKnew 1985; Kestenbaum and Kron 1987; Liebowitz and Kernberg 1988; Nissen 1986). Clinical studies have demonstrated both the feasibility of conducting controlled clinical trials with depressed adolescents and the possible efficacy of group psychotherapy based on trials in the population. However, there has not yet been a controlled trial with random assignment, DSM-III diagnoses, and individual psychotherapy for this specific population.

Rationale for Modifying IPT with Adolescents

Because there is evidence for the efficacy of IPT for depressed adults, it seemed reasonable to try this approach with depressed adolescents based on findings that there is 1) a similarity in symptom patterns between depressed adults and adolescents (McGee et al. 1990; Robbins et al. 1989b; Ryan et al. 1987; Shain et al. 1990), and 2) a suggestion of continuity between child and adult depressive symptoms (Kandel and Davies 1986) and disorder (Harrington et al. 1990).

The brief nature of IPT makes it particularly responsive to the adolescent's reluctance to seek or stay in treatment, and its goals parallel the adolescent's developmental issues and the desire to focus on the here and now. The focus on the present and on future, rather than past, issues and the focus on the identification and resolution of disputes seem appropriate for adolescents, who often are in disputes with a parent, school, or friends. Because adolescence is a time of major life choices in education, work, and establishment of intimate relationships, a treatment that helps the adolescent identify and master interpersonal problems seemed timely. IPT-A has been developed for the treatment of the nonpsychotic, non-suicidal depressed adolescent outpatient who is not engaging in daily drug abuse or antisocial activities of a violent nature. IPT-A is not, however, designed to handle adolescents in crisis.

Description of Interpersonal Psychotherapy for Adolescent Depression

Developing the Manual for Use With Adolescents

Prior to conducting a controlled clinical trial, it was necessary to develop a manual of the modified IPT to provide a basis for training therapists and to ensure that the treatment being tested was standardized so that it could be replicated in future studies. The revised techniques were used with depressed adolescents seeking treatment at an outpatient clinic at a university hospital.

Therapy sessions, conducted by an experienced child clinical psychologist under the supervision of the developer of IPT, were videotaped. These experiences are being used to further modify the manual. The manual is intended to assist experienced therapists in their clinical practice. The modification for adolescents should be read in conjunction with the manual for adults (Klerman et al. 1984).

Goals

The overall goals and problem areas in IPT-A are similar to those that are encountered in IPT as previously defined. A fifth problem area, the single-parent family, has been added because of its frequent occurrence and the conflicts it engenders for adolescents. The treatment has been adapted to address developmental issues most common to adolescents. These issues include separation from parents, exploration of authority in relation to parents, development of dyadic interpersonal relationships with members of the opposite sex, initial experience with death of a relative or friend, and peer pressures.

The Initial Phase

The initial sessions are devoted to establishing the treatment contract, dealing with the depressive symptoms, and identifying the problem areas. There are six tasks that the therapist needs to accomplish in the initial phase of treatment:

1. Address the depression by completing a diagnostic assessment that includes reviewing the symptoms with the patient, giving the syndrome a name, explaining depression and its treatment, giving the patient the sick role, and evaluating the need for medication.
2. Assess the type and nature of the patient's social and familial relationships (i.e., the interpersonal inventory) and relate the depression to the interpersonal context.
3. Identify the problem area(s).
4. Explain the rationale and intent of the treatment.
5. Set a treatment contract with the patient.
6. Explain the patient's expected role in the treatment.

Because of the high comorbidity of childhood depression with drug abuse, and the serious dangers of suicidal behavior (frequently impulsive in nature), both the depression and the drug abuse are fully evaluated. Until further studies can substantiate the efficacy of medication in depressed adolescents, the cautious and supervised use of medication with depressed adolescents should be advised. Accordingly, the present authors use medication with depressed adolescents when depressive symptoms are unremitting and unresponsive to a 4-week course of supportive and psychotherapeutic interventions.

The responsible parent, usually the mother, is brought into the diagnostic process and is educated about the depression, its nature, its course, and treatment options. Both the parent and the adolescent are involved in discussing the various treatment options as part of the education about depression.

The Sick Role

As part of the psychoeducational component of IPT, depression as a clinical disorder is explained, and an effort is made to demystify the experience. The adolescent is encouraged to think of himself or herself as in treatment and is given the sick role. There is often a tendency to withdraw socially as part of the depressive syndrome and to experience symptoms (e.g., fatigue, weakness, drowsiness) that may be used to justify avoidance of usual social expectations. When the patient first becomes depressed, he or she may receive sympathy or reassurance. However, if the symptoms persist, sympathy may turn to hostility and criticism. The adolescent is encouraged to maintain the usual social roles in the family, at school, and with friends. The parent is advised to be supportive and to encourage the adolescent to engage in as many normal activities as possible, although it is recognized that the patient may have difficulty performing up to par. Together, the assignment of the sick role and psychoeducation can help reverse negative behaviors by family members.

Frequency and Timing of Sessions

The telephone is used with adolescents to maintain contact and ensure greater flexibility in the timing and spacing of sessions. During the first 4 weeks of treatment, the therapist may check in with the adolescent, or vice versa, by telephone once or twice a week to provide additional support for engagement in the therapeutic process. These contacts may help establish trust between the therapist and the adolescent in that the adolescent can perceive the therapist as being concerned and involved. Similarly, the adolescent is encouraged to call if the need arises. Telephone contacts as a substitute for sessions are responsive to the adolescent's increased need to resume normal activities with recovery.

Involving the School

It is important for the therapist to maintain an alliance with the school system. The therapist and school may find it necessary to work out an individual academic program to reintegrate the school-avoidant adolescent back into school and to assess the effectiveness of the therapeutic intervention. The therapist can assume the patient-advocate role with the educational system, educating teachers about the effects of a depressive episode on school functioning. The therapist should generally maintain contact with the school, obtaining information from school personnel on the patient's behavior and academic performance to better inform the treatment regarding the most pressing problems or evidence of improvement. Similarly, the school should be made to feel that they can call the therapist with any questions regarding behavioral observations of the patient. It is very important to know how the patient is functioning in one of his or her major roles so that the therapist can monitor the effectiveness of the interventions.

Involving the Parents

The therapist must also maintain an alliance with the parents when treating adolescents. It is important for the therapist to help the parents take the patient's problem seriously and to adjust to the notion of having an adolescent who is having difficulties, in addition to helping them accept any role they may be playing in the adolescent's difficulties. If there is a hostile dispute between the adolescent and parent(s), or the adolescent has been coerced into coming for treatment, the therapist should help the adolescent and the parent(s) see that the treatment is an effort to resolve the dispute in a time-limited therapy. This approach may alleviate the tension and increase compliance with treatment. Parents may also be directly involved in the therapy sessions with the adolescent, depending upon the nature of the interpersonal problem. This is further discussed under the appropriate problem area.

Concluding the Initial Phase

The initial phase is concluded when there is a therapeutic contract and the therapist has formulated the diagnosis and treatment plan (i.e., identified the problem area[s] and explained these concepts to the patient and parents). The middle phase can begin once an agreement has been reached on the treatment plan.

The Middle Phase

The middle phase of IPT-A is focused on the identified problem area(s) (i.e., grief, interpersonal role disputes, role transitions, interpersonal deficits, and single-parent families). The task of the middle phase is to associate the depressive symptoms with the interpersonal problems identified in the initial phase of treatment.

Grief

Grief itself is not considered a problem unless it is prolonged or becomes abnormal. In normal bereavement, a person may experience sadness, changes in appetite and/or sleep, and difficulties in day-to-day functioning. However, the symptoms tend to resolve without treatment in 2 to 4 months. There are three types of pathological mourning—distorted grief, delayed grief, or chronic grief—that can lead to depression either immediately following the loss or at some later time when the patient is reminded of the loss (Raphael 1983).

Loss of a loved one at any age is painful. Loss of a parent during adolescence necessitates premature separation and individuation in addition to the usual tasks of mourning. Common reactions include withdrawal and depressed feelings, a display of pseudomaturity, identification with the deceased, or regression to earlier developmental stages (Krupnick 1984). The adolescent also may experience feelings of abandonment. The difficulties may manifest themselves in behavioral problems rather than affective symptoms. The therapist must be alerted to problems of drug or alcohol abuse, sexual promiscuity, or truancy (Raphael 1983).

The strategies of IPT-A in the treatment of grief are essentially the same for adults and adolescents, but the goals are modified (see below). The therapist helps the adolescent or adult discuss the loss, as well as identify and experience the associated feelings. As the patient begins to grieve appropriately and the symptoms dissipate, the loss should be better understood and accepted, and the patient should then be freed to pursue new relationships.

Interpersonal psychotherapy for adolescents has two goals in dealing with grief: 1) to help the adolescent with abnormal grief, and 2) to help the normal adolescent cope with grief as a prevention strategy to avert future depressive episodes. The authors believe the role of IPT in the treatment of normal grief reactions in adolescents is to assist the adolescent in separating from the deceased by recognizing the limitations of the deceased and by accepting the loss of idealization of and dependency on the deceased (Raphael 1983). IPT-A similarly addresses the depression associated with abnormal grief reactions that results from failure to go through the various phases of the normal mourning process. In specifically addressing the impact of loss in adolescents, one must consider the adolescent's role in the family system, the nature of the relationship lost, the remaining social support network, and the adolescent's psychological maturity.

The role of IPT-A for grieving adolescents has the additional task of reducing the risk of suicide attempts. Adolescents whose loss has been a result of suicide either in their family or among peers are at a greater risk for a suicide attempt (Gould and Davidson 1988). It is important to prevent their acceptance of suicide as a viable option for coping with problems. Specific strategies include discussion of more adaptive ways the deceased could have chosen to address problems, and development of more adaptive coping mechanisms for the adolescent.

The Case of J.M.

J.M., a 12-year-old male, presented for treatment because of increasing problems in school and at home since his 4-year-old sister had been killed by a bus 4 months previously. J.M. described a decrease in concentration at school, an inability to make decisions, increased irritability at home with his younger brother, feelings of guilt over his relationship with his deceased sister, increased tearfulness, feelings of wanting to be dead so he could be with his sister, and loss of interest in usual activities. He met criteria for uncomplicated bereavement.

J.M. reported many guilty feelings about how he should have conducted his relationship with his sister (e.g., spent more time with her, taken her more places, not teased her as much). He was very worried about the grief his mother was experiencing and did not want to upset her by telling her about his own feelings of loss. He expressed the wish that it had been him who had been killed because his mother had another son but not another daughter.

J.M. felt a lack of control over his life and generalized this to his academic performance: he no longer felt that his effort affected the results on his tests and thus decreased his efforts at school. Because of his inability to talk with anyone about his feelings, J.M. grew increasingly irritable, particularly with his younger brother, who, J.M. felt, was getting more attention because he had been at the scene of the accident.

The first intervention made by the therapist was to have J.M. discuss his feelings about his sister, their relationship, and the accident in an attempt to correct his misconceptions about his responsibility for what happened. In addition, the therapist talked with J.M. about his feelings of being unloved by his mother and treated differently than his brother, and his feelings of insecurity about his place in the family. J.M.'s mother was already in treatment to deal with her own grief over the accident. Subsequent sessions focused on how J.M.'s feelings about life in general had changed since the accident and how they might be affecting things such as his school performance and his relationship with his brother. J.M., with the help of the therapist, explored his feelings of guilt, loss, abandonment, and anger, and his fear about something else happening to the family. Through expression of these feelings, J.M. experienced some relief from the anger and guilt feelings, and improved his ability to talk about what he was feeling rather than to act it out through disruptive behavior at home and at school. J.M. felt a decreased need to punish himself for his sister's death and made a concerted effort to improve his schoolwork, with much success.

Interpersonal Role Disputes

An interpersonal dispute is defined as a situation in which the individual and at least one significant other person have nonreciprocal expectations about their relationship. In adults, role disputes frequently arise between a marital couple, and they sometimes may occur between a parent and child. Adolescents' role disputes commonly occur with parents over issues of sexuality, authority, money, and life values (Miller 1974).

One particularly common interpersonal role dispute that occurs between adolescents and parents is the conflict between a parent with traditional values and an adolescent who is trying to behave in ways that are consistent with his or her peers. Often these conflicting values lead to different expectations for the adolescent's behavior. This conflict can also arise in the normal adolescent's rebellion against parental authority in an effort to continue the separation process from his or her family.

Adolescents often act out their disputes with disruptive, antisocial, or self-punishing behavior (Miller 1974). It is important to attempt to associate these behaviors with feelings and to encourage the expression of the feelings directly. The adolescent sees the parent as a role model to identify with or disavow (Miller 1974). (For example, sexual promiscuity in girls may be associated with noninvolved fathers and an inadequate role model in the mother.) The adolescent is helped to resolve the dispute through identification and understanding of feelings toward the parent(s) and establishment of his or her own values.

The general strategies for treating interpersonal disputes are essentially the same for adolescents as they are for adults: identify the dispute, make choices about negotiations, reassess expectations for the relationship, clarify role changes, and/or modify communication patterns for resolution of the dispute. What differs in treating role disputes of adolescents is the nature of the problems and the involvement of the parents. The therapist needs to explain to the adolescent and the parents how the interpersonal role disputes contribute to depressive symptoms and how resolution of these disputes can alleviate the symptoms. It can be useful to bring in the parent(s) with whom there is a dispute and to facilitate the negotiations of the relationship in the session with the therapist. Improvements may take the form of a change in the expectations and behavior of the patient and/or the other person, or satisfactory dissolution of the relationship. The latter outcome is not fostered in cases of disputes with parents. There are times when less-than-optimal goals have to be accepted for the treatment, particularly if the parent(s) is resistant to the treatment. In such a case, the adolescent's expectations may be reasonable and those of the family may be unreasonable. Consequently, the goal of IPT is to help the adolescent clarify his or her expectations for the relationship, evaluate which expectations are realistic, and find strategies for coping with the unreasonable and immutable expectations of the parent(s). The therapist attempts to preserve workable family relationships, but if unable to do so, he or she attempts to provide alternative care.

The Case of S.J.

S.J., a 16-year-old 11th-grade student, was referred for treatment by the school after expressing suicidal ideation on a school questionnaire. The school notified the parents that he might be depressed and in need of treatment. S.J. came in with his mother, who reported that she did not see any signs of depression in her son. S.J. reported that he was having early and middle insomnia, increased appetite, decreased concentration in school and a drop in grades, increased irritability and fighting with his father, frequent headaches, and suicidal ideation after arguments with his father. He met the DSM-III-R criteria for a major depression.

S.J.'s mother was a very passive woman who felt quite helpless in the face of her husband's rigid rules and short temper. She initially felt unable to challenge her husband's unrealistic restrictions on S.J.'s activities. S.J. reported much anger and sadness over the fact that his parents did not trust him to participate in after-school football, to work out at a local gym, or to go to the movies with friends from school on the weekends. His father required that S.J. be in the house immediately after school ended and did not allow him out on weekends except to socialize with one cousin. The lack of trust and social isolation was very upsetting to S.J. When he tried to challenge his father, they would have heated arguments and almost come to blows. In the aftermath of his anger, S.J. would feel like killing himself.

SJ's father refused to participate in the treatment, so most of the work was done with S.J. alone, with infrequent visits with the mother. The identified problem was role disputes, as S.J.'s parents did not want him to function as an adolescent but rather wanted to keep him close to home, thwarting his independence. They had many conflicts over S.J.'s goals after high school, disagreeing with his desire to go away to college. The therapist, given the unlikelihood of change in the father, focused on S.J.'s expectations for his relationship with his father: which expectations were realistic and which were not, what type of relationship he could have with his father, and who could fulfill some aspects of the role his father could not fulfill for him. At the same time, the therapist addressed S.J.'s feelings of guilt over his relationship with his father, reviewed the positive aspects of his behavior to improve self-esteem, discussed ways to diffuse his anger toward his father, and tried to work with the mother to help her feel strong enough to make some decisions with the father about giving S.J. more trust and freedom.

S.J.'s mother slowly did begin to play a larger role in making the rules for her son's behavior. With the therapist's emphasis on what a responsible boy he was, she gradually loosened some of the restrictions. S.J. reported decreased feelings of anger and blame, increased self-confidence to seek out other relationships with other adults to fulfill some of his needs, improved communication skills, and decreased depressive symptoms. The relationship with his father remained tense, but with his revised expectations S.J. had more tolerance for the limitations of the relationship.

Role Transitions

Role transitions are defined as the changes that occur as a result of progression from one social role to another. A person can experience a depression when there is difficulty coping with life changes associated with a role change. The transition may result in impaired social functioning if it occurs too rapidly or is experienced by the individual as a loss. Adolescents and adults experience role transitions differently.

Normal role transitions are expected and anticipated by adolescents and their families as rites of passage and are typically handled successfully (Miller 1974). Normal role transitions for adolescents include 1) passage into puberty, 2) shift from group to dyadic relationships, 3) initiation of sexual relationships or desires, 4) separation from parents and family, and 5) work, college, or career planning. Problems arise when parents are unable to accept the concomitant changes to the transition or when the adolescent himself or herself is unable to cope with the changes. Problems that can occur include loss of self-esteem, failure to meet one's own and others' expectations, increasing pressures and responsibilities, and inability to separate from family and vice versa (Erikson 1968).

Role transitions also can be thrust upon adolescents as a result of unanticipated circumstances. Unforeseen or imposed role transitions include becoming a parent or a change in family role due to divorce, remarriage, death, illness, impairment in parent, or separation from parent. The ability of adolescents to cope with unforeseen circumstances rests on their prior psychological functioning and social supports.

Role transitions can be perceived as a loss to the adolescent, particularly if he or she felt more competent in the former role. Consequently, the adolescent's psychological reaction to the transition can resemble that of mourning. The adolescent may similarly need to review his or her former role and the feelings associated with it, and discuss why the transition was made and the feelings such as fear that are associated with the new role. This will enable the adolescent to formulate a way in which he or she can better adapt to the new role and view it as a gain rather than a loss.

The strategies for addressing role transitions in adolescents do not differ significantly from those used with adults. If the role transition problems involve changes in family roles and difficulties in separation and family pressures, the therapist may include the parents in several sessions. The therapist would include the parents to help support the adolescent in giving up his or her role, or, if necessary, to help the family adjust to the normative role transition so that they do not restrict the adolescent's development and impair his or her functioning. It is not only the adolescent, but other family members who have a difficult time accepting the concomitant changes in their adolescent. The parents must be educated about normal developmental tasks for an adolescent, the feelings these tasks may elicit in them, and ways to cope with their feelings. The therapist needs to evaluate their concerns and fears, normalize these if possible, and put them in the appropriate context. Therefore, if the family is having an easier adjustment to the transition, it will hopefully facilitate an easier transition for the adolescent.

The Case of F.S.

F.S., a 15-year-old 10th-grader, was the second of three children who lived with her mother and siblings. Although her parents had never lived together, her father lived nearby, and she enjoyed a good relationship with him. F.S. presented to the outpatient depression clinic with symptoms of sad mood, increased irritability, social withdrawal, decreased concentration, decreased grades, loss of interest in friends, loss of appetite, early and middle insomnia, increased heart rate, and tingling in hands periodically when at home. Her symptoms had been present for approximately 2 months and had been precipitated by a breakup with a boyfriend that had resulted in conflict with her mother. F.S. met the DSM-III-R criteria for major depression.

F.S. described her parents, particularly her mother, as very old-fashioned in regard to dating. If she introduced her mother to a boy, it was assumed that F.S. would likely date him until they got married when she finished school. F.S. had brought home a boy, but had decided that she did not like him and ended the relationship. This resulted in her mother getting angry about the way F.S. conducted her social life and increased restrictions on her social life. While her mother was away for 2 weeks, F.S. met another boy whom she liked and began to see him after school. When her mother came home, F.S. was too afraid to discuss her new relationship and her views on dating with her mother. Her concealment of her relationship increased her anxiety and feelings of depression about her deceitful behavior and her anticipation that her mother would not understand other dating practices.

The identified problem area was role transitions. The therapist focused on F.S.'s transition from a little girl to an adolescent girl who was beginning to date. Discussion focused on examining her parents' concerns, what F.S.'s expectations were for dating, and how to communicate with her mother and father about her need for increasing independence while still remaining under their guidance and supervision. The therapist and F.S. frequently role-played how she might tell her mother about her new boyfriend, elicit her mother's concerns, and discuss them rationally so that a mutually agreeable plan could be worked out.

Although her parents were unable to attend sessions, F.S. was able to communicate to her parents about her desire for a relationship. She told them that she felt that the fact that she was in a relationship should not preclude her from remaining a part of the family as their daughter. She also expressed her views on dating and worked out a compromise that was acceptable to her parents as well as to her. As her communication with her parents improved, the conflict and anxiety decreased, and her concentration and mood improved, as did her grades. She felt more comfortable talking with her mother about her relationship and getting her advice while making the transition from same-sex to opposite-sex dyadic relationships.

Interpersonal Deficits

Interpersonal deficits are identified when an individual appears to lack the requisite social skills to establish and maintain appropriate relationships within and outside the family. Both adults and adolescents may have similar deficits, but interpersonal deficits in an adolescent can impede his or her achievement of developmental tasks. These tasks are primarily social and include making same-age friends, participating in extracurricular activities, becoming part of a peer group, beginning to date, and learning to make choices regarding exclusive relations, career, and sexuality (Hersen and Van Hasselt 1987). As a result of interpersonal deficits, the adolescent may be socially isolated from peer groups and relationships, which can lead to feelings of depression and inadequacy. These feelings of depression can in turn lead to increased social withdrawal and result in a lag in interpersonal skills when the depression resolves.

The strategies for treating interpersonal deficits in adults and adolescents do not differ significantly. The focus is on those interpersonal deficits that are more a consequence of the depression rather than on personality traits that result in isolation. The therapist approaches a problem of interpersonal deficits by reviewing past significant relationships and exploring repetitive or parallel interpersonal problems. New strategies for approaching situations are identified and discussed. The patient is then encouraged to apply these strategies to current issues. In treating adolescents, the therapist may utilize role-playing of identified problematic interpersonal situations, enabling the adolescent to explore and practice new communication skills and interpersonal behaviors (e.g., learning how to make friends). Practicing situations in the session and encouraging further practice between sessions in small increments can engender a sense of social competence in the adolescents that can be generalized to other situations.

The Case of C.Y.

C.Y. is a 16-year-old high school student who presented to the clinic with depressive symptoms that she had been experiencing for over a year. She complained of early insomnia, loss of appetite, low self-esteem, depressed mood, and poor school performance. She met the criteria for dysthymic disorder. C.Y. reported having several relationships with boys the previous year that had resulted in her feeling badly about herself.

Feeling that she was unable to negotiate the school social scene, C.Y. experienced increasing social withdrawal and school refusal. She complained of feeling like she did not know how to fit in and interact with peers.

C.Y.'s main problem area was identified as that of interpersonal deficits. As a result of several unhappy encounters with boys her age, she began to feel badly and awkward about herself, distrusting her instincts about people and causing her to withdraw, which in turn only increased her sad mood. During the course of therapy, the therapist focused on ways of initiating and maintaining relationships, ways of evaluating a relationship and deciding if it is what she wants, how to assert herself in a relationship so that she does not do something against her wishes, and how to be more active and less passive in her relationships. The therapist and C.Y. role-played different social situations to practice her skills and increase her self-confidence.

During the course of treatment C.Y. switched to a new school, so she was encouraged to try out many of the role-plays and skills in her new school. As her new classmates attempted to draw her out of her shell, and armed with new skills, C.Y. gained more confidence in herself. She was able to make new friends and to decide which activities she did and did not want to participate in. Consequently, she felt more successful socially. Her mood and sleep improved, as did her school attendance and concentration. She felt more in control of what would happen to her in her relationships and therefore was more selective about her companions and enjoyed the relationships more. As her communication skills improved, she became more effective in her relationships at home as well as at school.

Single-Parent Families

Single-parent homes arise out of divorce, separation, incarceration, out-of-wedlock births, death by medical illness or violence, the AIDS crisis, and the increase in crime and drug abuse. Each of these situations presents unique emotional conflicts for the adolescent and the custodial parent. Depending upon the circumstances, children of single-parent families can function without significant problems, or they can experience a myriad of problems, including depression.

Researchers have found that higher levels of interparental conflict following a divorce or separation are associated with longitudinal increases in depressed mood, anxiety, and physical symptoms in adolescents (Mechanic and Hansell 1989). The departure of the parent is often characterized by uncertainty as to whether or not the parent will return, whether or not the parent is even still alive, feelings of abandonment, and difficulties in accepting the negative behaviors of the parent. The intensity of the depressive reaction is likely to be related to the degree of separation, its abruptness, and whether it has happened before (Jacobson and Jacobson 1987). Not only is the child's relationship with the absent parent affected, but the relationship with the remaining parent is also frequently altered. Reactions to these events often include depressed mood, increased sexual behavior, and increased conflicts with the custodial parent over discipline and independence.

Several tasks for the treatment of such adolescents with IPT-A have been identified.

1. Acknowledgment that the departure of the parent was a significant disruption in their lives
2. Addressing feelings of loss, rejection, abandonment, and/or punishment by the departed parent
3. Clarification of remaining expectations for their relationship with the absent parent
4. Negotiation of a working relationship with the remaining parent
5. Establishment of a relationship with the removed parent
6. If possible, acceptance of the permanence of the current situation.

In discussing the feelings associated with the parent's departure, it can be helpful to have the custodial parent participate in a session. The focus of the session is to discuss the parent's recollection of the spouse and to correct any misconceptions the adolescent may have about the parents. It may also be helpful to have a session with the parent alone specifically to discuss parenting issues of adolescents, including appropriate discipline and restrictions on their behavior.

The Case of P.Z.

P.Z., a 15-year-old girl, lived alone with her mother. Her parents had been divorced since she was 3 years old. Her father lived nearby and visited regularly. P.Z. presented with decreased concentration and school performance, increased irritability and crying, headaches, depressed mood, suicidal ideation, social withdrawal, loss of appetite, and early and middle insomnia, in addition to panic attacks with symptoms of light-headedness, heart racing, tingling in her hands, shortness of breath, saliva tasting sweet, and feelings of nausea.

At the time she presented to the outpatient clinic, P.Z. and her mother were sharing a room in her grandmother's apartment because of financial troubles they were having. She and her mother were getting into increasing conflict, as were she and her grandmother. P.Z. felt as though she never had any quiet or a place to herself. Her mother felt similarly and was in the process of finding them another place to live. During this time P.Z. continued her contact with her father and told him about their living conditions and the resulting stress. In the fourth week of treatment, she and her mother moved to their own apartment, but P.Z. was very worried about how they could afford it and what that pressure was going to do to her mother. She felt guilty about complaining to her mother. She expressed much anger at her father because he would always want to come over and joke around with her, but he had not been making his child support payments or giving her an allowance as had been mandated by the courts. She felt the need to stand up for her mother and to try to convince her father to make the payments. He would respond by telling her she favored her mother over him. P.Z. felt very trapped in her relationship with him and guilty that she had angry feelings toward him.

The therapist identified her problem area as related to being part of a single-parent family due to the divorce of her parents and having a father who was jealous over his wife's relationship with his daughter. P.Z.'s father refused to participate in the treatment, which he felt was not necessary. P.Z. wanted to pull away from her relationship with him because of the conflicting feelings she had toward him. P.Z.'s mother did participate in several sessions. The therapist focused on discussing and clarifying P.Z.'s expectations for her relationship with her father and what she perceived were her mother's expectations that she felt she needed to defend. Her mother participated in these sessions to help clarify for her daughter her feelings about her ex-husband and what type of relationship she wished for P.Z. to have with her father despite the circumstances, and to relieve P.Z. of feeling the need to defend her needs to the father. Together, different ways of communicating P.Z.'s feelings to her father and mother were explored, and the differences in feelings she may have between her custodial and noncustodial parent were normalized. P.Z. was able to delineate more realistic expectations for her relationship with her father and to resume her visits with him with these new terms in mind. With increased clarification of the issues between her and her parents and improved communication and negotiation of her place in regard to her parents' custody arrangement, P.Z.'s depression and anxiety symptoms resolved.

The Termination Phase

Termination should be addressed at the beginning of treatment and then periodically during the course of therapy. Many patients are unaware of having any feelings about the end of treatment; others may hesitate to acknowledge that they have come to value the relationship with the therapist. Patients should be advised that a slight recurrence of symptoms as termination approaches is common and that it is not unusual for patients to have feelings of apprehension, anger, or sadness. The appearance of such feelings does not portend a return to depression. To support the patient's ability to cope with problems, the therapist should highlight the patient's skills and external supports. The final session can be used to discuss areas of future difficulty and review strategies for problem resolution. Early warning signs of distress, situations of stress, and methods of coping should be identified and discussed.

The handling of termination as described above is similar for adolescents and adult patients. For adolescents there are the following additional issues. Termination of treatment with the adolescent also means terminating work with the adolescent's family. The final session of IPT-A may be a family session with the patient, parent(s), and other family members who may have been involved in the treatment process. The goals of this final session include a review of the patient's presenting symptoms, the interpersonal conflicts, the identified problem area as it relates to the goals of therapy, achievement of the therapy goals, and a discussion of the changes in the family interactions and functioning as a result of the therapy. Symptoms and conflicts should be presented in four categories: those symptoms specific to the depressive episode, those symptoms secondary to the depressive episode, those areas of conflict that are more enduring and representative of personality style, and those areas of conflict between parent and adolescent that are part of a normal developmental process. The patient and family also should be made aware of the possible recurrence of some symptoms shortly after termination. Management of further treatment, if indicated, and management of future recurrent episodes of depression should be discussed.

The distinction between a regression that will resolve in a few weeks and a recurrence of symptoms should be clarified. The latter should be tolerated by the family, who should provide support to the adolescent during this transition from dependence on the therapist to independence. If the adolescent's symptoms do not resolve in a few weeks, the therapist should be contacted to determine if further treatment is necessary. If it is clear at termination that the adolescent needs further treatment, this is the time to arrange for appropriate referral. Long-term treatment may be indicated for patients with long-standing personality problems, chronic or recurrent depression, or a history of not responding to treatment.

Special Issues

The therapist often encounters special issues in his or her work with adolescents. These include indications for medication, non-nuclear families, the suicidal patient, the assaultive patient, school refusal, substance abuse, notification of protective service agencies in cases of physical and sexual abuse, learning disabilities, and adolescents with sexual identity problems. These issues, which apply to some but not all adolescents and can cross all problem areas, will be discussed in the following subsections.

Antidepressant Medication in Conjunction With IPT-A

The decision to use antidepressant medication in depressed adolescents is a clinical and medical one made by a child/adolescent psychiatrist in collaboration with the treating clinician. Antidepressant medication is not contraindicated during IPT-A; in fact, it may be a useful adjunct treatment for severely depressed adolescents whose symptoms do not remit during the initial phases of treatment. Adolescents who can be treated on an outpatient basis are rarely started on antidepressant medication before the fourth week of treatment. Information regarding their depression, based upon self-report and clinician-rated scales, is systematically reviewed every 4 weeks or sooner if the treating clinician thinks it is necessary to do so. If by the fourth week of IPT-A treatment the adolescent is still significantly depressed based on these reports, then antidepressant medication is recommended as an adjunctive treatment to IPT-A. Indications for medication by the fourth week include persistent depressed mood, insomnia, poor concentration, school refusal, social isolation, hopelessness, and persistent thoughts of death.

The decision to use medication is discussed in a joint session with the psychiatrist, therapist, patient, and parents. Prescriptions are given to the parents or to another responsible adult, who will then be instructed on appropriate administration of the medication. If there are two treating therapists (one for medication and one for therapy), a plan of weekly communication throughout the course of dual treatment should be agreed upon to keep each other abreast of changes in mental status, compliance with each aspect of the treatment, and any reported side effects of the medication. The adolescent and parent should be informed what role each therapist plays in the treatment. Appointments should be coordinated to maximize the adolescent's participation in both aspects of the treatment.

Non-nuclear Families

For various reasons, adolescents live in alternative arrangements (i.e., *non-nuclear families*), which include homes of other relatives, foster homes, and group homes. Reasons for these alternative arrangements include death, abandonment, interventions by protective service agencies, irreconcilable differences, and illness. For the therapist, the task with these adolescents is to engage the relative, foster family, or leader from the group home as he or she would engage the parents. As with the parents, these persons are important in the adolescent's daily life and must be educated about the nature of depression and ways to support the adolescent in his or her recovery and, if necessary, participate in the treatment to facilitate changes in the home environment that will play a role in the adolescent's recovery.

Suicidal Patient

Although completed suicide in adolescence is a rare event, suicide attempts and suicidal ideation are highly prevalent (Shaffer et al. 1988). Evaluation for suicidality is a critical part of the initial evaluation, and suicidality should be monitored throughout the treatment. The adolescent should be asked if he or she has thoughts about death, about wanting to die, and about killing himself or herself. The therapist should be very specific in his or her questioning and obtain specific answers. The therapist should assess the intention and lethality of the patient's past suicide attempts, current suicidal ideation, and future plans. Based upon this assessment, and taking into account the stability of the home and family, the therapist must determine whether the adolescent is an acute suicide risk. If the therapist is uncertain, a second opinion should be sought. Any adolescent who is an acute suicide risk is not a candidate for IPT-A and will usually require psychiatric hospitalization.

The suitability of an adolescent with suicidal ideation for IPT-A will depend upon his or her capacity to establish and maintain a therapeutic alliance with the therapist. The cornerstone of this alliance is the adolescent's assurance that he or she will not make a suicide attempt and will notify the therapist or go to an emergency room immediately if the urge becomes compelling. The task of the therapist is not only to monitor the adolescent's suicidality but also to address the inappropriate use of suicide as a means of communicating feelings of anger or distress or as a means of solving a conflict.

Assaultive Patient

Although the frequency of having an adolescent patient who is homicidal is rare, there are occasions when some adolescents may be so upset that they know no other way of venting their frustration than through aggressive and violent behavior. Assessment of the patient for thoughts of hurting other persons should be done in conjunction with the assessment of suicidal behavior. As in the assessment of suicide, it is very important for the therapist to ask highly specific questions about the intent and the feasibility of going through with the action. Based on this assessment the therapist must determine whether the adolescent is at risk of harming another person. If so, the therapist (by law in some, but not all, states) must hospitalize the patient and has a duty to warn the intended victim of the patient's wishes.

An adolescent who is a serious risk for homicidal behavior is not a candidate for IPT-A. An adolescent who expresses anger and hostility in vague threats to others may be a candidate for IPT-A if he or she is able to establish a therapeutic alliance with the therapist, feel capable of controlling his or her behavior, and feel capable of making an agreement with the therapist that the violence will not be acted upon while in treatment. The therapist should also educate the adolescent as to more appropriate methods of communicating anger or upset and ways to diffuse his or her anger.

School Refusal

As a result of feelings of fatigue, poor concentration, and anhedonia, some depressed adolescents are unable to attend school regularly. Moreover, when they have been out of school for a week or two, they may conclude that they are too far behind to catch up and are embarrassed to go back to school after their absence, and consequently remain home for an extended period of time. It is important that the therapist question the adolescent and parent about school attendance during the initial evaluation. The therapist's role should be to stress the importance of returning to school and to enlist the assistance of the parents and school in ensuring the adolescent's return. The therapist should explain to the adolescent that although he or she may not feel like going back and may be embarrassed, the embarrassment will dissipate after the first day and he and she will feel better by being productive in school. The adolescent should be told that his or her concentration will improve as the depression resolves. Throughout the treatment the therapist should continue to check on the adolescent's school attendance and performance and be in contact with the school as necessary.

Substance Abuse by the Adolescent

Part of a screening and history of an adolescent should include a complete history of drug and alcohol use/abuse. Other family members should be interviewed about the adolescent's drug use even though they may be ignorant of such abuse. If necessary, the adolescent should be referred for drug treatment before IPT-A is started. To participate in IPT-A, the adolescent must not be abusing or using any substances and must make a commitment to a maintenance of a drug-free life. If the therapist feels that the drug abuse is a primary problem and the depression is secondary to the drug abuse, the adolescent should be referred to a drug treatment center. The therapist can help the adolescent deal with peer pressure and family dynamics that lead to drug use, and engage another family member who may be another source of support in the patient's abstinence from drugs.

Protective Service Agencies

Protective service agencies have the purpose of protecting the welfare of children when their environment is harmful or neglectful. Each state has its own agency for accepting and dealing with reports, and its own laws governing when and how to report a case. A child may already be in the jurisdiction of a protective service agency when he or she begins therapy, or it may be the duty of the therapist to report the child to the protective service agency if information about possible harm to the child is uncovered in the course of treatment. The therapist contacting a protective service agency can disrupt the therapeutic alliance with the child or parent. The therapist must be alert to this possibility and must work with the adolescent and parent to help them understand that the service was notified to alleviate a stressful situation for both child and parent and provide help. The therapist should emphasize that the protective service agency is a means to provide the adolescent with increased social support so that the family can function better.

Sexual Abuse

As with all of these special issues, the therapist should carefully evaluate the adolescent for any past or current history of sexual abuse. Frequent symptoms that might indicate a past history of abuse include depression, suicide, sexual promiscuity, severe anxiety about sex, and conduct problems (Browne and Finkelhor 1986). Evaluating for abuse requires sensitivity and time. The adolescent may not reveal the abuse during the initial visit, but rather may reveal it during the course of treatment as he or she begins to trust the therapist. If the abuse is currently ongoing, the therapist is required by law to contact the protective service agency for children so that the agency can intervene with the family and provide the appropriate social services to the family or to the adolescent. If the abuse is current, the adolescent may not be appropriate for treatment with IPT-A, because IPT-A is not designed to deal with the acute or long-term consequences of sexual abuse. If the abuse was in the past, the therapist still needs a detailed history of the interpersonal context in which the abuse occurred so that an accurate picture of the familial relationships can be created.

Learning Disabilities

Depression is commonly associated with cognitive impairments during its acute stages. A psychosocial history will help the therapist distinguish between long-standing learning disabilities and impairments secondary to the depressive episode. This task is made more difficult when the patient has long-standing depressive symptoms or a personality style that presents with what appear to be cognitive limitations. Psychological or educational testing can be useful in identifying learning disabilities. When learning disabilities are diagnosed, special educational resources are necessary and the therapist will need to arrange for this in conjunction with the school system. Cognitive impairments secondary to the depression will resolve when the depressive symptoms resolve. The child and parents should be made aware of the etiology of the child's impairments and revise their expectations accordingly.

Adolescents With Sexual Identity Problems

Adolescence is a time when the person begins to form intimate dyadic relationships, usually with partners of the opposite sex, and for some adolescents with partners of the same sex. Exploration of sexual relationships with different partners is common. Those adolescents who find their sexual interest is exclusively with partners of the same sex can feel isolated and alone. Those adolescents who feel attracted to both same and opposite-sex partners may feel confused about their sexual orientation. The role of the therapist is to help the adolescent explore his or her sexual feelings and concerns about his or her orientation in a nonjudgmental context. In addition, it may be appropriate to identify the association between the adolescent's state of confusion and his or her depression. It also is possible that the adolescent is comfortable with and has accepted his or her sexual orientation. In such a situation, the therapist must be supportive of the decision. It is important for the therapist to keep these discussions confidential unless the adolescent has a desire to share the information with others.

Crisis Management

During the course of any type of psychotherapy with an adolescent a crisis can occur, and it can be a direct result of the adolescent's familial or social environment. The crisis can pose a direct threat to the adolescent's treatment and must be handled swiftly and decisively to protect the adolescent and the treatment. The following events are considered to be a crisis: physical or sexual abuse, a change in suicidal ideation or a suicide attempt, suicidal behavior in a friend or family member, running away, illness in the adolescent, illness or death in the family, pregnancy, violence occurring at home or outside the home, drug use, legal difficulties, homicidal ideation, or abrupt termination by the adolescent or the adolescent's family.

The first task facing the IPT-A therapist is to determine the etiology of the crisis. What is the cause of the particular crisis? The IPT-A therapist needs to elucidate the events surrounding the crisis and assess the adolescent's reaction and the family's response to the crisis. It must first be determined whether the crisis is a response to the therapist or to issues being addressed in the therapy. Did the therapist miss early warning signs that such a crisis was likely, or was the patient or family concealing information that would have allowed the therapist to expect and prevent the crisis? Alternatively, the event may have been unpredictable and a response to events out of the control of therapist, patient, and family.

The second but simultaneous task in crisis management for the therapist in IPT-A is to bring the patient in for an emergency session as soon as possible. In the case of suicidal or homicidal ideation, if an appointment cannot be set up soon enough, the patient should be sent to the closest emergency room. When meeting in the emergency session, the therapist must determine the need for and level of family involvement. When dealing with an adolescent who is under 18 years of age, it is mandatory for the therapist to notify the parent if there is a significant risk to the patient. The level of involvement will vary with the different types of crises and the nature of the patient's relationship with the family members. The therapist must be careful to elicit the entire story from the adolescent regarding the precipitant and the accompanying emotions. After hearing the whole story, the therapist must again assess whether the risk of the patient getting hurt or of hurting others is great enough to warrant hospitalization. In addition, the therapist must evaluate whether there is a need to involve other agencies or parties, such as medical or legal consultations or protective services for children, in evaluating or intervening in the crisis.

If the therapist determines that the adolescent is able to remain in outpatient treatment, the IPT-A treatment contract should be reexamined and revised as necessary. Items in the contract that may change include frequency of the sessions, frequency of phone calls between therapist and patient, and the identified problem area that is the focus of the treatment. At times the crisis may suggest that a significant problem area was overlooked, or there may be an interaction between two problem areas. The therapist may also choose to meet more frequently in the weeks following the crisis until it is apparent that the patient's situation has stabilized.

Management of the individual crises varies with each situation. The most significant decision the therapist must make is whether to hospitalize the patient and/or whether IPT-A must be terminated and another form of treatment begun. If the decision has been made to involve the family, it would be important to meet with the family separately as well as conjointly with the patient to see how the problem is understood and how it can best be resolved. The therapist might conduct several sessions with the family to assist in the negotiation of the precipitant for the crisis and then resume individual treatment with the patient. If the protective service agency was notified, the therapist will work with the agency to try and change the patient's situation.

Further Work

Using the present modifications of the IPT manual for treatment of adolescents, the authors are currently conducting an open clinical trial of IPT-A for adolescents with a range of depressive disorders, including major depression, dysthymia, adjustment disorder with depressed mood, and depressive disorder not otherwise specified. Results of the pilot trial will be used to further modify the manual, to develop scripts and videotapes illustrating the therapeutic procedures, and to conduct a larger controlled clinical trial. The intent is to make the manual available to investigators interested in conducting such trials. Data available on the treatment of depressed adolescents using drugs and/or psychotherapy are more than a decade behind comparable data available for the treatment of depressed adults. It is the authors' hope that these efforts will accelerate the production of a rational, scientific basis for treatment of adolescent depression.

References

American Psychiatric Association: Diagnostic and Statistical Manual of Mental Disorders, 3rd Edition. Washington, DC, American Psychiatric Association, 1980

American Psychiatric Association: Diagnostic and Statistical Manual of Mental Disorders, 3rd Edition, Revised. Washington, DC, American Psychiatric Association, 1987

Angold A, Weissman MM, John K, et al: Parent and child reports of depressive symptoms in children at low and high risk for depression. J Child Psychol Psychiatry 28:901, 1987

Bemporad JR: Psychodynamic treatment of depressed adolescents. J Clin Psychiatry 49:26–31, 1988

Brent DA, Kolko DJ, Allen MJ, et al: Suicidality in affectively disordered adolescent inpatients. J Am Acad Child Adolesc Psychiatry 29:586–593, 1990

Browne A, Finkelhor D: Impact of child sexual abuse: a review of the research. Psychol Bull 99:66–77, 1986

Campbell M, Spencer EK: Psychopharmacology in child and adolescent psychiatry: a review of the past five years. J Am Acad Child Adolesc Psychiatry 27:269–279, 1988

Chevron E, Rounsaville B, Rothblum ED, et al: Selecting psychotherapists to participate in psychotherapy outcome studies: relationship between psychotherapist characteristics and assessment of clinical skills. J Nerv Ment Dis 171:348–353, 1983

Christie KA, Burke JD, Regier DA, et al: Epidemiologic evidence for early onset of mental disorders and higher risk of drug abuse in young adults. Am J Psychiatry 145:971–975, 1988

Clarke G, Lewinsohn PM: The Coping With Depression Course: a group psychoeducational intervention for unipolar depression. Behavior Change 6:554–569, 1989

Cytrn L, McKnew DH: Treatment issues in childhood depression. Psychiatric Annals 15:401, 1985

Earls F: Prevalence of behavior problems in three-year-old children: a cross-national replication. Arch Gen Psychiatry 37:1153–1157, 1980

Erikson EH: Identity, Youth, and Crisis. New York, WW Norton, 1968

Fendrich M, Warner V, Weissman MM: Family risk factors, parental depression and psychopathology in offspring. Developmental Psychology 26:40–50, 1990

Fleming JE, Offord DR: Epidemiology of childhood depressive disorders: a critical review. J Am Acad Child Adolesc Psychiatry 29:571–580, 1990

Fleming JE, Offord DR, Boyle MH: The Ontario Child Health Study: prevalence of childhood and adolescent depression in the community. Br J Psychiatry 155:647–654, 1989

Garber J, Kriss MR, Koch M, et al: Recurrent depression in adolescents: a follow-up study. J Am Acad Child Adolesc Psychiatry 27:49–54, 1988

Garrison CZ, Sluchter MD, Schoenbach VJ, et al: Epidemiology of depressive symptoms in young adolescents. J Am Acad Child Adolesc Psychiatry 28:343–351, 1989

Geller B, Chestnut EC, Miller D, et al: Preliminary data on DSM-III associated features of major depression disorder in children and adolescents. Am J Psychiatry 142:643–645, 1985

Geller B, Cooper TB, Graham GL, et al: Double-blind placebo-controlled study of nortriptyline in depressed adolescents using a "fixed plasma level" design. Psychopharmacol Bull 26:85–91, 1990

Gould M, Davidson L: Suicide contagion among adolescents, in Advances in Adolescent Mental Health, Vol 3: Depression and Suicide. Edited by Stillman AR, Feldman RA. Greenwich, CT, JAI Press, 1988, pp 29–59

Harrington R, Fudge H, Rutter M, et al: Adult outcomes of childhood and adolescent depression. Arch Gen Psychiatry 47:465–473, 1990

Hersen M, Van Hasselt VB: Behavior Therapy With Children and Adolescents: A Clinical Approach. New York, Wiley, 1987

Jacobson G, Jacobson DS: Impact of marital dissolution on adults and children: the significance of loss and continuity, in The Psychology of Separation and Loss: Perspectives on Development, Life Transitions, and Clinical Practice. Edited by Bloom-Feshbach J, Bloom-Feshbach S. San Francisco, CA, Jossey-Bass, 1987, pp 316–344

Kandel DB, Davies M: Epidemiology of depressed mood in adolescents. Arch Gen Psychiatry 39:1205–1212, 1982

Kandel DB, Davies M: Adult sequelae of adolescent depressive symptoms. Arch Gen Psychiatry 43:255, 1986

Kaplan S, Hong GK, Weinhold C: Epidemiology of depressive symptoms in adolescents. Journal of the American Academy of Child Psychiatry 23:91–98, 1984

Kashani JH, Sherman DD: Childhood depression: epidemiology, etiological models and treatment implications. Integrative Psychiatry 6:1–21, 1988

Kashani JH, Shekim WO, Reid JC: Amitriptyline in children with major depressive disorder: a double-blind crossover pilot study. Journal of the American Academy of Child Psychiatry 23:348–351, 1984

Kashani JH, Carlson GA, Beck NC, et al: Depression, depressive symptoms, and depressed mood among a community sample of adolescents. Am J Psychiatry 144:931–934, 1987

Kashani JH, Burbach DJ, Rosenberg TK: Perception of family conflict resolution and depressive symptomatology in adolescents. J Am Acad Child Adolesc Psychiatry 27:42–48, 1988

Kestenbaum CJ, Kron L: Psychoanalytic intervention with children and adolescents with affective disorders: a combined treatment approach. J Am Acad Psychoanal 15:153–174, 1987

Klerman GL, Weissman MM, Rounsaville BJ, et al: Interpersonal Psychotherapy of Depression. New York, Basic Books, 1984

Kovacs M, Feinberg TL, Crouse-Novak MA, et al: Depressive disorders in childhood, I: a longitudinal prospective study of characteristics and recovery. Arch Gen Psychiatry 41:229–237, 1984a

Kovacs M, Feinberg TL, Crouse-Novak MA, et al: Depressive disorders in childhood, II: a longitudinal study of the risk for a subsequent major depression. Arch Gen Psychiatry 41:643–649, 1984b

Kovacs M, Paulauskas S, Gatsonis C, et al: Depressive disorder in childhood, III: a longitudinal study of comorbidity with and risk for conduct disorders. J Affective Disord 15:205–217, 1988

Kramer E, Feiguine R: Clinical effects of amitriptyline in adolescent depression. Journal of the American Academy of Child Psychiatry 20:636–644, 1981

Krupnick J: Bereavement during childhood and adolescence, in Bereavement: Reactions, Consequences, and Care. Edited by Osterweis M, Solomon F, Green M. Washington, DC, National Academy Press, 1984, pp 99–141

Lefkowitz MM, Tesiny EP: Assessment of childhood depression. J Consult Clin Psychol 14:25–39, 1985

Lewinsohn PM, Clarke GN, Hops H, et al: Cognitive-behavioral treatment for depressed adolescents. Behavior Therapy 21:385–401, 1990

Liebowitz JH, Kernberg PF: Psychodynamic psychotherapies, in Handbook of Clinical Assessment of Children and Adolescents, Vol 2. Edited by Kestenbaum CJ, Williams DT. New York, New York University Press, 1988, pp 1045–1065

McGee R, Feehan M, Williams S, et al: DSM-III disorders in a large sample of adolescents. J Am Acad Child Adolesc Psychiatry 29:611–619, 1990

Mechanic D, Hansell S: Divorce, family conflict, and adolescents' well-being. J Health Soc Behav 30:105–116, 1989

Miller D: Adolescence: Psychology, Psychopathology, Psychotherapy. New York, Jason Aronson, 1974

Nissen G: Treatment for depression in children and adolescents. Psychopathology 19:156–161, 1986

Offer D: The Psychological World of the Teenager: A Study of Normal Adolescent Boys. New York, Basic Books, 1969

Offer D, Ostrov E, Howard KI: The mental health professionals' concept of the normal adolescent. Arch Gen Psychiatry 38:149–152, 1981

Offord DR, Boyle MH, Szatmari P: Ontario Child Health Study, II: six-month prevalence of disorder and rates of service utilization. Arch Gen Psychiatry 44:832–836, 1987

Orvaschel H, Weissman MM, Kidd KK: Children and depression: the children of depressed parents; the childhood of depressed patients; depression in children. J Affective Disord 2:1–16, 1981

Puig-Antich J, Weston B: The diagnosis and treatment of major depressive disorder in childhood. Annu Rev Med 34:231–245, 1983

Puig-Antich J, Lukens E, Davis M, et al: Psychosocial functioning in prepubertal major depression disorders, II: interpersonal relationships after sustained recovery from the depressive episode. Arch Gen Psychiatry 42:511–517, 1985

Puig-Antich J, Perel JM, Lupatkin W, et al: Imipramine in prepubertal major depressive disorders. Arch Gen Psychiatry 44:81–89, 1987

Raphael B: The Anatomy of Bereavement. New York, Basic Books, 1983

Reinherz HZ, Stewart-Berghauer G, Pakiz B, et al: The relationship of early risk and current mediators to depressive symptomatology in adolescence. J Am Acad Child Adolesc Psychiatry 28:942–947, 1989

Reynolds WM, Coats KI: A comparison of cognitive-behavioral therapy and relaxation training for the treatment of depression in adolescents. J Consult Clin Psychol 44:653–660, 1986

Richman N, Stevenson JE, Graham PJ: Prevalence of behavior problems in 3-year-old children: an epidemiological study in a London borough. J Child Psychol Psychiatry 16:277–287, 1975

Robbins DR, Allessi NE, Colfer MV: Treatment of adolescents with major depression: implications of the DST and the melancholic clinical subtype. J Affective Disord 17:99–104, 1989a

Robbins DR, Allessi NE, Cook SC, et al: The use of the Research Diagnostic Criteria (RDC) for depression in adolescent psychiatric inpatients. J Am Acad Child Adolesc Psychiatry 21:251–255, 1989b

Rutter M, Graham P, Chadwick OFD, et al: Adolescent turmoil: fact or fiction. J Child Psychol Psychiatry 17:35–56, 1976

Ryan ND: Pharmacotherapy of adolescent major depression: beyond TCAs. Psychopharmacol Bull 26:75–79, 1990

Ryan ND, Puig-Antich J: Affective illness in adolescence, in Psychiatry Update: The American Psychiatric Association Annual Review, Vol 5. Edited by Frances AJ, Hales RE. Washington, DC, American Psychiatric Press, 1986, pp 420–450

Ryan ND, Puig-Antich J, Cooper TB, et al: Imipramine in adolescent major depression: plasma level and clinical response. Acta Psychiatr Scand 73:275–288, 1986

Ryan ND, Puig-Antich J, Ambrosini P, et al: The clinical picture of major depression in children and adolescents. Arch Gen Psychiatry 44:854–861, 1987

Ryan ND, Meyer V, Dachille S, et al: Lithium antidepressant augmentation in TCA-refractory depression in adolescents. J Am Acad Child Adolesc Psychiatry 27:371–376, 1988a

Ryan ND, Puig-Antich J, Rabinovich H, et al: MAOIs in adolescent major depression unresponsive to tricyclic antidepressants. J Am Acad Child Adolesc Psychiatry 27:755–758, 1988b

Shaffer D, Garland A, Gould M, et al: Preventing teenage suicide: a critical review. J Am Acad Child Adolesc Psychiatry 27:675–687, 1988

Shain BN, Naylor M, Alessi N: Comparison of self-rated and clinician-rated measures of depression in adolescents. Am J Psychiatry 147:793–795, 1990

Smucker MR, Craighead WE, Craighead LW, et al: Normative and reliability data for the Children's Depression Inventory. J Abnorm Child Psychol 14:25–39, 1986

Strober M: Depression in adolescents. Psychiatric Annals 16:375–378, 1985

Strober M, Carlson G: Bipolar illness in adolescents with major depressive disorder: clinical, genetic, and psychopharmacological predictors. Arch Gen Psychiatry 39:549–555, 1982

Strober M, Green J, Carlson G: Phenomenology and subtypes of major depressive disorder in adolescence. J Affective Disord 3:281–290, 1981

Strober M, Freeman R, Rigali J: The pharmacotherapy of depressive illness in adolescence, I: an open label trial of imipramine. Psychopharmacol Bull 26:80–84, 1990

Weissman MM, Gammon GD, John K, et al: Children of depressed parents: increased psychopathology and early onset major depression. Arch Gen Psychiatry 44:847–853, 1987a

Weissman MM, Jarrett RB, Rush JA: Psychotherapy and its relevance to the pharmacotherapy of major depression: a decade later (1976–1985), in Psychopharmacology: The Third Generation of Progress. Edited by Meltzer HY. New York, Raven, 1987b, pp 1059–1069

Wells VE, Deykin EY, Klerman GL: Risk factors for depression in adolescents. Psychiatr Dev 3:83–108, 1985

Wilkes TCR, Rush JA: Adaptations of cognitive therapy for depressed adolescents. J Am Acad Child Adolesc Psychiatry 27:381–386, 1988

Interpersonal Psychotherapy in the Treatment of Late-Life Depression

Ellen Frank, Ph.D.
Nancy Frank, A.C.S.W.
Cleon Cornes, M.D.
Stanley D. Imber, Ph.D.
Mark D. Miller, M.D.
Susan M. Morris, L.S.W.
Charles F. Reynolds III, M.D.

Depression is an illness that knows no age limits; its symptoms afflict young and old alike. Affective disorders constitute the most common psychiatric problem in late life. Ten to fifteen percent of community resident elders are suffering from depression at any one point in time, which amounts to approximately one million older Americans (Blazer and Williams 1980; Butler and Lewis 1982). Although those over 65 years of age account for only about 11% of the United States population, they commit 25% of all suicides. Unlike loss, sadness, or grief, depression can be a life-threatening disorder, not only because of the increased suicide risk but also because depression is associated with a greater

The development of maintenance interpersonal psychotherapy was supported in part by National Institute of Mental Health Grants MH-43832, MH-00295, and MH-30915.

risk for morbidity from cardiac disease, malnutrition, and a variety of other causes.

In light of the many losses, role transitions, and frequent isolation of elderly persons in the United States, it would appear that the traditional problem areas of interpersonal psychotherapy (IPT) are likely to have broad application in this age group. Furthermore, the relatively less structured nature of IPT (as compared with other manual-based treatments for depression) would appear to be particularly well suited to the greater flexibility required in psychotherapeutic interventions with elderly persons. The active stance of the IPT therapist and the problem-oriented focus of the intervention are appealing to older persons who may require, at least initially, direct help in problem resolution and who view work toward short-term goals as consistent with the limited time they may see remaining in which to make changes in their lives.

Various authors have reported successful application of IPT in the treatment of depression in late life. Sloane et al. (1985) and Schneider et al. (1986) indicated early positive outcome with IPT in preliminary reports of a comparative study with nortriptyline. In a separate study by investigators in New Haven (Rothblum et al. 1982; Sholomskas et al. 1983), similar positive results for IPT were reported in pilot work with depressed elderly outpatients. The efficacy and safety of IPT itself for the treatment of depression have been well documented in the National Institute of Mental Health (NIMH) Treatment of Depression Collaborative Research Program (Elkin et al. 1989).

The four specific problem areas addressed by IPT—grief, interpersonal disputes, role transitions, and interpersonal deficits—are particularly relevant to the lives of older individuals. Elderly persons are at high risk to suffer delayed grief and mourning following multiple deaths of loved ones, friends, and acquaintances, and may have severe problems with loneliness secondary to these losses. Role transitions of various types can occur with the onset of a depressive episode. These include changes related to deteriorating health, wealth, and status; decreasing support systems and reduced contact with friends and family; retirement or loss of job; changing familial roles, including the "empty nest syndrome" and the transition to being grandparents or even great-grandparents; and medical disorders, pain, and disabilities that lead to decreased activities and withdrawal from constructive and formerly satisfying activities. Interpersonal conflicts in the lives of the elderly may be related to increased dependency on others; to decisions about where to live; to changes in the financial situation; to chronic, unresolved grievances; or to general preparation for an end period of life. Interpersonal deficits are often connected to long-standing patterns of isolation and loneliness, or to decreased energy and motivation to make new friends.

In this chapter we describe the origins of interpersonal psychotherapeutic work with elderly persons by the original New Haven–Boston group and then move on to describe our experience with its use in the Late Life Depression Prevention Program at the Western Psychiatric Institute and Clinic in Pittsburgh, Pennsylvania. We are using *interpersonal psychotherapy for late life depression* (IPT-LL) and *interpersonal psychotherapy for the maintenance treatment of recurrent depression in late life* (IPT-LLM) in the context of a controlled trial examining the relative efficacy of interpersonal psychotherapy, nortriptyline, and the combination in preventing new episodes of major depression among individuals of ages 60 to 80 who have a history of recurrent episodes (see Figure 7–1).

In the context of this study, all patients are receiving IPT-LL along with nortriptyline in the acute treatment phase. Once patients have maintained a stable remission for 16 weeks, they are randomly assigned to either monthly sessions of IPT-LLM in combination with nortriptyline, IPT-LLM and placebo, medication clinic visits and nortriptyline, or medication clinic visits and placebo.

Early Descriptions of Interpersonal Psychotherapy With Elderly Persons

As Sholomskas and his colleagues (1983) have pointed out, IPT (Klerman et al. 1984) readily lends itself to adaptation for use with patients experiencing depression in late life. Sholomskas et al. do, however, point to certain changes that must be made if IPT is to be adapted successfully to use with older patients. They note that although IPT was originally intended to be conducted in sessions of 50 to 60 minutes' duration, more flexibility may be needed with elderly persons. The therapist must also be more flexible in terms of his or her willingness to meet the dependency

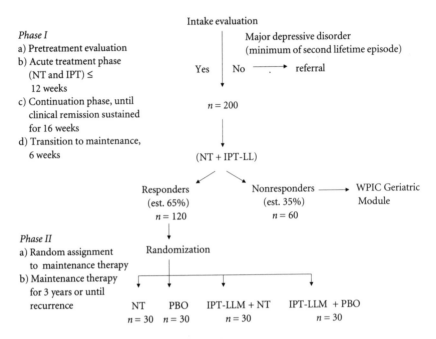

Figure 7–1. Maintenance therapies in late-life depressed patients.
NT = nortriptyline; PBO = placebo; IPT = interpersonal psychotherapy;
IPT-LL = interpersonal psychotherapy for late-life depression;
IPT-LLM = maintenance interpersonal psychotherapy for late-life depression.

needs of older patients, especially when these are expressed as requests for practical help with life management. While with younger patients the therapist might attempt to help the patient to alter dramatically or even terminate a profoundly troubled relationship, in working with elderly persons a more appropriate goal may be to help the patient to tolerate that relationship and to reduce its depressive effect upon the patient. Sholomskas et al. also note that older patients frequently produce gifts for the therapists and that accepting these gifts graciously (and, we assume, without overt interpretation) facilitates the therapeutic work.

In concluding their review, Sholomskas et al. (1983) make three general recommendations for the IPT therapist working with persons in late life: 1) make use of, and even emphasize, the active, non-neutral stance of the IPT therapist; 2) be prepared to help the patient find solutions for financial problems, transportation, health care, and so forth, to maximize the beneficial effects of therapy; and 3) be aware of the limitations of therapy with persons in late life in whom some problems simply are not amenable to resolution, including material, functional, and psychological losses, life-long psychopathology, and the existential issues of late life.

Within the Late Life Depression Prevention Program at Western Psychiatric Institute and Clinic, we have instituted a program of care for elderly persons with recurrent unipolar depression. We have also had considerable experience in working with the "young old" (ages 50 to 65) in the context of a recently completed study of maintenance therapies in recurrent depression (Frank et al. 1990), which we carried out in our Depression Prevention Clinic between 1982 and 1990. Our experience suggests that many of the recommendations made by Sholomskas et al. for the adaptation of IPT to the patient in late life are correct, and these are elaborated on below. We have found that there are additional issues that require special consideration in working with depressed late-life patients, as will also be discussed in this chapter.

Adaptation of Interpersonal Psychotherapy to the Late-Life Patient

Session Length of IPT-LL

Some allowances must be made with respect to length of sessions when working with older patients. The physically well, remitting elderly patient may be considerably more talkative and may have more difficulty remaining focused than would his or her younger counterpart. The more physically frail and/or acutely depressed patient may not have enough energy to sustain an entire 1-hour session. We find that, typically, the therapist will want to work toward a goal of 45- to 50-minute sessions, gently helping the more talkative patient to focus more directly on therapeutic issues, and encouraging the less talkative patient to be more expansive. Depending upon the particular requirements of the setting in which IPT-LL is being used (e.g., private practice versus a carefully scheduled clinic environment), the therapist may be able to maintain flexibility on this point, or he or she may need to work harder on helping the patient to conform to the "50-minute hour."

Dependency Issues

Many older patients find themselves facing difficulties in managing the problems of daily living. Within the structure of our collaborative treatment program, in which patients are managed by a treatment team that includes a therapist, a psychiatrist, and a social caseworker, it is possible to differentiate the roles of IPT therapist and social caseworker. In many treatment settings this rather artificial distinction may not be necessary. Regardless of whether these needs are met by one person or two, certain principles apply. The IPT therapist's role is to work alone or with the caseworker to assess the validity of the expressed need, to encourage the patient to make use of the caseworker for help in meeting valid needs, to facilitate contact between the patient and the caseworker, and to work collaboratively with the caseworker to help the patient to increase independence where appropriate or to accept the need for help. The therapist and caseworker coordinate their efforts so as to avoid conveying different messages to the patient and to avoid splitting on the part of the patient. By clearly defining and attempting to adhere to relatively separate but carefully coordinated roles for the therapist and caseworker, the late-life patient's true dependency needs can be met successfully, and the capacity for independence can be maximized, as in the following example:

> Ms. D., a 73-year-old foreign-born widow of somewhat limited intelligence, was literate in her first language, Polish, but she never achieved literacy in English. She was nonetheless quite capable, when well, of negotiating the public transportation system and making use of the phone system. Following the death of her husband, who had been literate in English, Ms. D. transferred many of her dependency needs to her IPT therapist and social caseworker, requesting help with a large number of life-management tasks.
>
> The therapist and caseworker were able to agree that her request for help with the applications for public housing were legitimate, because these required a fairly sophisticated knowledge of English. On the other hand, her requests for help in making appointments at the medical center hospital for her various medical problems were not deemed legitimate, because she was able to use the phone book and, in particular, her own small phone directory that she kept in a mix of Polish and English.
>
> The IPT therapist and social caseworker collaborated in helping Ms. D. to understand the difference between these two kinds of requests. They pointed out that it would be unreasonable to expect her to be able

to complete the housing application on her own, but, using her own little phone directory, she was more than capable of calling to make her medical appointments. Both the IPT therapist and the caseworker reinforced Ms. D.'s successes at making her medical appointments and continued to clarify the difference between what she was capable of doing on her own and what constituted legitimate requests for help. In several instances, some experimentation was helpful with Ms. D. in order to test the limits of her abilities to negotiate on her own.

Tolerating Rather Than Ameliorating Role Disputes

Patients experiencing depression in late life often attribute many of their symptoms to chronically troubled relationships with a spouse, child, or some other close relative. It is not always clear whether the onset of the episode is related to an increase in the actual level of trouble in the relationship, to a decreasing tolerance on the part of the aging individual, or to some combination of the two. With a younger depressed patient, the IPT therapist would likely emphasize the alteration of maladaptive communication patterns in the relationship or, if the disputes were sufficiently severe and intractable, might explore the reasonableness of remaining in the relationship. With patients in late life the most practical therapeutic goal is often to increase the patient's tolerance for the distressing aspects of the relationship and to facilitate an appreciation for any positive aspects. The following case illustrates this point:

Ms. L. was a 62-year-old married woman who presented in an episode of major depression citing marital distress as her most troubling interpersonal problem. She described her husband as being a rigid, autocratic, self-absorbed man who was completely incapable of admitting that he was wrong or of making an apology. Their relationship was characterized by frequent explosive arguments, following which Ms. L. would invariably threaten to leave the marriage.

During the course of treatment, Ms. L. was first helped to be more direct in her communicative style with Mr. L., improving her ability to indicate directly what she wanted from him rather than indirectly hinting and leaving him to guess at what it was that she was really asking for. However, the arguments continued, and Mr. L. became no better at apologizing to Ms. L.

About midway through the treatment, the therapist realized, however, that on the day following one of these arguments, Mr. L. would invariably stop on his way home to pick up a bag of cookies or some small item for the home to give to Ms. L. The therapist helped Ms. L. to see these "peace offerings" as Mr. L.'s form of apology.

Shortly thereafter, Ms. L. came into her session stating that she realized that should she decide to leave Mr. L., she had, in fact, nowhere to go. As she put it, "What am I going to do, cry at my mother's grave?" Following this insight, Ms. L. began to decrease her threats of leaving the relationship. This added to decreasing the feelings of conflict in the relationship and appeared to help considerably in the remission of Ms. L.'s depressive symptoms.

Some older patients who present with chronically distressed relationships appear to the therapist to be in such relationships at least in part because of long-standing social-skills or interpersonal deficits of their own. Because of their intractable nature, such long-standing problems are probably not amenable to change even in longer-term maintenance treatment and would not be an appropriate focus for short-term IPT. Some patients have adequate social skills and a history of good interpersonal relationships outside the context of the one important, distressed relationship. These patients can often be helped to tolerate the distressed relationship through encouragement to decrease the amount of time spent with the upsetting individual (if this can be done without increasing the patient's feelings of guilt), and to increase the amount of time spent in fulfilling activities and satisfying interpersonal contacts.

Ms. J. is a 67-year-old woman who, after placing her very ill and irritable mother in a nursing home, found herself spending all day, every day at the nursing home. Although she was relieved of the nighttime responsibilities for her mother, her days were just as difficult as they had been prior to placing her mother in the nursing home, and she found herself becoming increasingly depressed.

Ms. J. was encouraged by her IPT therapist to take some part of each day to do things for herself. This was very difficult for Ms. J., who had always assumed that she could only feel good about herself if she were giving to others. To do something only for herself was, Ms. J. thought, a selfish act that would lower her self-esteem and thereby increase her depression. She was surprised to find, however, that when she did take part of each day and devote it to her own sewing or writing projects, she actually felt better. Occasionally, she was able to have her husband, a very patient minister, visit her mother in her place while she prepared a nice dinner for the two of them. Ms. J. found that decreasing the amount of time she spent with her mother gave her a greatly increased ability to tolerate the time she did spend with her.

Later, in the maintenance treatment phase, when Ms. J.'s mother came close to death, the relationship had improved to the point that Ms. J. was able to do very important grief work with her mother, helping her mother to resolve some of the guilt she still carried over the way she had treated a younger sister.

Transference Issues

It is clear in the original manual for interpersonal psychotherapy and in the Klerman et al. (1984) volume that the positive transference that develops during treatment is not to be interpreted, and that the acceptance of small gifts from patients during the course of IPT is entirely appropriate. This issue may become even more important in work with elderly persons. As with all overt indications of positive transference, we find that the therapist must learn to separate the manipulative gift from one that represents a sincere expression of gratitude. It is also important for the IPT therapist to be aware of what the gift may represent, whether it is a tin of cookies intended for the entire staff or an elaborate piece of woodwork that has been fashioned specifically for the therapist. The gift from the elderly person often has important meaning to the giver: it represents the fact that the patient is still a person capable of producing and giving.

With some older patients, particularly those who are in the process of recovering from an abnormal grief reaction, the therapist may, as in the following example, actually encourage the activity as a way of motivating the patient:

> Mr. P., a 76-year-old bachelor who had always been somewhat socially isolated, went into a deep depression following the death of his brother for whom he had been caring for the last 5 years. Once the depression began to remit, the therapist encouraged him to engage in a variety of activities, the most satisfying of which appeared to be a bookbinding course that he took at a local community center. In this instance, the therapist went so far as to give him books of her own to be rebound. This provided the patient with a highly therapeutic activity and, at the same time, an opportunity to express his gratitude to the therapist and other staff members.

Avoiding a Neutral Stance

It is probably the case that a therapist's passive or neutral stance is difficult for all depressed individuals to tolerate. Avoiding such a stance can be especially important with older patients, who may enter treatment with the assumption that the younger therapist is not genuinely interested in them. Likewise, long silences that may be appropriate in work with younger patients, especially as they remit, seem inappropriate with older patients, who may not be able to sustain conversation for a full 45 minutes. In our work with the depressed elderly we have found that it is generally preferable to terminate the session early rather than to fill the time period with extended silences.

The IPT therapist has never been constrained from giving direct advice to the patient, and this remains especially true in the use of IPT with elderly persons. Specific therapeutic suggestions regarding how to increase social contacts or address communication problems in a troubled relationship are entirely appropriate within the context of IPT with older patients.

Measuring Treatment Gains

As Sholomskas and colleagues (1983) observed early on in their use of IPT with elderly patients, therapeutic work with this population at times requires a special kind of patience and vision from the clinician. A therapist may be repeatedly called upon to look for and point out to the patient even the smallest gains that have been made. On the other hand, the older patient may, as in the following case, be satisfied and even delighted with much smaller gains and rewards than those that would be required to satisfy or enhance the self-esteem of younger patients:

Ms. M., a 68-year-old European-born woman, became depressed following the death of her husband. This was not really an abnormal grief reaction, but rather a role transition for this woman, whose activities had centered around her husband and her children, who were now living outside the city. Making use of her experience as a parent, she first engaged in volunteer work at a local day care center and then made connections with the University Council for International Visitors. She was able to create a volunteer position there in which she organized activities for the children of foreign visitors to the university. Here, she was able to make use of the fact that she remained fluent in several western European languages. Although this was an infrequent activity, it did bring tremendous satisfaction. As a result of the pleasure that the children had from these activities, and as a result of the recognition given her by the council, the level of satisfaction that Ms. M. received from this volunteer activity was very high, and her sense of accomplishment was sustained long after each of the activity sessions.

Other Adaptations

In addition to the specific changes in IPT suggested by Sholomskas et al. (1983), our experience with older patients suggests other important areas for awareness on the part of the therapist employing IPT-LL:

1. Completion of the interpersonal inventory
2. Prioritization of problem areas
3. Specific applications of IPT technique to late-life patients
4. Use of confrontation within the IPT problem areas
5. Clarification of countertransference issues
6. Exploration of early relationships
7. Personal grief work
8. Transition to less frequent sessions if maintenance therapy is contemplated

In addition, special work with late-life patients may be necessary in the presence of patients' grief reactions, other forms of grief not related to an actual death, and romantic and sexual relationships. Finally, special consideration must be given to assessing and managing suicide risk in elderly persons.

Completing the Interpersonal Inventory

As indicated in the original IPT manual and in the book by Klerman et al. (1984), once the initial work of dealing with the patient's depression has been accomplished through reviewing the depressive symptoms, giving the patient the sick role, and explaining depression as an illness, the therapist and patient can then move on to the interpersonal work requiring attention. To identify an appropriate problem area for treatment, the therapist must review current and/or past interpersonal relationships as they relate to the patient's current depressive symptomatology.

Two types of problems may arise for therapists working with elderly depressed patients that do not as frequently arise in the treatment of younger patients. The therapist may find that the elderly person has so few current relationships that most of the focus of treatment will need to be centered on past relationships. While this scenario often occurs with younger IPT patients with whom an interpersonal deficit is the focus of treatment, there is usually more reason to hope in younger patients that new relationships can be formed. It is critical to assess the extent to which the late-life patient's social isolation actually represents an interpersonal deficit, rather than a reflection of realistic problems in socialization based on physical or interpersonal losses.

A second problem that we have encountered in our work centers around the elderly patient who is intimately involved in a large multigenerational family with multiple conflicted relationships. In this instance, several sessions may be required to complete the interpersonal inventory. Furthermore, the therapist may find that the family is so large and the relationships so complicated that simply listening is not sufficient. In this instance, it is not inappropriate for the therapist to elicit the patient's assistance in drawing a family tree, pedigree, or sociogram as an aid in understanding the nature of the relationships.

Choosing a Problem Area

The therapist's next task is to select a problem area as the focus of treatment. As Sholomskas et al. (1983) indicated in their original description of IPT with late-life patients, often more than one problem area may be prominent when working with elderly patients, and it becomes necessary to examine the priorities for treatment intervention. The patient can be asked which of these problem areas seems to be most directly related to the onset of the most recent episode of depression; however, the therapist may have other ideas as to which area is most important to the patient's depression. Sometimes the area that is most vociferously minimized is actually the one in which the source of greatest distress seems to reside. Even if the therapist can feel fairly confident that the problem area most responsible for the patient's symptomatology has been identified, this area may not be the most amenable to change in an elderly patient. Because hopelessness is often a highly prominent feature of depression, particularly in elderly persons, it may be best to choose the interpersonal problem area most amenable to *rapid* change in order to decrease the patient's hopelessness.

Application of IPT Techniques Specifically to Late-Life Patients

There are eight general techniques to be used in interpersonal psychotherapy: exploratory techniques, encouragement of affect, clarification, communication analysis, directive techniques, use of the therapeutic relationship, behavior change techniques, and adjunctive techniques (Klerman et al. 1984). All of these techniques have some usefulness in the treatment of depressed late-life patients, but the way in which they are applied may be somewhat different. We review the way that four of these general techniques are adapted to working with late-life patients.

Exploratory techniques. Nondirective exploration is an important aspect of IPT regardless of the age of the patient. However, the extent to which one chooses to use silences with the elderly patient is minimal, because silence may be interpreted as lack of interest or rejection on the part of the therapist. The therapist may in fact need to be somewhat more overt in using nondirective exploration, taking into account the possible poor hearing capacity of the elderly patient. The sort of low-level supportive acknowledgment that encourages the younger patient to continue speaking may be completely missed by the elderly patient whose hearing is impaired. Thus, the unobtrusive gesture or vocalization that suffices for the younger patient may be inadequate for the late-life patient.

In our experience with older depressed patients, we have found that more direct elicitation of patient material is sometimes required for a number of reasons. Some older patients have a less clear idea than do their younger counterparts as to which aspects of their interpersonal lives may be relevant to the treatment of their depression. Furthermore, many older patients appear to assume that much of what they have to say would not be of interest to the therapist. Therefore, more direct elicitation is required with this population. Particularly in the early sessions, very specific questions that can give the patient an idea of what aspects of relationships or interchanges are of interest to the therapist seem to aid in indicating to the patient what type of material is useful to bring to later therapy sessions.

Encouragement of affect. Encouragement of affect must be handled with some care when working with depressed elderly persons. Our experience has been that relatively few of our older patients present in an emotionally constricted state. On the contrary, many patients are troubled by intense and diffuse negative affects. It is important to help these patients suppress these overwhelming feelings once the basis for the feelings has been understood. Even those older patients with relatively little insight seem to be able to understand that the repetitive experiencing and display of negative affect are not only counterproductive but may actually retard their recovery.

The older patient who presents with constricted affect represents a considerable challenge to the therapist, as is illustrated in the following example:

Ms. M. was a 66-year-old widow who was living independently in a home she and her husband built many years ago. She reported feeling depressed since her husband died 4 years earlier, but her symptoms worsened prior to presentation for treatment. At that time, she endorsed sleep difficulty, appetite disturbance, low energy, absence of pleasure, social isolation, irritability, and overall feelings of sadness and hopelessness. Her family was quite concerned about her and were extremely supportive but felt very helpless. Ms. M. herself was frightened by her depression and felt she should be able to control the symptoms, especially because she had no ideas about what could have caused them.

Ms. M. had been the eldest of three siblings born to a farm family. She was raised in a very strict Presbyterian home by caring but totally undemonstrative parents. Work and church comprised the basics of life. Ms. M. married a boy from a neighboring farm, also a strict Presbyterian, when both of them had finished college. The marriage was a good one, and Ms. M. reported that what she missed most was her husband's joking and teasing. She was a very private person who had never been able to talk about feelings or emotions, and her husband had provided an outlet for her.

Ms. M. did not feel that talking would help her depression. She was polite and reserved but passively adamant that talking about her feelings was an intrusion. The first four sessions focused on the interpersonal inventory, which Ms. M. reported matter-of-factly and with little affect. She was not hostile or angry, but extremely constricted and very private.

Ms. M. began to respond a little to the therapist's supporting any attempts she made toward getting out of the house and beginning some activities. At that point, the therapist asked her to bring in some pictures of herself and her husband to see if he could get at feelings of any kind.

For Ms. M., the photos provided the bridge that enabled her to talk about her feelings of loss and her desire for other relationships that might mirror the lightheartedness of her relationship with her husband. Therapy actually proceeded quite rapidly following this critical intervention.

Communication analysis.   Attempts to help late-life patients who are very set in their communicative styles can prove frustrating for both patient and therapist. We begin by assessing the extent to which patients are actually capable of altering their communication styles. When it appears that change is possible, we make one or two attempts to use this technique. If the patient seems to have difficulty understanding or incorporating this technique into future behavior, then we typically move on to other techniques with that particular patient.

Directive techniques.   Directive techniques have an important role in work with depressed elderly patients. Some directive techniques typically used in IPT fall into the realm of social casework—for example, helping the patient to find transportation, housing, or financial assistance. Other kinds of directive techniques are always appropriate for the therapist using IPT with a late-life patient. This is particularly true of education and decision analysis, which are especially applicable to many of the problems facing elderly persons. In our experience, the decision-analysis techniques are highly therapeutic with older patients if taken in small steps. It is also helpful, as in the following case, to use decision analysis in order to explore the extent to which a patient may or may not be ready to make a decision:

> Ms. L. was a 79-year-old widowed white female who was being pressured by her family and by members of her church to make a decision about whether or when she would be willing to enter the church's old-age home. When the therapist attempted to carry out decision analysis on at least two different occasions, she noted that the process generated extreme anxiety for Ms. L. The therapist concluded that other problems in Ms. L.'s life were so pressing, including some uncertainties about her medical status, that she was at this point truly incapable of participating effectively in a decision analysis regarding the issue of the old-age home. The therapist then intervened with the family and church committee, explaining that the patient needed to delay making this decision for at least several months until her medical status was clarified.

Confrontation

Although, on the surface, confrontation may appear to be an inappropriate technique for use with elderly patients, it has been our experience that these patients are as much in need of having their "blind spots" pointed out as are younger patients. The way in which confrontation is handled does differ, however, when working with older patients. The confrontation must be well timed and gentle, keeping in mind that the therapeutic relationship may be one of the few relationships the patient has with a younger person. Such relationships are often highly important to older persons. The IPT therapist seeks to "join" with the patient as much as possible when initiating a confrontation, perhaps trying to relate the issue at hand to something in his or her own experience and thereby deemphasizing the differences between the therapist's experience as a younger person and the patient's experience as an older person:

> Ms. S., a 76-year-old woman, was experiencing conflict in her relationship with her 51-year-old daughter. These conflicts centered around the older woman's tendency not to be patient enough to wait to see whether this daughter would use good judgment in various situations. Instead, she tended to flood the daughter with instructions as to how things should be done. On the other hand, the patient always reported real delight when she discovered her daughter's competence in situations when she had not been available to advise or had not been aware of an opportunity to instruct the daughter. In both instances, the therapist drew parallels to her own relationship with a teenage daughter with whom many of the conflicts were the same. Rather than pointing out how the *patient* was robbing herself of the opportunity for the satisfaction associated with seeing her daughter perform well independently, the therapist pointed out how they *both* were robbing themselves of such an opportunity. The therapist then went on to help the patient look for situations that might arise in the near future in which she could practice exercising this restraint and wait, albeit with some anxiety, for the satisfying results that they both anticipated.

Countertransference Issues

Countertransference issues can sometimes interfere with appropriate confrontation of older patients, particularly when the patient is approximately the age of the therapist's grandparents.

Mr. B., a 78-year-old white single male, lived with his 84-year-old sister and 82-year-old brother-in-law. The referral for IPT was made when symptoms of depression and anxiety increased significantly as Mr. B. made preparations to move into a retirement home. Mr. B. had lived with his parents until he left to serve in the army during World War II. He worked for the post office for 35 years, maintaining somewhat superficial friendships, and moved in with his sister following his parents' death. He retired at age 65 but remained active, going out daily and doing some messenger work for a local architect. Psychotherapy focused on two issues: role conflict with his sister and brother-in-law and the impending role transition, as plans for Mr. B. to move to a retirement home were well underway.

Mr. B. complained of tension at home and frequent arguments over financial matters initiated by his sister. He felt that these arguments and the ongoing high level of criticism were going to occur irrespective of any position he took. Conflict inevitably led to an increase in general anxiety and accompanying lower mood. He felt the anxiety was almost unmanageable and also expressed a "fear of being afraid." To cope with this high level of anticipatory anxiety, he tended to be indecisive and refrain from commitments. He acknowledged that retirement should be a time for relaxation and travel but found himself unable to make plans, because as soon as he made plans he might become anxious that he would be anxious and unable to go. The therapist experienced some difficulty initially, focusing too much on anticipatory anxiety and not enough on the relationships with his family.

There was considerable reluctance to confront this patient, clearly an age peer of the therapist's grandfathers. This countertransference was discussed in supervision, as the therapist's relationship with his grandfathers (both deceased) had been traditional and devoid of any conflicts. It had been easier for him to confront a peer or a parent than a grandparent whose age and family position the therapist saw as entitling the grandparent to a high level of respect. Once the therapist was more confident, he was able to confront Mr. B. about the nature of his relationships, and Mr. B. was able to examine more closely the relationship with his sister.

Exploring Early Relationships

Whereas the emphasis of IPT with younger and mid-life depressed patients (except, perhaps, in the case of delayed grief) tends to be on current relationships, our work with elderly patients has suggested that for many of these patients it is the exploration of early relationships that seems to hold the key to reducing their depressed mood. Thus, it would appear that the interpersonal inventory should give more than the usual emphasis to past relationships, especially those with deceased parents and siblings. The following case illustrates this point:

> Ms. B. was a 79-year-old white single college graduate with a history of anxiety, nervousness, medical problems, and recurrent depression. Her history also included problems with social isolation, alcohol abuse, medical problems, and difficulty maintaining close relationships. She had several heterosexual relationships but never married. She was an only child whose parents died when she was young and had little extended family. She felt that being raised by a rigid, critical mother significantly affected her self-esteem. She recalled positive parenting from her father, who died suddenly of a gall bladder illness when the patient was 15 years old. Her maternal grandmother died 2 years later, and her mother died when the patient was 24 years old. Ms. B. was able to work productively as a secretary, travel, and have relationships with men throughout a good part of her adult life.
>
> In the beginning sessions, while reviewing significant relationships, Ms. B. touched on her intense anger toward her mother, which she was able to talk about for the "first time." She reported that venting these feelings and the grief that was related to the loss of her mother and father significantly "relieved" her. This relief, coupled with some exploration of the ways in which she had in the past cut off relationships, enabled her to decrease her isolation and become increasingly involved socially.

Grief Reactions

One type of grief reaction that late-life patients may experience is the reaction following a loss that appears, at least superficially, to be much less important than previous losses. It may be the case that the patient has survived a number of earlier losses of major proportion without experiencing an episode of depression, but following what seems like a much less significant loss, the patient becomes unable to recover from the grief reaction. In this instance, we have found it helpful to explore other losses the patient has sustained, and attempt to understand whether the observed grief reaction is in fact a reaction to the most recent loss, or a cumulative reaction to earlier losses.

> Ms. A., who was in her early 60s, had been born in Eastern Europe and had come to the United States as a young girl, immediately after the death of her mother. This highly intelligent but entirely uneducated woman

married very shortly after her arrival in the United States, and the couple quickly had a son and a daughter. While these children were still school age, her husband was killed in a car accident on a business trip, leaving her with both small children to raise and absolutely no money. She managed this challenge with considerable skill, putting both children through college.

At the time she was referred for treatment, she was living alone, but retained good contact with both her children, who had since married. She dated her depression to the death of her sister a few months earlier from cancer and said that she found herself completely unable to recover from this loss.

With the help of the therapist, the patient was able to explore all of the unexpressed grief following her two earlier losses and to explore the various reasons (most of them, practical necessity for survival) that had precluded any extensive expression of grief following the deaths of her mother and her husband. Having had an opportunity in the therapeutic relationship to mourn each of these important losses, Ms. A. found that her depression remitted and she was able to resume her previously high level of functioning.

At times, a grief reaction may be the appropriate focus for an IPT intervention with the late-life patient, even though the individual in question has not died and is still under the patient's care. Those older patients who are caring for a spouse, parent, or other important relative who has become severely ill or demented or who has suffered a stroke are, in fact, experiencing grief reactions of considerable importance. The loved one whom the patient had originally known is lost to the patient at this point. Complicating the patient's ability to deal with this loss is the fact that the loved one is not actually dead and constitutes a considerable burden in the patient's life.

Important work can be done to help such patients make the most of what remains, to distance themselves emotionally from a situation that cannot be changed, and to grieve for the loss of the healthy partner or relative. This work serves to enable the patient to express the distress and burden being experienced. It may be difficult to encourage these patients to enter and participate in any sort of new social world. However, even minor changes in the patient's social experience, along with appropriate discussion of grief reactions and guilt feelings, may lead to remission of depressed affect.

Reducing the Frequency of IPT-LL Sessions

In our work with older patients, we have found that in many instances it is difficult to reduce the frequency of sessions with those patients who have come to look forward to their weekly psychotherapy sessions. If the treatment plan requires continuation or maintenance treatment, some patients may require a few sessions spaced 10 days apart before they are ready for biweekly sessions. Likewise, in moving from biweekly to monthly sessions, some patients may require a few sessions spaced at 3-week intervals before they are comfortable with monthly sessions.

Other Important Considerations

Romance and sex. In working with late-life patients, younger therapists, in particular, may be reluctant to address, and patients may be reluctant to express, romantic and sexual needs or the complications of their romantic relationships. In our experience, however, these can be more profound in elderly patients than they sometimes are in younger patients. In healthy individuals, sexual desire and capacity to obtain sexual gratification can and does persist through the 80s. Furthermore, the need for physical closeness undoubtedly persists until death.

Individuals who were able to sustain rejections and romantic losses on many occasions when younger may be much less resilient later in life, particularly as they may see any romantic relationship in which they are involved as "their last hope."

Ms. Z. was a 77-year-old woman who went through normal grief after the death of her husband, who had been an invalid for several years. Following his death, she became involved in a variety of community activities and, fairly soon thereafter, formed a relationship with a man who spent four to five evenings per week at her home and with whom she formed a "couple" for all of their social activities. This gentleman decided to take a vacation to California to visit his children. While on this vacation, he met another woman and married her. When he returned to his hometown, not only was the patient distraught over the rejection and the loss of her status as a "coupled" person, she was mortified at the embarrassment of being replaced by the other woman.

Ms. Z. presented for treatment virtually immobilized by depression, incapable of doing anything other than sitting on her sofa and staring into space. Following a few weeks of medication she was able to engage successfully in IPT and discuss the several losses sustained as a result of this relationship. Eventually, she was able to resume more or less normal functioning, although she never returned to the euphoric state that she described during the romance.

Suicide

All of the epidemiological data would suggest that, other than the teenage population, it is the elderly population, and particularly the isolated male elderly person, who are most vulnerable to suicide. Additional risk factors for the elderly depressed male include chronic painful medical conditions, abuse of sedatives or alcohol, and a previous history of suicide attempts. There are several instances in which the therapist needs to be particularly alert to suicide risk.

Patients who have met a number of challenges in recovering from their depression but who suddenly find themselves facing a new and different challenge are at increased risk for suicide. For example, a patient who has successfully worked through his or her role transition difficulties and who has made a good accommodation to retirement life suddenly is overwhelmed with paperwork and bills following a minor illness. The therapist must be aware of situations that may resemble the proverbial "straw that breaks the camel's back."

Another risk situation to which therapists need to be particularly alert involves the patient who is truly overburdened with care or responsibilities. Patients who have been able for a considerable period of time to sustain major caregiving responsibilities sometimes rapidly and suddenly deteriorate in their ability to care for an ailing loved one for reasons that may not be clear. Therapists must always be alert to such verbalizations as "I just can't go on caring for him any longer. It's too much for me." Such remarks may be important indicators of the need for both additional physical assistance to such patients with their caregiving responsibilities, and additional intensity of therapy, which may involve major shifts in the problem focus in order to improve the quality of the patient's life and interpersonal experiences.

A third situation requiring the attention and concern of the IPT therapist is the elderly patient who appears to be working *very* hard at retaining his or her remitted status. When the patient seems to be constantly struggling to remain well, we need to be alert to the possibility that such patients may simply grow weary of having to work so hard to overcome their depression.

Termination in IPT-LL

Under ordinary circumstances, termination in IPT-LL can be handled using the guidelines outlined by Klerman and colleagues (1984), keeping in mind that for some older patients the importance of the therapeutic relationship may be somewhat greater than for younger patients who have many social relationships. For the elderly patient who is socially isolated or has few meaningful social relationships, we find that the IPT-LL therapist must be aware that more than usual grief may be associated with the end of the therapeutic relationship.

Interpersonal Psychotherapy as Maintenance Therapy in Late-Life Depression

Background

Within the last decade, a number of investigators (Glen et al. 1984; Kane et al. 1982; Prien et al. 1984) have begun to confront the question of how the gains made in the study of acute treatments could be applied to the maintenance treatment of patients with recurrent affective disorders. At present, the number of maintenance pharmacotherapy trials far exceeds those involving psychotherapy. The large number of treatment failures and the relatively high dropout rates (Frank et al. 1985) in most maintenance pharmacotherapy trials have led to an interest in what psychotherapy might add, both in terms of improvement in treatment adherence and in terms of preventing recurrences of affective illness.

For example, one collaborative investigation of maintenance pharmacotherapy for patients with recurrent depression (Prien et al. 1984) indicated that 50% of those patients who were assigned to active imipramine or to the combination of imipramine and lithium experienced a recurrence over the course of the 2.5-year maintenance trial. Furthermore, in at least one site of this investigation, even those patients who remained remitted throughout the course of the maintenance treatment phase failed to approach the general healthy population on measures of social adjustment during their remissions (D. J. Kupfer and E. Buzzinotti, personal communication, 1982). Given Weissman et al.'s (1974) finding that medication affects depressive symptoms while psychotherapy affects social adjustment, one cannot help but wonder how the results of this collaborative investigation might have differed had some or all patients also been offered psychotherapeutic intervention.

In an attempt to investigate the possible relationship between deficits in social adjustment and the unsatisfactory preventive capacity of maintenance pharmacotherapy for 50% of patients with recurrent depression, the Late Life Depression Prevention Program at the Western Psychiatric Institute and Clinic decided to explore the relative efficacy of a psychotherapeutic intervention, alone or in combination with pharmacotherapy, in preventing recurrence of illness in a population at high risk for frequent recurrent depressive episodes (Frank et al. 1990). In order to do so, it was necessary to find or create a psychotherapeutic intervention that 1) had efficacy in the treatment of depressive illness, 2) could be reliably reproduced by a group of five to seven therapists, 3) could be discriminated from a "medication clinic" control condition, and 4) was appropriate to long-term maintenance treatment in a population likely to have marked deficits in social adjustment. We chose to adapt IPT developed by Klerman et al. (1984) for use in a long-term maintenance trial.

We found that when mid-life patients with recurrent depression were maintained on the same relatively substantial dose (median = 215 mg) of imipramine that was used to treat their index episode, there was no significant advantage to the addition of maintenance IPT (IPT-M). Indeed, the probability of remaining well throughout the 3-year maintenance trial was approximately 80% for patients treated with imipramine, with or without IPT-M. However, there was a significant effect of IPT-M alone or with placebo when compared with medication clinic visits with the placebo ($P = .04$). For more details concerning this study see Chapter 4.

Maintenance interpersonal psychotherapy may have an even greater role to play in the treatment of elderly persons. First, because both biological "resistance" and intentional noncompliance are likely to be greater in this population, antidepressant medication may be less completely protective, allowing psychotherapy more "room" to add to prophylaxis. Second, many clinicians may prefer to discontinue medication in older patients once the index episode is fully resolved, especially in cases with whom there is some risk of cardiotoxicity, or when the patient is taking multiple other medications for chronic medical conditions.

The overriding goal of IPT as adapted to maintenance treatment is to maintain remission of the depressive symptoms. The length of maintenance treatment is measured in years rather than weeks. In the case of the late-life protocol we are currently conducting (i.e., IPT-LLM), the length of treatment is 2 years; in actual clinical practice it may be considerably longer.

In developing IPT-LLM, we retained the four problem areas that distinguish IPT and continued to emphasize a largely "here and now" orientation; however, we assumed that the number of problem areas likely to become the focus of one patient's maintenance treatment would be greater than is typically the case with short-term IPT. In summary, while IPT-LLM employs all of the strategies of IPT, it differs from IPT in its goals and its timing, and in the number of problem areas typically addressed with an individual patient. In addition, because of the length of treatment, the IPT-LLM therapist, while not attempting to restructure personality in the traditional psychoanalytic sense, often focuses on long-standing patterns of interpersonal behavior that appear to be nonadaptive for the patient.

The Goals of IPT-LLM

The IPT-LLM process begins with older patients with a history of recurrent depression who are in a remitted state, and has as its goal the maintenance of that remitted state. For this reason, the therapist remains constantly alert to early signs of interpersonal problems similar to those that the patient and therapist earlier identified as having been associated with the onset of the index episode, as well as signs similar to those in the preceding earlier episodes of depression. Therapeutic efforts are directed toward enhancing those strengths that appear to have been present before the onset of the index episode or that became apparent as the patient began to recover. The patient is instructed to watch for early warning signs in the noninterpersonal realm. This is accomplished by focusing discussion on the particular somatic and cognitive symptoms that have marked the early stages of prior episodes. When somatic, cognitive, or mood changes are reported to the

IPT-LLM therapist, the therapist and patient work together to develop a plan to try to avert a new episode, basing their strategies largely in the interpersonal realm and focusing on interpersonal techniques for improving the patient's mood and functioning.

Problem Areas With IPT-LLM

In the short-term IPT experience, typically only one major problem area can be fully addressed. In IPT-LLM, which is intended to last over the course of several years, it is virtually impossible to restrict the therapy to a single problem area, nor would the therapist want to do so. During the course of acute treatment, invariably a number of interpersonal themes emerge but do not become an important focus of treatment. The therapist, however, notes these additional themes. As IPT-LLM proceeds, these themes will often reemerge, and they can then become a focus of therapeutic attention. In almost all instances, maintenance treatment will include some focus on each of the IPT problem areas.

Role Transitions in IPT-LLM

Individuals faced with *role transitions* are helped to grieve for the lost role and then to view the new role in the most positive, least restricted manner. They are encouraged to see the new role, if not as an opportunity for growth, at least as an opportunity to search for new strengths in themselves. The role of the IPT-LLM therapist is to help patients regain their self-esteem and sense of mastery in relation to the demands of their new role. This emphasis on self-esteem and mastery is especially critical with older patients. Patients are guided to a realistic rather than exaggerated view of what has been lost in the transition and are encouraged to develop a social support system and a repertoire of social skills that can be called upon in the new role.

In working on role transitions with patients in late life, the therapist depends upon the same techniques that would be helpful with this kind of problem in younger patients. The therapist uses exploratory techniques to understand the meaning of the lost role and the patient's fears or concerns about the new role. Encouragement of affect is used to further understand the feelings associated with the lost role as well as those associated with the assumption of the new role. Clarification may be a particularly important technique when patients, despite their basic negative feelings about the role transition, actually express some interest in or positive attitude about the new role. In general, communication analysis does not have a part in role transition work in IPT-LLM, nor does the therapist typically use the therapeutic relationship; however, behavioral techniques are usually critically important in this work, particularly education and decision analysis.

Ms. A., a 71-year-old married woman, had a rapid and successful recovery from her index episode of depression in IPT-LL. Approximately 1 year into maintenance treatment, her 75-year-old husband decided that he would finally give up his still nearly full-time practice as an internist. Dr. A. had planned well for his retirement and had a variety of interests that sustained him during the first few months of his retirement. These included continuing to expand his medical knowledge through the reading of recent articles; working in his garden, in which he had always taken great pride; and catching up on his extensive correspondence with medical school friends.

Ms. A. was surprised about 5 or 6 weeks into Dr. A.'s retirement to find her mood becoming increasingly sad, because after years of relative unavailability on Dr. A.'s part, he was almost constantly with her or nearby. It was not that Dr. A. was a bother or that Ms. A. perceived him as being "underfoot." She did, however, express to her therapist that because she had looked forward to having him around for so long, she felt constrained in pursuing her normal social activities. Thus, she was more likely to turn down invitations to play bridge or shop with her female friends. Yet, she denied that this was the source of her sad feelings. The therapist then began to explore the sources of Ms. A.'s positive feelings prior to her husband's retirement. Within a few minutes, the therapist was able to identify the tremendous sense of pride that Ms. A. had had in being "the doctor's wife" and that she missed several aspects of that role. She prided herself on being able to "hold" her husband's patients when they called looking for him in an emergency and on the efficient way in which she relayed messages from his answering service. She had enjoyed being asked medical questions at her frequent luncheon and bridge parties and noted that these seemed to have stopped since her husband had retired. She indicated that she actually had very little information as to the financial provisions for their retirement and that although she had complete faith in her husband's medical abilities, she worried about how well he had provided for their retirement years and what the loss of income might mean to them.

Over the next five or six maintenance sessions, Ms. A.'s therapist was able to address each of these concerns. First, she helped Ms. A. to focus on other sources of skill and adequacy that she retained since her husband's retirement. Second, the therapist helped Ms. A. explore the financial provisions for their retirement years directly and at the same time obtain more knowledge about the couple's current financial affairs. In the event that Dr. A. should die, the patient would be more competent and have less to worry about with respect to her own finances. As soon as this work began, Ms. A.'s mood began to improve, and within 5 weeks Ms. A. reported feeling 110% of her normal self.

A majority of the IPT-LLM patients we have treated thus far, in addition to exploring the sort of role transition typically explored in IPT-LL, have needed to address the role transition they may have made from depressed individual to well individual. For some, this is a relatively easy transition. However, for those who have had many years of recurrent episodes, the experience of remaining well for a long period of time is a new one, both for the patient and for his or her spouse and children as well.

Helping older individuals to adjust to long-term remission presents something of a challenge. Because both older patients and their family members and friends have a long history of viewing the patient in a stereotypical way, it takes considerably more inventiveness on the part of the therapist to help the patient to view himself or herself in this new manner. It also requires more therapeutic creativity to help the patient to help others to respond to him or her on the basis of his or her newly found energy and interest in things rather than on the basis of his or her old patterns of behavior.

Mr. N. had been a public school teacher and then a low-level school administrator throughout his entire adult life. Although several clear episodes of depression were evident throughout this time, he operated on a more-or-less dysthymic baseline. His wife was perfectly comfortable pursuing her own interests while Mr. N. was busy at his job, but she felt constrained to provide companionship and activity as soon as the school day ended and throughout the weekend.

Mr. N. developed an episode of depression and entered IPT treatment approximately 6 months prior to his scheduled retirement from the school system. In an effort to expand Mr. N.'s horizons and to help him prepare for the large amount of time that would be available to him during his retirement, the IPT therapist encouraged him to expand his existing interest in swimming. As Mr. N. experienced what was probably the first complete remission of his life, his energy was sufficient that he was able to be competitive in the Senior Olympics. One year into his maintenance treatment he was the winner of the statewide competition. Indeed, Mr. N.'s leadership in his position as a Senior Olympics organizer provided sufficient self-esteem and confidence that he assumed important leadership positions in the Veterans of Foreign Wars, of which he had been a member for many years.

With these two activities actually taking up more time than Mr. N. had previously devoted to his professional activities, Ms. N. now found herself with no one to "babysit" after school and weekends. It was Ms. N. who had to make the adaptation to Mr. N.'s newly found personality because her entire life had previously been structured around her husband's dependency needs. At first, she was extremely irritable when he was not home when she expected him to be. However, with the help of the IPT therapist, Mr. N. was able to point out to his wife that she could now enjoy this time either by coming to join him in some of his activities or by finding new activities of her own.

Interpersonal Disputes in IPT-LLM

When an interpersonal dispute is present, the IPT-LLM therapist helps the patient identify the nature of the dispute, guides him or her in making choices about a plan of action, and encourages the patient to modify maladaptive communication patterns if that is possible. When such modification cannot be accomplished or is not desirable, the patient is encouraged to reassess expectations for the relationship.

Because patients in IPT-LLM are seen over such a long period of time, it is practically inevitable that some role disputes will emerge. Whether these are in the context of marriage, family (often spanning two or three generations), work, or social settings varies from patient to patient; however, IPT techniques are easily applied as these interpersonal disputes occur. Our experience in using IPT-LLM, thus far, has indicated that one or two relationships in the patient's life typically emerge as those that are occasionally or chronically fraught with difficulty. Having the opportunity to work with the patient on these relationships over a long period of time enables both the therapist and the patient to recognize characteristic negative, destructive patterns of interaction and to modify them.

As is the case in IPT and IPT-LL, the strategy most frequently employed by the IPT-LLM therapist in working on interpersonal or role disputes is the *communication analysis.* Such analysis often yields evidence of both very disturbed and very long-standing patterns of communication. In some instances, particularly if both parties are highly motivated to improve the quality of the relationship, communication analysis can be used successfully to modify the role dispute. However, as indicated earlier in this chapter, the strategy of choice in older patients often is to encourage them to reassess their expectations for the relationship and to facilitate their better tolerating the relationship as it presently exists.

Interpersonal Deficits in IPT-LLM

For patients whose interpersonal deficits do not ameliorate with the resolution of the depressive episode during acute IPT treatment, the IPT-LLM therapist works to reduce the patient's social isolation and enhance the quality of any existing relationships. This can be particularly difficult in work with the late-life patient because his or her social isolation may result from a combination of interpersonal deficits and reality-based factors such as lack of transportation and reduced mobility. If this is the case, the therapist may use directive techniques or work in collaboration with a caseworker to increase the patient's access to transportation and maximize mobility. The goal should be to attempt to involve the patient in group social activity or, perhaps, if the patient is sufficiently well and energetic, in some form of volunteer activity within his or her community.

In the acute treatment phase of our work, when there are no current meaningful relationships, the focus of treatment may be on past relationships, the relationship with the therapist, and the tentative formation of new relationships. The therapy session is used to model appropriate interpersonal behaviors. In IPT-LLM, as in Stage-2 work described with IPT patients showing interpersonal deficits (Klerman et al. 1984), much more emphasis is placed on helping the patient to apply the learning occurring in treatment to outside situations to facilitate the development of new relationships. Each attempt at a new relationship, successful or unsuccessful, is analyzed in terms of correctable deficits in the patient's communication skills.

Many patients need encouragement to decrease their social isolation, increase their social interaction, and, in general, to pay more attention to their interpersonal needs. Others need to form more independent, self-reliant styles in order not to feel constantly at the mercy of other persons in their environment. The long course of IPT-LLM provides a secure base from which patients can experiment with these new styles of relating and to which they can bring their questions and concerns about the success of the experimentation.

Grief Reactions in IPT-LLM

Grief reactions were rarely a major focus of our IPT-M work with mid-life patients, but that is not the case in work with late-life patients. Indeed, with the latter patients, grief experiences of one kind or another are almost a constant feature of their lives. Grief work with IPT-LLM patients can take any of four forms: 1) anticipatory grief work for losses (through death and through other means) that appear likely to occur during or after the period of projected IPT-LLM treatment; 2) help with normal grieving, including some explicit education about the difference between normal grief reaction and a depressive episode; 3) grief work for losses other than those that occur through death, including loss of function or mobility; and 4) work on morbid grief reactions.

Much work can be done over the course of a maintenance treatment to help patients to *anticipate* losses of many sorts that appear likely to occur during and after the course of treatment. While both anticipatory and current grief work can focus on the loss of an important loved one, it can also include grief work for the patient's own loss of function, mobility, and so forth. When the death of an important significant other does occur, it is particularly helpful if the IPT-LLM therapist can clarify the distinction between a normal grief reaction and a depressive episode.

Ms. T., a 61-year-old married woman with a largely seasonal pattern to her recurrent depressive illness, had a history of almost 40 years of winter depressions dating back to her early adult life. The only well years were those winters during which she was pregnant with her four children. Otherwise, she would become profoundly sad, anergic, and disinterested during the winter months and would not recover until some time in May. At that time, she would become the family organizer and social secretary for her large extended family throughout the summer months. She never failed to hold large Memorial Day and July 4th celebrations, and she had, for almost 30 years, finished her energetic summer months with the planning of an enormous family reunion that took place each Labor Day weekend.

When Ms. T. entered IPT-LL treatment, she simply assumed that her essentially seasonal affective illness was the "way things were" and that she merely experienced a more exaggerated form of the "winter blahs" that are experienced by most individuals. Following successful treatment with a combination of nortriptyline and IPT beginning in January, her energy returned by mid-February, and she subsequently experienced 2 years of continuous good health despite the fact that her husband was becoming increasingly ill and dependent upon her during that time. Because she had more than enough energy to care for him and enjoy all of the activities that interested her, his progressive physical deterioration was taken in stride.

In April of Ms. T.'s third year in the clinic, Mr. T. suffered a stroke that left him completely aphasic. By mid-May, Ms. T. was reporting several of her early symptoms of depression. She was quite surprised by this because, in her mind, depression came only in the winter, irrespective of any precipitating life events. When she and her IPT-LLM therapist had an opportunity to discuss the possible factors that might be contributing to Ms. T.'s depression, it became apparent that Ms. T. was profoundly grief-stricken as a result of the loss of her previously responsive partner, yet felt she had no "permission" to mourn. Working with her IPT-LLM therapist, Ms. T. was able to mourn the loss of her communicative and supportive relationship with her husband.

Terminating IPT-LLM

Throughout the course of maintenance treatment, the IPT-LLM therapist makes frequent reference to the termination point. Approximately three to four sessions prior to the end of maintenance, the IPT-LLM therapist begins the real work of termination. As in other forms of IPT, the therapist begins with a review of what the patient has accomplished over the course of treatment. The therapist then moves on to help the patient acknowledge the end of treatment as a time of potential grieving, and, finally, works with the patient to help him or her recognize his or her independent competence. Because treatment takes place over such a long period of time in IPT-LLM, it may be helpful for the therapist to review the treatment notes so as to have a clear recall of precisely how far the patient has come. The potential for some grief is high, particularly with those patients who are otherwise somewhat socially impoverished, and the therapist may wish to adjust his or her behavior to a slightly more distant stance in the last five to six sessions so that this loss may not be felt quite so intensely. The real emphasis should be on the objective evaluation of the patient's newly acquired skills.

References

Blazer DG, Williams CD: Epidemiology of dysphoria and depression in an elderly population. Am J Psychiatry 137:439–444, 1980

Butler RN, Lewis M: Aging and Mental Health, 3rd Edition. St Louis, MO, CV Mosby, 1982

Elkin J, She JT, Watkins SD, et al: National Institute of Mental Health Treatment of Depression Collaborative Research Program: general effectiveness of treatments. Arch Gen Psychiatry 46:971–982, 1989

Frank E, Prien R, Kupfer DJ: Implications of noncompliance on research in affective disorder. Psychopharmacol Bull 21:37–42, 1985

Frank E, Kupfer DJ, Perel JM, et al: Three-year outcomes for maintenance therapies in recurrent depression. Arch Gen Psychiatry 47:1093–1097, 1990

Glen AIM, Johnson AL, Shepherd M: Continuation therapy with lithium and amitriptyline in unipolar depressive illness: a randomized, double-blind, controlled trial. Psychol Med 14:37–50, 1984

Kane JM, Quitkin FM, Rifkin A, et al: Lithium carbonate and imipramine in the prophylaxis of unipolar and bipolar II illness. Arch Gen Psychiatry 39:1065–1069, 1982

Klerman GL, Weissman MM, Rounsaville BJ, et al: Interpersonal Psychotherapy of Depression. New York, Basic Books, 1984

Prien RF, Kupfer DJ, Mansky PA, et al: Drug therapy in the prevention of recurrences in unipolar and bipolar affective disorders: a report of the NIMH Collaborative Study Group comparing lithium carbonate, imipramine, and a lithium carbonate–imipramine combination. Arch Gen Psychiatry 41:1096–1104, 1984

Rothblum E, Sholomskas A, Berry C, et al: Issues in clinical trials with the depressed elderly. J Am Geriatr Soc 30:694–699, 1982

Schneider LS, Sloane RB, Staples FR, et al: Pre-treatment orthostatic hypotension as a predictor of response to nortriptyline in geriatric depression. J Clin Psychopharmacol 6:172–176, 1986

Sholomskas AJ, Chevron ES, Prusoff BA, et al: Short-term interpersonal therapy (IPT) with the depressed elderly: case reports and discussion. Am J Psychotherapy 37:552–566, 1983

Sloane RB, Staples FR, Schneider LS: Interpersonal therapy versus nortriptyline for depression in the elderly, in Clinical and Pharmacological Studies in Psychiatric Disorders. Edited by Burrows G, Norman TR, Dennerstein L. London, John Libbey, 1985, pp 344–346

Weissman MM, Klerman GL, Paykel ES, et al: Treatment effects on the social adjustment of depressed patients. Arch Gen Psychiatry 30:771–778, 1974

CHAPTER 8

Interpersonal Psychotherapy for Depressed HIV-Seropositive Patients

John C. Markowitz, M.D.
Gerald L. Klerman, M.D.
Samuel W. Perry, M.D.
Kathleen F. Clougherty, M.S.W.
Laura S. Josephs, Ph.D.

At least a million American adults are infected with the human immunodeficiency virus (HIV) (Centers for Disease Control 1990). Most are physically asymptomatic and likely to remain so for a decade or more following infection. Yet HIV-seropositive individuals appear to be at increased risk for developing depression, at least in part because of the stress of awareness of the infection and the social pressures accompanying it.

We adapted interpersonal psychotherapy (IPT) to develop pilot data for a treatment study of depressed HIV-seropositive patients at Cornell University Medical College, research subsequently funded by the National Institute of Mental Health. Our promising early results require replication. The ongoing study compares relative efficacies of 1) IPT, 2) cognitive-behavior therapy, 3) desipramine plus clinical management, and 4) clinical management alone in treating HIV-seropositive outpatients with major depression or dysthymia. This research thus will assess the efficacy of antidepressant interventions previously studied in HIV-seronegative patients (Elkin et al. 1989).

Rationale for Using Interpersonal Psychotherapy With HIV-Seropositive Patients

Comorbidity of Depression With HIV Infection

Mood disorders are probably more common among individuals infected with HIV than they are in the general population. The Epidemiologic Catchment Area study found a 6-month prevalence of 5.8% and a lifetime rate of 8.3% for DSM-III (American Psychiatric Association 1980) mood disorders (Regier et al. 1988). Perry and colleagues (1990), assessing psychiatric diagnosis among 207 physically asymptomatic subjects seeking serological testing, found that 14% had a current mood disorder and 42.7% had a history of mood disorder; rates were highest among the subgroup that subsequently tested seropositive for HIV. Atkinson and colleagues (1991) found 7.2% of 55 HIV-seropositive Navy men met criteria for current major depression; lifetime prevalence for major depression was 32.6% for subjects in Centers for Disease Control (CDC) Stages II and III (i.e., seropositive but asymptomatic) and 44.4% for those in Stage IV (acquired immunodeficiency syndrome [AIDS]). These findings are not surprising given the stress of learning that one is HIV-seropositive—an emotional, if not actual, death sentence to an individual whose friends and lovers may already be dead or dying from HIV.

Depression carries significant morbidity and mortality (Wells et al. 1989). Damaged relationships, impaired work function, inertia, somatic symptoms, and a grim prospect of the future are often due to *depressive* symptoms, although the individual may mistakenly attribute them to HIV. Depressed HIV-seropositive patients therefore need psychiatric intervention beyond the supportive management given acutely or terminally ill patients. Some patients fear potential immunosuppressive effects of antidepressant medications and avoid group therapy to preserve confidentiality, enhancing the importance of individual psychotherapy as a treatment modality. Yet psychotherapy of HIV-seropositive individuals has received little research (Kelly et al. 1989; Perry et al. 1991).

Our experience derives largely from work with patients who are gay or bisexual, or with female partners of bisexual men (see Table 8–1). Depressed patients who contract HIV through intravenous drug use constitute a distinct, probably more difficult-to-treat population for whom IPT may require further modification (Rounsaville et al. 1983, 1985; see Chapter 12). Our intended patient is the depressed HIV-seropositive gay or bisexual patient with relatively few physical symptoms, or who is in any case not so debilitated by AIDS that therapy is rendered purely supportive and palliative.

Psychiatric Aspects of Human Immunodeficiency Virus

Human immunodeficiency virus enters the central nervous system (CNS) in conjunction with systemic infection and is neurotoxic as well as im-

Table 8–1.   Demographic characteristics of depressed HIV-seropositive patients ($N = 24$)

Age	36.9 ± 13.0 (range 17–61)
Sex	
Male	18 (75%)
Female	6 (25%)
Ethnicity	
White	17 (71%)
Black	5 (21%)
Hispanic	1 (4%)
Asian	1 (4%)
HIV risk factors	
Gay male	13 (54%)
Bisexual male	4 (17%)
Intravenous drug user	3 (13%)
Heterosexual partner	3 (13%)
Transfusion recipient	1 (4%)
IPT problem areas	
Grief	7 (29%)
Dispute	6 (25%)
Role transition	8 (33%)
Deficits	3 (13%)

munosuppressive. HIV itself, as well as the secondary infections and tumors comprising AIDS, can produce cognitive changes ranging from subtle neuropsychological impairment to frank dementia (Markowitz and Perry 1992). Among its myriad neuropsychiatric presentations is subtle neuropsychological impairment characterized by slowed cognitions, apathy, and social withdrawal that can mimic "functional" depression (Markowitz and Perry 1992; Perry 1990). In general, the greatest difficulty in differential diagnosis of our patients has been in deciding the etiology of symptoms of fatigue, cognitive slowing, and social withdrawal, which might be caused either by depression or by progression of HIV infection.

Failure of immune defenses can result in organic mood disorders consequent to secondary opportunistic infections and tumors of the CNS, or systemic illness (Markowitz and Perry 1990). Depressive syndromes can arise from drug and alcohol use, which is prevalent among HIV-seropositive patients (Perry et al. 1990), and from medications, such as zidovudine (AZT), that are used to treat HIV and its sequelae (Markowitz and Perry 1992).

Comorbid medical and psychiatric disorders must therefore be carefully considered in diagnosing a HIV-seropositive individual as depressed. The medical history and physical examination are important assessments prior to embarking on psychotherapy, and continuing awareness of changes in mental and medical status and medical treatment are necessary during the course of IPT (Markowitz and Perry 1990). Developing expertise about HIV and AIDS is important for both patient and therapist in this treatment.

Psychosocial Factors

Individuals who are HIV-seropositive are vulnerable to a variety of psychosocial stresses.

Stigma. HIV has evoked much irrational fear and societal prejudice, its carriers not infrequently viewed and treated as modern-day lepers who perhaps deserve their illness as punishment for sexual (or drug-abusing) misdeeds (Kalman et al. 1987). Instead of receiving the concern and compassion generally accorded someone with a serious illness, the HIV-seropositive individual may be met with suspicion, revulsion, and condemnation if his or her medical status is revealed. Learning of one's HIV infection often makes the already stigmatized person feel still more socially rejected and isolated.

Effect on the community. HIV also reverberates in the social milieu. For gay individuals whose vital interpersonal supports are other gay persons, as for intravenous drug–using persons recovering from chemical dependency in a support network of their fellows, the experience is of a community under siege—a subculture rapidly losing vast numbers of its members. In couples where both partners are seropositive, one partner may nurse the other through illness and then, upon their partner's death, be left alone to cope with his or her own physical decline. Loss of a sexual partner and other social supports are key precipitants of depression (Brown and Harris 1978). A distinct but also difficult problem affects the HIV-seropositive individual who does not feel part of a "high risk" community and therefore feels isolated in his or her seropositivity.

Dealing with the family of origin. For some gay men, telling family members of HIV seropositivity is the simultaneous revelation of their homosexuality. Some remain isolated from families, who learn the truth only at the funeral. The gay community has itself provided an alternative support network, most visible in such organizations as the Gay Men's Health Crisis in New York City. Yet the crisis of HIV seropositivity also provides an opportunity for gay men to reconcile with families and to gain needed support from them.

Coping with medical aspects of HIV seropositivity. An individual developing physical symptoms endures the stress of coping with illness—with its drain on his or her sense of well-being, energy, and financial resources and its negative impact on body image and sense of attractiveness—and the threat of death. Even if an individual is physically healthy, HIV infection prefigures future illness in all of its grim ramifications. Furthermore, knowledge that one is HIV-seropositive means either curtailing one's sexual activity or experiencing inevitable, if sometimes unconscious, guilt over the possibility of transmitting the virus to others.

Discovery of HIV seropositivity often entails a young, previously healthy individual becoming a patient. Coping with HIV seropositivity requires finding a doctor willing to treat HIV-seropositive patients; under-going periodic blood tests and anticipating their results; sometimes taking medication even when physically asymptomatic; and dealing with the hy-pochondriacal fear that any subtle physical symptom might signal the onset of AIDS. These patients frequently remark that they are in limbo, not yet sick but awaiting the inevitable.

In treating HIV-seropositive patients, IPT therapists must understand these stresses as comprising the interpersonal context in which depression develops, as well as providing relevant and important focuses for IPT. All four of the problem areas associated with the onset of depression—grief, interpersonal role dispute, role transition, and interpersonal deficits—are readily found in depressed HIV-infected patients.

The emergence of a mood disorder in the context of HIV infection adds those psychosocial issues associated with depression itself. Klerman et al. (1984) described the reaction of those in the depressed individual's interpersonal environment to his depression: "The usual response of oth-ers to normal sadness, disappointment, and depression, and to grief and mourning, is sympathy, support, encouragement, and offers of assurance. However, as time goes on, this positive response often gives way to frustra-tion, friction, and withdrawal" (p. 62). In the case of the depressed HIV-se-ropositive individual, the reaction of others to his or her depression may compound rejection already felt as a consequence of HIV.

Treatment of Depression in HIV-Seropositive Patients

Fernandez and Levy (1990) state that pharmacotherapy of depressed HIV-seropositive patients "continues to be guided by intuition and clinical experience" (p. 617). Anecdotal reports support use of tricyclic antidepres-sants, monoamine oxidase inhibitors, lithium, and psychostimulants. To our knowledge there has been only one randomized, double-blind phar-macotherapy study, which showed imipramine to be superior to placebo in treating depressed HIV-seropositive subjects (Manning and Frances 1990).

Evidence for psychotherapeutic intervention with HIV-seropositive patients includes our pilot data (see below) and the work of Kelly et al. (1989) and Perry et al. (1991). Our ongoing study with Samuel Perry, M.D., is the first randomized comparative treatment study of focused psychotherapies (i.e., IPT, cognitive-behavior therapy, and standard care) with medication (i.e., desipramine).

Modifying Interpersonal Psychotherapy for HIV-Seropositive Depressed Patients

Our psychotherapeutic approach, IPT for HIV-seropositive patients (IPT-HIV), does not fundamentally differ from the IPT of depressed outpatients as described by Klerman et al. (1984) and throughout the present volume. Our approach does, however, modulate the treatment to the needs of HIV-seropositive patients. IPT-HIV remains a time-limited, brief therapy in which the patient is diagnosed, the sick role is granted, and depressive symptoms are related to one or more of four interpersonal problem areas, particularly grief, role transition, or role dispute. The therapist thereafter helps the patient to recognize and mediate social roles that have been affected by and may contribute to depression.

IPT-HIV works through affective engagement on an interpersonal focus, followed by renegotiation of the interpersonal difficulty, which simultaneously relieves depression. Hence, the goal of IPT-HIV is to use the interpersonal perturbations surrounding HIV seropositivity and the onset of depression as a mechanism for treating depression.

Interpersonal therapists are health care professionals with at least 2 years of postgraduate clinical experience and facility in psychodynamic psychotherapy. An IPT-HIV manual[1] and videotaped recording of IPT sessions ensure consistency of technique within and across treatments (Rounsaville et al. 1984). Because therapists appear to be most effective when affectively engaged with the patient, we discourage a checklist or "cookbook" approach to the manual, which might distract the therapist from interaction with the patient.

Interpersonal psychotherapy might have been developed with the depressed HIV-seropositive patient in mind. Not only do its problem areas

---

[1] See J. C. Markowitz, G. L. Klerman, L. Josephs, et al.: *Manual for Interpersonal Therapy With Depressed HIV-Seropositive Patients.* New York, Cornell University Medical College, unpublished manuscript.

neatly fit the patients' situations, but its brief temporal framework also appeals to them. These patients unanimously describe a subjective *time pressure*: the sense of time running out and of careers and relationships being abruptly amputated, with every second counting. Every decision must be productive: as one patient stated, "If you're going to eat a meal or see a movie, it had better be good." IPT offers a brief commitment and the opportunity to evaluate and maximize the remainder of one's life course. Once anxiety and hopelessness have been addressed by patient and therapist, the sense of urgency engendered by HIV infection promotes active engagement in therapy.

This sense of time pressure particularly affects more seriously ill patients, who may correctly judge their longevity to be more limited. Paradoxically, the development of physical HIV-related illness can unavoidably interrupt therapy. By visiting physically incapacitated patients at home or in the hospital, the IPT therapist may alleviate the sense of precious time being wasted, maintain momentum and continuity of psychiatric care, and greatly further the treatment alliance.

It is dangerous to generalize about prototypical HIV-seropositive *individuals*, given the enormous variability among those infected with the virus. Yet our clinical experience suggests that at least some aspects of their *interpersonal environment* overlap, and this environment is crucial to IPT. Whereas HIV-seronegative depressed patients often present in the wake of a single psychosocial stressor (e.g., complicated bereavement, the loss of a job or relationship, or onset of a serious illness), our HIV-seropositive patients almost invariably described a host of problems (i.e., all of the above). They discovered their HIV seropositivity because a lover was already ill or dead, lost their primary relationship upon revealing their HIV serostatus, and had lost dozens of friends and colleagues to AIDS. The cumulative weight of these interdependent events was considerable—and, indeed, worth pointing out to the patient.

Most HIV-seropositive individuals, despite stress, do not develop depression. That those whom we saw did become depressed often seemed due to chronically limited interpersonal repertoires: these individuals seemed on the whole to have less flexibility in interpersonal functioning than many HIV-seronegative depressed patients. This was not to say, however, that they could not learn new skills with guidance from their IPT therapist.

Setting and Structure of Treatment

Sessions are videotaped in therapists' offices and last 50 minutes. Patients provide written informed consent for the study and for videotaping. In the comparative treatment study at Cornell, treatment consists of up to 17 sessions over 17 weeks, with sessions twice weekly in the first 2 weeks and weekly thereafter for 10 weeks, and the remaining 3 sessions completed within 4 months of beginning treatment. These treatment guidelines are explicitly presented to the patient at the outset. Videotapes are reviewed in supervision to ensure adherence to technique.

Initial Sessions

The first few sessions of IPT encompass multiple goals.

Collecting data. Patients may not recognize depression as such, attributing neurovegetative symptoms and hopelessness to HIV infection or simply accepting these symptoms unthinkingly. The exposition of the therapeutic drama requires carefully diagnosing the patient's disorder and then representing it as a discrete, treatable disorder. The Hamilton Depression Rating Scale (Ham-D; Hamilton 1960) provides symptomatic guidelines; in the current study, patients with Ham-D scores of greater than 13 are eligible for treatment. Even when, as in this study, the patient has already met criteria in order to have been randomized to treatment, diagnosis by the therapist is an important therapeutic gambit.

Psychiatric evaluation includes history of present illness, previous psychopathology and psychiatric treatment, family history of psychiatric disorders, and mental status examination. Particular attention is paid to the quality, duration, expectations, and outcome of the patient's important past and present relationships, the interpersonal inventory. Medical and medication histories are also crucial for HIV-seropositive patients, including a full review of medical systems, duration of known seropositivity and HIV-related symptoms, and prescribed medications and other "remedies" for HIV.

Taking the interpersonal inventory. The *interpersonal inventory*, a catalog of the patient's important relationships, begins with childhood but focuses on the recent past and present. The therapist explores patterns of interpersonal behavior, including expectations of others, the nature of interactions, and the patient's perceived role in life. This includes relationships with lovers and friends, parents and siblings, and with co-workers in the occupational setting. The state of current relationships and recent changes in them deserve detailed attention.

The therapist should also determine how the patient has spent his or her leisure time in the past, and how the patient's use of this time has changed. Key questions are what the patient wants from relationships, and whether these goals are realistically achievable. Birthdays, anniversaries, holidays, and particularly deaths are noteworthy during the course of treatment for their interpersonal impact. Deaths in the gay community and among intravenous drug–using persons are complicated by the fact that funerals are sometimes disguised or suppressed by family: several patients reported that friends seemed simply to disappear and only later were discovered to have died.

Establishing the problem area. We have had little difficulty in finding IPT problem areas to fit the situations of our depressed patients. The challenge has been to define a single problem area, or two at most, that best meets the patient's situation, and to address the interpersonal difficulties he or she most needs to change. The patient's input and agreement are necessary to this determination.

Interpersonal deficits constitute the problem area least fully developed and hardest to work with. This area represents the case of last resort: any other problem area provides a preferable focus. To the extent that the role transition of coming to terms with HIV infection is ubiquitous among these individuals, avoiding concentrating on interpersonal deficits is less difficult than among HIV-seronegative patients.

Legitimizing the sick role. Part of initiating therapy is legitimizing the patient role. The patient is given the "sick role" (Parsons 1951), which provides the patient exemption from certain social obligations and pressures, defines him or her as needing help, and requires the patient's cooperation in recovering from the disease state as quickly as possible. Defining the patient as suffering from a discrete psychiatric disorder allows symptoms to be distinguished as ego-dystonic rather than seen as defective attributes of the self. To extend understanding of the sick role to those around the patient, we are developing a brochure explaining depression and HIV seropositivity in an interpersonal context.

The patient may or may not have had previous experience in psychotherapy. He or she needs to understand the patient role in IPT, which includes choosing topics and offering material for sessions, with an emphasis on thoughts and feelings about interpersonal life events (see Chapter 1 for differences between IPT and other psychotherapies).

Making the interpersonal formulation.   Once convinced of the diagnosis of depression, the therapist presents the constellation of somatic, cognitive, and emotional symptoms as a recognizable and treatable diagnosis. DSM-III-R (American Psychiatric Association 1987) may be employed as evidence. The therapist lists the elicited signs and symptoms of depression, indicates that they confirm the diagnosis, and then weaves into a recapitulation of the patient's story the interpersonal events relevant to the problem areas on which he or she proposes therapy should focus:

> These symptoms are part of depression, and that depression is related to what has been happening in [the specific interpersonal situation]. Although your situation *feels* hopeless, enduring, and untreatable, it isn't; that feeling is simply a symptom of depression, which is in fact a highly treatable and common disorder. More than 8% of the U.S. population develops a significant depression in their lifetime. Depression nearly always improves with treatment. Depression affects and is affected by interpersonal relationships. [It is helpful here to point out social withdrawal, losses, disputes, or transitions in the patient's own case.] Interpersonal therapy, a brief treatment based on this connection, has been shown to be as effective as medication or any other treatment in treating the kind of depression you have. We'll try to understand current stresses and relationships in your life that may be contributing to depression.

Therapist and patient must explicitly agree on the interpersonal focus for the treatment.

A significant difference between IPT-HIV and other forms of IPT is that the patient is given *two* medical diagnoses, depression and HIV infection, both of which are treatable, although depression may cause the patient to doubt this assessment. Indeed, a crucial role transition for the HIV-seropositive patient is acceptance of an *ongoing* patient role, because medical follow-up will be necessary even if further psychiatric treatment is not. A confident, pragmatic, and effective approach to depression underscores that HIV, too, can be confronted and treated.

Establishing a therapeutic alliance.   HIV-seropositive individuals, based on their experience of social bias against homosexuality or substance abuse compounded by prejudice about HIV, are frequently wary of therapists. Therapists may be feared to represent traditional morality. Patients may have felt rejected by past therapists who were fearful of their seropositive status, or ignored by physicians running HIV protocols who were overworked, detached, or discouraged by the many deaths they attended. Many patients have felt frustrated by doctors who are unable to give unequivocal answers about the effectiveness and likely longevity of medical treatments. Consequently, it is important to explore previous interpersonal relationships with caregivers. The IPT therapist, while frankly acknowledging the inability to predict the variable course of HIV infection, can offer confident answers about treatment and outcome of depression.

As the therapist gathers information about the patient's life and forms hypotheses about interpersonal associations with depression, he or she works to establish a supportive, encouraging alliance. This involves clarity about the nature and limits of the therapeutic relationship and a sense of mutual endeavor (albeit focused squarely on the patient). Psychoeducation and the instilling of hope are further aspects of initiating treatment that help to build trust.

Incorporating psychoeducation.   Psychoeducation should not be restricted to the nature of depression and likely course and effectiveness of its treatment, but should also include germane information about HIV, medication effects, and so forth. Despite widespread educational efforts regarding HIV, many relatively sophisticated HIV-seropositive patients still harbor misconceptions or irrationally misinterpret what they have heard. Waiting in dread for results of T-cell counts, they tend to attribute exaggerated meaning to clinically trivial shifts. A matter-of-fact, confident tone, backed by reference to appropriate research, can help the patient learn to structure and deal with HIV. Part of the IPT experience thus involves patients becoming experts on HIV. (In fact, one patient helped edit the family brochure mentioned above.)

Therapists treating HIV-seropositive patients need familiarity with the HIV literature so that they can respond to patient questions and correct their distortions. Basic issues include the following (Perry and Markowitz 1988):

- The prevention of reinfection with HIV and transmission to others
- The ways HIV is *not* transmitted
- The variable course of HIV infection, ranging from acute fulminant infection to asymptomatic status for 12 years or more
- The difference between HIV infection and AIDS
- The availability of appropriate medical interventions

Exploring options and instilling hope. Hopelessness is a key feature of depression, and awareness of HIV infection provides HIV-seropositive patients with concrete evidence that their situation is bereft of hope. From the start, it is crucial that the therapist impart hope: depression is a treatable illness, and IPT is an effective treatment; there always *are* options, even if hard to see when depressed. Although being HIV-seropositive has clear negative consequences—which ought not to be trivialized—learning of HIV infection also presents the opportunity to alter one's life trajectory in potentially positive and affirmative ways (Viederman 1983). This change in life-style can satisfy important fantasies that would otherwise have gone unrealized. For example, one seropositive patient simultaneously alleviated his depression and fulfilled a lifelong dream by deciding to move to Europe to expand his career.

Middle Sessions

The middle phase of therapy begins with agreement on a treatment contract. This stage of IPT has two goals: 1) alleviating depressive symptoms and 2) assisting the patient to explore and rethink the interpersonal problems on which the treatment centers.

The therapist begins sessions with the statement, "Tell me how you have been since we last met" (Or, if the focus is on an interpersonal dispute: "How have you been doing with your lover since we last met?") This opening helps preserve the focus on current interpersonal issues. It also clarifies that the therapist will take an active, interested role and maintain thematic continuity from session to session. In contrast, a dynamic therapist might say nothing or may ask about thoughts and feelings, a cognitive therapist would arrange an agenda and query depressive cognitions, and a supportive therapist might simply ask how the patient is feeling.

The patient is likely to respond to the opening in one of two ways, reporting either depressive symptoms or interpersonal events. If he or she describes depressive symptoms, the therapist can relate these to contemporary interpersonal events and the appropriate problem area. Symptoms should be paid careful attention, elicited in detail, and, in a psychoeducational mode, acknowledged as symptoms of the depressive disorder. (This approach assumes that they are not clearly attributable to HIV.) The patient can then be reassured that his or her symptoms are amenable to treatment:

> Lack of energy and difficulty concentrating are symptoms of your depression; so is the lack of sleep. Those symptoms certainly can interfere [at the office/with your relationship]. They'll improve as the treatment begins to take effect.

A bridging statement then connects this to an interpersonal framework. Whereas a cognitive therapist might address automatic thoughts connected with the work situation, the IPT intervention might be, "Your symptoms seem to fluctuate depending upon how you're getting along with [your boss/your lover]." If the patient offers an interpersonal issue, the therapist should listen, explore the material, and eventually tie the theme to symptomatic fluctuation. Fidelity to the IPT problem area has been an important predictor of therapeutic outcome (Frank and Kupfer 1991).

Applicability of IPT Problem Areas

The sections that follow modify the application of the four IPT problem areas (Klerman et al. 1984) to the treatment of HIV-seropositive patients based on clinical experience and pilot research to date, including the 33 pilot cases reported below. The "here and now" framework of IPT helps maintain a helpful focus in the face of a potentially lethal infection, implying to the depressed patient that life is not over. The IPT approach avoids abetting depressive ruminations on the "there and then," including self-blame for contracting HIV. It mobilizes internal resources by encouraging a sense of mastery of the situation, and external supports by facilitating interpersonal relationships, without ignoring the reality of HIV infection.

Problem areas sometimes emerge in the course of therapy. For example, a patient working on a role transition revealed late in the course of treatment a long-standing covert dispute between himself and his lover in what he had previously declared an unproblematic relationship. AIDS-related deaths of friends or lovers during the course of IPT may reinforce the need for grieving. Therapists should search for latent or masked problem areas and then concentrate the therapy on those that are most salient.

Grief. Depression has long been associated with object loss. In IPT, grief is defined as the death of a loved one in a spousal or sexual relationship, in one's biological family, or in one's circle of friends. Other losses, such as the loss of a job or health, should be considered role transitions. Uncomplicated grief is not considered a mental disorder (Lazare 1979): most mourners do not require professional help, particularly if they are bolstered by interpersonal supports.

Having seen sexual partners, friends, and others in their social network die from AIDS, many HIV-seropositive individuals experience *anticipatory mourning* (i.e., grief) for their own lost future health and foreshortened longevity. For a number of our patients, life seemed to have halted when they recognized their seropositive status, even in the absence of physical symptoms. Therapists confront this lassitude—whether it be part of a grief reaction, interpersonal dispute, or role transition—along the following lines:

> You're acting as if you're mourning your own death—as if your life is over. Yet you have [almost] no symptoms of physical illness and may not have any for years. What you're suffering from is depression; that is what is making your life seem hopeless and ended. But in fact you have options, and depression is treatable. Let's talk about what you can do with your life.

Almost all of our patients knew friends who had died or were dying of AIDS, and many had sexual partners who learned of their own HIV seropositivity more or less simultaneously with the patients. Patients also reported affective numbing from sheer numbers of losses in their circle of friends. Several reported having lost *several hundred* friends, acquaintances, and business contacts. This knowledge complicated the patients' personal predicaments.

Treating complicated bereavement requires facilitating the process of mourning. Depressive symptoms are reviewed, their onset is related to the death of significant others, and the relationship between patient and deceased is reconstructed. The patient's experience of events leading up to the death, his or her response to the death itself, and the patient's subsequent attempts to grieve bear careful examination. Unmet expectations—things the patient would like to have said—and positive and negative feelings about the lost other are aired. As grieving proceeds in and outside of the IPT sessions, the patient can gradually be encouraged to explore new, compensatory relationships.

> Mr. A., a 42-year-old gay white male businessman, had been depressed since his lover's death from AIDS 3 years before. He had nursed this older man, 14 years his senior, for 3 years prior to his death and had known of his own HIV infection for 4 years. His depressive symptoms had intensified 1 month before seeking treatment, following the end of a relationship with another, exploitative lover. He felt hopeless, avoided friends and the telephone, and noted insomnia, weight loss, and compulsive behaviors. His HIV infection was currently asymptomatic, although he had been hospitalized a year before with Pneumocystis carinii pneumonia and had not complied with subsequent medical recommendations.
>
> The case was formulated as a combination of unresolved grief and role transition. Sessions focused on complicated bereavement, recognizing the more recent breakup as exacerbating Mr. A.'s sense of loss of his first lover, and on the role transition to accepting and appropriately addressing his HIV infection. Initial sessions helped the patient to mourn his first lover while reviewing strengths and weaknesses of that relationship. He reestablished contacts with friends, and his symptoms rapidly improved. He voiced newly identified anger at his second, manipulative lover, who was also sick with AIDS. By termination Mr. A. recognized the limitations of both relationships and how much he had grown: "If by chance I could go back [to either relationship], I wouldn't." Although still wary of prescribed medication, he sought appropriate medical follow-up and was no longer depressed.

Disputes.   Discovery of HIV infection frequently causes or increases tension in sexual relationships and may end them entirely. Being disowned by family or friends or discriminated against in various settings may precipitate or worsen depression. Effective treatment includes addressing and ameliorating these interpersonal problems. The IPT therapist often relates depression to a dispute in a key intimate relationship that has reached an impasse. Resolving the dispute may involve reconciling two lovers who had believed their differences insuperable, or helping a patient to leave a partner and mourn the loss of the relationship. This framework may have particular utility for treating sexual partners, HIV positive and negative, of HIV-seropositive individuals.

Treatment of a dispute requires 1) identification of the dispute, 2) the temporal and situational association of symptoms with worsening of the interpersonal relationship, 3) exploration of options within that relationship, and 4) choice of the option most viable to the patient. It is important to help the patient to see that there are indeed options: that the partners may be able to compromise, that the relationship may be tolerable with slight modification, or that the patient in fact feels that it is in his or her best interests to end the relationship but has avoided doing so lest HIV seropositivity preclude finding another partner. Mild interpersonal disputes may require simple negotiation between partners; disputes that have reached an impasse generally require more work. We found no fundamental differences requiring alteration in technique necessary to treat HIV-seropositive depressed patients in gay relationships or in relationships with individuals who formerly used intravenous drugs.

Mr. B., a 47-year-old gay male, had considered himself infected since the early 1980s and tested HIV-seropositive 1 year ago. He had been depressed for a year while sharing a studio with C., his intermittent partner of 13 years. He resented the latter's presence and distrusted his commitment, but felt terribly alone when they were apart. Mr. B. supported his HIV-seropositive lover financially and worried more about C.'s medical status than his own.

His depression was formulated as an interpersonal role dispute that had reached an impasse. In weekly sessions he acknowledged both his anger at C. and the anxiety, guilt, and loneliness he felt without him. After considering his options, he arranged to have C. leave for 2-month intervals, allowing Mr. B. to experiment with other relationships without feeling entirely abandoned. He then explored alternative contacts despite worries of rejection due to his age and HIV seropositivity. Not all contacts were successful, but the attempts themselves strengthened his self-esteem and sense of independence. Mr. B. ultimately negotiated a reconciliation with his partner, who showed renewed interest after Mr. B. reduced his demands on the relationship. Symptoms of depression entirely resolved.

There are unwritten codes for relationships, among which is the expectation that partners expect one another to disclose their risk of HIV infection. We have numerous clinical examples of couples where one partner has known of his change in serology but failed to inform or to change behavior patterns that endangered his mate. An interpersonal dispute of importance to sexual partners of HIV-seropositive individuals concerns *transgressions*. A transgression occurs when a partner breaks explicit or implicit rules of a relationship, and usually this involves a breach of trust. Sexual infidelity is a common interpersonal transgression; financial indiscretions and child abuse are other examples.

Concealing HIV infection from a partner adds a new, lethal dimension to breach of trust. We have found that when this is revealed, the partner, instead of reacting with rage, tends to become guilty. This may be because the "object" of anger is dying, because of an underlying sense of self-blame, or because of the usual difficulty depressed patients have in expressing anger. A crucial therapeutic point is that the victim needs to challenge the transgressor and assert his or her moral injury and right to justice. The therapeutic goal with such patients is not simply catharsis, but rather mobilization of anger toward the transgressor who has betrayed expectations.

Ms. D., a 27-year-old single white Catholic photographer, presented with major depression during the past "hellish" year. A year before, her fiancé and lover of 3 years had persisted in unprotected intercourse with her despite his positive HIV antibody test and progressive physical symptoms; he then abruptly abandoned her for a male lover with the revelation that he had AIDS. Stunned, she was initially slightly angry but felt guilty for her anger toward a dying man. She spent much of the year listening to his complaints, intermixed with sadistic comments, and periodically took care of him. She acquiesced to his maintaining their joint checking account and retaining some of her possessions. She tested HIV-seronegative 6 months after their last sexual contact. Nine of her friends had died of AIDS.

Ms. D.'s depression was conceived as a response to betrayal—an interpersonal role dispute needing resolution. Expressing anger was foreign to her own and her family's interpersonal repertoire. Over 16 sessions, Ms. D. verbalized her outrage and anger toward both her ex-lover and her father, whom her ex-lover resembled. She dramatically confronted both of them during the same week, asserting her anger and moral right. She resolved much "unfinished business" (e.g., the checking account) and denounced her ex-lover's continuing unprotected sexual activity with other partners. Although this confrontation yielded considerable satisfaction, she afterward felt depressed and directionless for a week. Following this, however, the symptoms resolved. She sought a career advancement, moved to a better apartment, and, showing new awareness of her former pattern of letting others take advantage of her, significantly improved her relationships with friends.

This case describes a still HIV-seronegative partner at risk for HIV infection, but has clear application to HIV-seropositive patients.

Transitions (especially becoming an AIDS patient). Discovery of HIV seropositivity is a critical event in the life of the seropositive patient. It opens—or, for many whose test results simply confirmed prior expectation, accelerates—a period of transition. Knowledge of infection often leads to reevaluation of relationships and career goals, and to reconsideration of one's core identity and mortality. A 30-year-old individual who suddenly realizes that he may have 10 or fewer years to live may well become overwhelmed and depressed.

Mourning of one's own AIDS-related death is almost inevitably an issue, even if not the focus of therapy. As such, role transitions are unavoidably present for HIV-seropositive patients. Key social patterns may be suppressed; for example, some gay men who previously depended upon sexual encounters to meet others may find themselves without a mechanism for introduction. The common reaction of restricting previous high-risk activities such as substance use or unprotected sexual contacts is frequently carried to an extreme, such as abandoning sexual activity altogether (even antedating depressive loss of libido). Among the goals of IPT should be restoration of activities that are not dangerous, and acknowledgment of the loss of pleasurable aspects of past activities, even when they have been maladaptive.

Thus the most common role transition associated with HIV infection is acceptance of being seropositive, and with it transition to a potential or actual patient sick role. Developing AIDS is an anticipated further role transition. There may be fantasies of moral retribution and punishment, because the social imagery of HIV and AIDS, like that of syphilis and other sexually transmitted diseases, often includes punishment for sexual transgressions. The social component of this role transition includes realistic fears of discrimination by employers, insurance companies, landlords, and acquaintances. In recognition of a chronic disease state and shortened life expectancy, patients shift career trajectories. Relationships with lovers, family, and co-workers may change. HIV-seropositive individuals feel they are in "viral isolation": contaminated, less attractive, and bound to be rejected because of their serostatus. "I think of myself mainly as a man with a virus," said one patient, implying his inseparability from HIV. He had suspended his entire life upon discovering his serostatus; an emblem of his improvement in IPT was his reclaiming of possessions he had put in storage 3 years earlier. Such patients frequently withdraw rather than reveal the secret of their HIV infection.

Treatment hinges on recognizing and labeling the transition state, and helping patients to mourn the loss of the pre-HIV role and to see the positive aspects of the new situation. The discovery that patients are not helpless, that they can cope with and control aspects of their new role, and that it is depression rather than HIV per se that has been holding them back, renews self-esteem and self-acceptance.

> Mr. E., a 32-year-old gay artist, became depressed following the breakup of his sole significant relationship. Previously physically healthy, he developed Pneumocystis carinii pneumonia (PCP) and was hospitalized during the course of therapy. Although he recovered, he felt the ongoing threat of illness "destroyed everything," ruining any opportunity to advance occupationally or to meet a new lover.
>
> IPT focused on his feelings of having been rejected by his ex-lover, an older man with whom he remained in contact, as well as on the gains he had achieved in having that relationship. Treatment facilitated mourning this relationship and addressed his fears of having to depend on anyone either for emotional or—given his HIV status and PCP—physical support. He then enumerated future options, among them lonely isolation and risk of future rejections and opportunities. Having acknowledged his fears of dependency, Mr. A. noted rapid improvement in his depression; his relationship with his former lover deepened, and he was able to explore new career directions and involvement with men his own age.

Mr. F., a 34-year-old black salesman and former intravenous drug user now on methadone maintenance, developed an insidious morbid depression months after notification of HIV-seropositive status. He began to question the value of "turning my life around only to die," contemplating a return to drug use and lethal overdose. In IPT sessions depressive symptoms were reviewed, the depression was related to serostatus notification, and positive and negative aspects of old (i.e., intravenous drug–using) and new (i.e., asymptomatic HIV-seropositive) roles were recognized. The therapist and patient also explored what was lost by seroconversion, rational and irrational feelings about this loss, and new opportunities despite this undeniable loss. They abreacted these feelings and encouraged the development of social support systems and the new skills necessary to manage the patient's infection.

Former substance abusers who are seropositive face *two* transitions: sobriety/recovery and HIV. This may present an overwhelming amount of material to cover in a brief therapy, especially if a patient has social and cognitive deficits related to substance abuse. If they have been chronically using drugs, former substance-abusing individuals may fear intimacy in and outside of the therapeutic situation.

Mr. G., a 41-year-old gay actor, had been rejected by his religious family as a teenager and had begun using alcohol and other drugs at roughly the same time. He soon progressed to intravenous cocaine. Several of his lovers died of AIDS. He became aware of his HIV status and became depressed shortly after successful drug and alcohol detoxification and rehabilitation some 2 years before entering our study. He was celibate and avoided social contacts in the interim.

IPT focused on his double transition in adjusting to being sober and HIV-seropositive. His speech was initially pressured and his affect shallow; but when this was addressed he gradually relaxed and became more engaged. He realized to his dismay that "the things I thought I'd worked through" (i.e., anxiety about intimacy and shame about his homosexuality) had simply been covered by drug use. Recognizing parallels between fighting addiction and fighting HIV, Mr. G. was able to mobilize himself, improving his romantic situation and changing his career in more satisfying directions while maintaining abstinence. His Ham-D score fell from 20 to 3.

The approach used with Mr. G. was to combine the two transitions: he found it helpful to compare living with the HIV virus to the never-ending, day-by-day (but gradually easing) process of alcohol recovery. It was also important to address his discomfort in the therapeutic situation before proceeding to other interpersonal situations.

For these patients IPT eased transition to acceptance of HIV seroconversion and improved interpersonal functioning by encouraging mourning of the loss of a past role. The patient and therapist were able to recognize the distress of acknowledging HIV-seropositive status and to attempt to optimize function within the new role context without ignoring realistic liabilities.

Deficits.   Interpersonal deficits represent the problem area of last resort. Helping the patient to reestablish adaptive coping mechanisms following grief, a role dispute, or role transition is less daunting than addressing long-standing characterological deficits. Chronic deficits socially isolate some individuals prior to their HIV seropositivity and depression; their relationships may be limited to transient or anonymous encounters. Interpersonal deficits may predispose to depression and hinder recovery. The paucity of relationships limits interpersonal material for therapy. Any of the other three problem areas is a preferable focus; fortunately, HIV seropositivity itself means that the problem area of role transition can be invoked in almost all cases.

Gay men and intravenous drug users with a history of only marginal relationships may see HIV-seropositive status as emblematic of their underlying inadequacy, isolation, and dysfunction. Several gay men with narcissistic character features who suffered from HIV-related physical symptoms, including the disfigurement of Kaposi's sarcoma, reported a sense of corporeal and concomitant psychic disintegration. One man described feeling "like a half-squashed roach with two legs still moving."

The therapist focuses on one of the other three problem areas whenever possible, while using the crisis of HIV infection as an opportunity to challenge the patient to conquer interpersonal barriers (cf. case of Mr. E. above). In cases where interpersonal deficits present an unavoidable focus, the therapist may sometimes uncover less-than-fulfilling but still meaningful relationships that patients can learn to use for support or to improve to their greater satisfaction. The therapeutic relationship has particular importance in treating these patients, providing a test environment for correcting distortions and developing their interpersonal skills.

Final Sessions

Termination. In terminating, the patient is asked to give up the relationship with the therapist as the patient moves toward recognition of independent competence to deal with problem areas. The therapist announces termination at least three to four sessions before the end and then elicits patient responses to it. Termination is recognized as a time of potential sadness, but also as a graduation from the sick role to social competence.

HIV-seropositive patients generally face many chronic difficulties that are likely to persist. Most, if not all, face an deterioration in physical status posttreatment and may be assumed to be at risk for recurrence of depressive symptoms. By reestablishing coping mechanisms and improving social supports and functioning, IPT may help patients deal with medical setbacks without depressive relapse—an area that needs further study. In the termination phase of IPT, fears of relapse are countered by reviewing symptoms of depression, summarizing/consolidating the problem area and how the patient has addressed it, and suggesting that he or she may be able to use these newly acquired skills should new problems arise. Patients should leave knowing that they always have options, even if depression seems to mask these possibilities, and that by dealing with interpersonal issues that have given them difficulty in the past, they may avert depression in the future.

Booster sessions. Difficulties arise in terminating with severely physically ill and potentially terminal patients. IPT was designed as a brief intervention, yet there are patients with whom it feels clinically inappropriate to terminate—dying patients being a prime example. In such cases, termination might be received as abandonment and a betrayal of the trust built during treatment. When termination seems clinically contraindicated, an alternative is to continue monthly IPT booster sessions with the same therapist (Frank et al. 1990). In fact, our patients have accepted termination with little difficulty.

Preliminary Research

Our observations above derive from clinical experience with more than 40 depressed HIV-seropositive patients. We here report outcome data on 24 depressed patients who met DSM-III-R criteria for nonpsychotic major depression or dysthymia. One patient was HIV-seronegative 6 months after repeated unprotected sexual contact with an AIDS patient; two others met criteria for frank AIDS but were relatively asymptomatic at the time of entry into the study. All others met criteria for CDC Stages II/III (i.e., essentially asymptomatic HIV infection) (CDC 1987). They had been aware of their HIV infection for periods varying from months to years.

One therapist (J.C.M.) formally treated six cases in individual IPT. Sessions were videotaped for supervision (by G.L.K.) to ensure adherence to technique. All subjects gave written informed consent. A 24-item Ham-D score of 18 was required for entry, and this rating was reassessed at Sessions 7 and 16. A Ham-D score of ≤ 6 was considered successful treatment.

A coauthor (S.W.P.), consulting the IPT manual, treated 18 cases in IPT without videotaping. The six formal cases were a nonrandom sample selected from an ongoing study of counseling for HIV testing recruited by newspaper advertisement and referral from physicians at New York Hospital. The remainder came from the coauthor's private practice. IPT was conducted in accordance with the IPT manual. Outcome was judged by global clinical impression, patients' subjective assessment, and, in the first six cases, by Ham-D score at baseline, midpoint (i.e., Session 7), and endpoint (i.e., Session 16).

Pilot results. The 24 patients had a mean age of 36.9 ± 13.0 (range 17–61; see Table 8–1). Predominantly white (71%) and male (75%), they reported a variety of HIV risk factors. Twenty-two showed evident improvement, and 21 (88%) recovered from depression. One patient left therapy after five sessions; those who completed the study received a mean 16 sessions (range 7–27). Six subjects showed a decrease in Ham-D score from 25.5 ± 6.8 initially to 11.8 ± 6.5 in Session 7, to 6.2 ± 5.0 at termination. The IPT problem areas focused upon were grief (29%), role disputes (25%), role transition (33%), and deficits (13%).

These pilot results were drawn from a nonrandom patient sample and cannot be contrasted with alternative treatment (or no treatment), and thus should be interpreted cautiously. Our ongoing comparative treatment trial may provide a more rigorous replication. Nonetheless, these preliminary findings are auspicious and suggest that IPT may be a useful treatment for depressed HIV-seropositive patients.

References

American Psychiatric Association: Diagnostic and Statistical Manual of Mental Disorders, 3rd Edition. Washington, DC, American Psychiatric Association, 1980

American Psychiatric Association: Diagnostic and Statistical Manual of Mental Disorders, 3rd Edition, Revised. Washington, DC, American Psychiatric Association, 1987

Atkinson JH, Grant I, Chandler J, et al: Psychiatric diagnoses in early HIV infection. Paper presented at the 144th annual meeting of the American Psychiatric Association, New Orleans, LA, May 1991

Brown GW, Harris T: Social Origins of Depression: A Study of Psychiatric Disorder in Women. London, Tavistock, 1978

Centers for Disease Control: Revision of the CDC surveillance case definition for acquired immunodeficiency syndrome. MMWR 36:3S–15S, 1987

Centers for Disease Control: HIV prevalence estimates and AIDS case projections for the United States: report based upon a workshop. MMWR 39:1–31, 1990

Elkin I, Shea MT, Watkins JT, et al: National Institute of Mental Health Treatment of Depression Collaborative Research Program: general effectiveness of treatments. Arch Gen Psychiatry 46:971–982, 1989

Fernandez F, Levy JK: Psychiatric diagnosis and pharmacotherapy of patients with HIV infection, in American Psychiatric Press Review of Psychiatry, Vol 9. Edited by Tasman A, Goldfinger SM, Kaufmann CA. Washington, DC, American Psychiatric Press, 1990, pp 614–630

Frank E, Kupfer D: Maintenance interpersonal psychotherapy for recurrent unipolar depression. Paper presented at the 144th annual meeting of the American Psychiatric Association, New Orleans, LA, May 1991

Frank E, Kupfer DJ, Perel JM, et al: Three-year outcomes for maintenance therapies in recurrent depression. Arch Gen Psychiatry 47:1093–1099, 1990

Hamilton M: A rating scale for depression. J Neurol Neurosurg Psychiatry 25:56–62, 1960

Kalman TP, Kalman CM, Connelly M, et al: Homophobia revisited. Hosp Community Psychiatry 38:996, 1987

Kelly JA, St Lawrence JS, Hood HV, et al: Behavioral intervention to reduce AIDS risk activities. J Consult Clin Psychol 57:60–67, 1989

Klerman GL, Weissman MM, Rounsaville BJ, et al: Interpersonal Psychotherapy of Depression. New York, Basic Books, 1984

Lazare A (ed): Outpatient Psychiatry. London, Williams & Wilkins, 1979

Manning DW, Frances AJ: Combined Pharmacotherapy and Psychotherapy for Depression. Washington, DC, American Psychiatric Press, 1990

Markowitz JC, Perry SW: AIDS: a medical overview for psychiatrists, in American Psychiatric Press Annual Review of Psychiatry, Vol 9. Edited by Tasman A, Goldfinger SM, Kaufmann CA. Washington, DC, American Psychiatric Press, 1990, pp 574–592

Markowitz JC, Perry SW: Effects of human immunodeficiency virus on the central nervous system, in American Psychiatric Press Textbook of Neuropsychiatry, 2nd Edition. Edited by Yudofsky SC, Hales RE. Washington, DC, American Psychiatric Press, 1992, pp 499–518

Parsons T: Illness and the role of the physician: a sociological perspective. Am J Orthopsychiatry 21:452–460, 1951

Perry SW: Organic mental disorders caused by HIV: update on early diagnosis and treatment. Am J Psychiatry 147:696–710, 1990

Perry S, Jacobsberg LB, Fishman B, et al: Psychiatric diagnosis before serological testing for the human immunodeficiency virus. Am J Psychiatry 147:89–93, 1990

Perry S, Fishman B, Jacobsberg L, et al: Effectiveness of psychoeducational interventions in reducing emotional distress after human immunodeficiency virus antibody testing. Arch Gen Psychiatry 48:143–147, 1991

Regier DA, Boyd JH, Burke JD, et al: One-month prevalence of mental disorders in the United States: based on five epidemiologic catchment area sites. Arch Gen Psychiatry 45:977–986, 1988

Rounsaville BJ, Glazer W, Wilber CH, et al: Short-term interpersonal therapy in methadone-maintained opiate addicts. Arch Gen Psychiatry 40:629–636, 1983

Rounsaville BJ, Chevron ES, Weissman MM: Specification of techniques in interpersonal psychotherapy, in Psychotherapy Research: Where Are We and Where Should We Go? Edited by Williams JBW, Spitzer RL. New York, Guilford, 1984, pp 160–172

Rounsaville BJ, Gawin F, Kleber H: Interpersonal psychotherapy adapted for ambulatory cocaine abusers. Am J Drug Alcohol Abuse 11:171–191, 1985

Viederman M: The psychodynamic life narrative: a psychotherapeutic intervention useful in crisis situations. Psychiatry 46:236–246, 1983

Wells KB, Stewart A, Hays RD, et al: The functioning and well-being of depressed patients: results from the Medical Outcomes Study. JAMA 262:914–919, 1989

Interpersonal Psychotherapy for Dysthymic Disorders

Barbara J. Mason, Ph.D.
John C. Markowitz, M.D.
Gerald L. Klerman, M.D.

Dysthymic disorder, now known as *dysthymia,* was introduced as a diagnostic category in DSM-III in 1980 (American Psychiatric Association 1980). Subsequently, there has been considerable research on clinical and epidemiological aspects of the disorder. The Epidemiologic Catchment Area study reported a diagnosis of dysthymia in 3.1% of adults surveyed in the United States (Weissman et al. 1988a, 1988b). The reported prevalence of dysthymia is even greater among psychiatric outpatients, with estimates ranging from 26% to 36% (Keller and Shapiro 1982; Keller et al. 1983; Markowitz et al. 1992; Rounsaville et al. 1980). In a recent medical outcomes study, dysthymia was associated with more significant morbidity and impairment of quality of life than most medical illnesses studied (Wells et al. 1989). The prevalence and morbidity of dysthymia indicate that it is an important public health problem.

Prior to DSM-III, dysthymia was generally viewed as "depressive neurosis" or "depressive personality." These chronic depressions were commonly treated with lengthy courses of psychotherapy and were considered

This work was supported by the National Institute of Mental Health Grants 3/103 and 19069. Appreciation is expressed to Eve Chevron, M.S.W., for consultation and supervision of selected IPT cases. Desipramine was provided by Rorer Pharmaceuticals. Statistical consultation was provided by Seth Thompson, M.Phil., and Andrew Leon, Ph.D.

225

to be relatively treatment refractory (Akiskal et al. 1980). DSM-III made the conceptual innovation of grouping dysthymia with the affective disorders, included somatic symptoms of depression in the symptom list, and specified a minimum duration of 2 years of fairly steady symptomatology.

In DSM-III-R (American Psychiatric Association 1987) the attempt was made to distinguish between severity of dysthymia and major depression by requiring two more symptoms for major depression than for dysthymia. However, studies have found depression to have a distorting effect on the recall of events (Beck et al. 1979; Zimmerman et al. 1988). Patient recall of two versus four symptoms over two previous years may be unreliable and may represent an artifactual overlap of diagnostic criteria (Kocsis and Frances 1987). In our experience, dysthymic patients often seek treatment when their illness has increased in severity (e.g., see Table 9–1). They commonly present with "double depression" (Keller and Shapiro 1982), that is, the superimposition of acute symptoms on chronic symptoms.

In DSM-III-R the distinction was made between *primary dysthymia*, in which the mood disturbance is not related to a preexisting, chronic nonmood Axis I or Axis III disorder, and *secondary dysthymia*, in which the mood disturbance is apparently related to a preexisting, chronic, nonmood Axis I or Axis III disorder. The DSM-III-R further distinguished between early-onset (i.e., before age 21) and late-onset (i.e., at age 21 or later) dysthymia. In our experience, many dysthymic patients report having been depressed "all my life," "for as long as I can remember," or, as one patient reported to Dr. Klerman, "since the sperm hit the egg."

Treatment Approaches for Dysthymia

Antidepressant Medication

Grouping dysthymia with the affective disorders in DSM-III had treatment implications. A number of investigators reported promising results using antidepressant medication for dysthymia (Akiskal et al. 1980; Harrison et al. 1986; Paykel et al. 1982; Rounsaville et al. 1980; Ward et al. 1979). Most recently, in a double-blind trial of tricyclic antidepressant medication, Kocsis et al. (1988a, 1988b) found highly satisfactory results with imipramine in patients meeting criteria for dysthymia, many of whom had a long-standing disorder and prolonged prior psychotherapy. Moreover, the placebo response rate in this study, as well as in subsequent reports from other investigators (Barrett 1984; McCullough et al. 1988), was less than 13%, indicating that expectancy is not a powerful determinant of treatment response in dysthymia. However, significant numbers of dysthymic patients (40% as reported by Kocsis et al. 1988b) either fail to respond to vigorous drug treatment or cannot tolerate medication trials because of side effects or development of bipolar symptoms (Akiskal 1981). Effective psychotheraputic interventions are clearly desirable for such patients.

Dynamic Psychotherapy

There have been only a few reports of psychosocial (Becker et al. 1987; Corney 1981; de Jong et al. 1986; Gonzalez et al. 1985) or psychotherapeutic (Jacobson 1971; Weissman and Akiskal 1984) interventions with dysthymia. At the same time, there have been many clinical discussions of psychodynamic treatment of chronic depression based on case reports (Arieti and Bemporad 1978; Bemporad 1976; Chodoff 1972; Klerman et al. 1984). Unfortunately, no reports exist of controlled or systematic studies of dysthymic patients treated with psychodynamic psychotherapy.

Cognitive-Behavior Therapy

A trial of a cognitive-behavioral intervention found that significantly more patients having an acute major depression based on Research Diagnostic Criteria recovered (75%) than did subjects with (chronic) intermittent depression (43%) or "double depression" (27%) (Gonzalez et al. 1985). However, McCullough (1991) reports that 9 out of 10 dysthymic patients treated in a naturalistic study with cognitive-behavior therapy were in remission for the disorder at follow-up of 2 or more years. De Jong and colleagues (1986) studied the effects of social competence training and cognitive restructuring interventions on 30 unmedicated inpatients meeting DSM-III criteria for both dysthymic disorder and major depression who had families negative for mood disorder. A 2- to 3-month trial of combined activity scheduling, social competence training, and cognitive restructuring yielded a higher response rate (60%) than cognitive restructuring alone (30%) or a waiting-list control condition (10%). Follow-up data on a subsample of patients ($n = 14$) at 6 months suggested stability of these treatment effects. Becker and colleagues (1987) reported preliminary results on 36 dysthymic subjects randomly assigned to social skills training or crisis supportive psychotherapy and to nortriptyline or placebo. Self-report and clinician ratings showed equally significant improvement for all treatment conditions.

Although the above studies are not comparable in methodology, the outcomes reported are generally better with cognitive-behavior therapy than would be expected from a placebo effect, thus offering tentative support for the use of a brief, focused therapy in the treatment of dysthymia.

The Role of Interpersonal Psychotherapy in the Treatment of Dysthymia

Interpersonal psychotherapy is a time-limited psychotherapy that, like cognitive-behavior therapy, has performed comparably to antidepressant medication in the treatment of outpatients with acute major depression (Elkin et al. 1989; Klerman et al. 1984). The goal of IPT is to treat depression by focusing on difficulties in the patient's interpersonal relationships, using the four problem areas defined by Klerman et al. (1984) as frequently associated with depression: grief, role disputes, role transitions, and social skills deficits. The interpersonal emphasis of IPT makes it particularly well suited to treating the decreased social facility and social withdrawal associated with dysthymia (Cassano et al. 1990; Kocsis et al. 1988a; Stewart et al. 1988), and the affectively toned features of the dependent, avoidant, and self-defeating personality disorders often found occurring comorbidly with dysthymia (Kocsis et al. 1986; Koenigsberg et al. 1985; Markowitz et al. 1992).

Effects of Dysthymia on Interpersonal Functioning

Kocsis et al. (1988a) found dysthymic patients to be significantly impaired compared with published findings of a community sample using the Social Adjustment Scale (SAS; Weissman and Bothwell 1976), with deficits noted in family and marital functioning, leisure time, and work. Imipramine treatment significantly diminished the social and vocational impairment of these dysthymic subjects after 6 weeks compared with placebo, although some residual impairment persisted in comparison with community scores. Cassano et al. (1990) also found dysthymic patients to have deficits on the SAS that exceeded those of patients with episodic depression on some SAS subscales.

Although dysthymic individuals may work diligently and maintain a facade of normalcy (Akiskal 1983), the chronicity and early onset that are common features of the disorder generally impede their learning to interact socially. The low energy and poor self-image associated with dysthymia may result in a lack of confidence in dating and the social assertiveness necessary for occupational advancement. Because IPT addresses interpersonal disorders and deficits, this form of therapy appears particularly appropriate for treating dysthymic symptomatology. Its focus on social functioning may teach new skills to dysthymic patients so that they can feel, often for the first time in their lives, in control of, rather than controlled by, their moods.

Comorbidity of Dysthymia

Various studies suggest that dysthymia rarely appears as an uncomplicated disorder (Barlow et al. 1986; Klein et al. 1988; Kocsis et al. 1990; Kovacs et al. 1984; Markowitz et al. 1992; Weissman et al. 1988a), with major depression the most common of the comorbid Axis I disorders, and social phobia and other anxiety disorders also seen. In most cases, dysthymia predated the development of other Axis I disorders.

A variety of Axis II disorders have also been associated with dysthymia. In DSM-III it is suggested that dysthymic disorder might be associated with borderline, histrionic, and dependent personality disorders. In DSM-III-R, associations between narcissistic and avoidant personality disorders and dysthymia are also suggested. A chart review of 2,462 psychiatric patients revealed that 34% of the 68 dysthymic patients had Axis II comorbidity: 16% classified atypical-mixed–other, 8% borderline personality disorder, and 8% dependent personality disorder (Koenigsberg et al. 1985). Kocsis et al. (1986) found a 47% prevalence of personality disorder in a sample of outpatients with dysthymic disorder, with atypical-mixed (13%) and dependent (11%) personality disorders the most common comorbid Axis II diagnoses. Markowitz et al. (1992) found that dysthymic outpatients were significantly more likely to meet criteria for avoidant, dependent, borderline, and self-defeating personality disorders than were nondysthymic outpatients.

Comorbidity may be important to the treatment of dysthymia in several respects. Clusters of comorbid diagnoses may predict response to pharmacological and psychotheraputic treatments. Axis II diagnoses, particularly the affectively toned behaviors associated with avoidant, dependent, and self-defeating personality disorders, may reflect the effects of chronically depressed mood on personality and thus identify interpersonal disturbances that IPT might address.

Modifying Interpersonal Psychotherapy for Treatment of Dysthymia

As part of a program of research at Cornell University Medical College on the clinical and therapeutic aspects of chronic depression and dysthymia, it was decided to explore the efficacy of IPT as a treatment of dysthymia. This modality was chosen because of its previously demonstrated efficacy in acute and recurrent depressions (Elkin et al. 1989; Frank et al. 1989; Klerman and Weissman 1991; Klerman et al. 1984) and because of the many interpersonal difficulties and social disabilities associated with dysthymia (Cassano et al. 1990; Kocsis et al. 1988b; Stewart et al. 1988). No systematic exploration of IPT's potential value in chronic depressions, such as dysthymia, had previously been undertaken.

Interpersonal psychotherapy was offered to patients with DSM-III-R primary dysthymia who presented for outpatient treatment on a double-blind study of tricyclic antidepressant medication for dysthymia but either refused to accept medication or failed to respond to medication after 10 weeks of treatment. IPT was conducted according to the technical specifications described in the IPT manual that was developed for treatment of major depressive disorder by Klerman et al. (1984). This initial study had two goals: 1) to determine whether IPT can be used to effectively treat dysthymia, and 2) to identify areas in which standard IPT techniques might be modified to better treat dysthymic patients. Treatment consisted

of 16 weekly 50-minute sessions focusing on the four interpersonal problem areas that were identified by Klerman et al. (1984) as frequently being
associated with depression: 1) grief, 2) interpersonal role disputes, 3) role
transitions, and 4) interpersonal deficits.

The results from this study to date support the efficacy of IPT for the
treatment of dysthymia. (See section on preliminary research below for a
quasi-experimental comparison of outcome data from nine dysthymic
patients treated with IPT and nine treated with desipramine.) With regard
to the second goal of the study, the basic structure of IPT was equally useful
for the treatment of dysthymia as for acute depressions, although certain
nuances relating to the differences between the disorders required consideration. In this section we focus on a qualitative examination of differences
between dysthymic patients and patients with major depression that may
require modification of IPT stategies.

Clinical Features of Dysthymic Patients

When patients present for treatment of primary dysthymia of early onset,
their symptoms may have persisted for as long as they can remember. In
addition to depressed mood, Mason et al. (1989) found that dysthymic
patients commonly suffer from chronic guilt, passive suicidal ideation,
fatigue, anxiety, somatization, low libido, pessimism, feelings of helplessness and worthlessness, difficulty concentrating, irritability, worry, indeci-
siveness, disturbed sleep, and social withdrawal. McCullough et al. (1988)
reported that a sample of untreated dysthymic patients maintained dysfunctional coping styles, destructive interpersonal patterns, introverted
and neurotic personality patterns, and an external locus of control orientation whereby the consequences of one's behavior are not viewed as stemming from one's own actions, but are instead perceived as resulting from
fate, luck, and/or chance.

Dysthymic individuals are often excellent workers, able to throw
themselves into work, particularly if it does not involve much interpersonal contact, while struggling to retain the facade of normalcy. Inwardly,
however, they feel inferior, inadequate, and unhappy. Hopelessness and
helplessness in the face of their moods are so persistent that dysthymic
individuals often do not distinguish these feelings from their core character. Thus, the treatment of dysthymia involves not only the treatment of

symptomatology but the need to undo the effects of illness from personality and core identity.

Differences Between Dysthymic Patients and Patients With Major Depression That Pertain to IPT

We have observed three central ways in which dysthymia differs from major depression, each having implications for the modification of IPT for dysthymia: 1) the lack of an acute precipitant, 2) the greater characterological effects of the mood disorder, and 3) the paucity of euthymic memories.

The Lack of an Acute Precipitant

It is common for dysthymic individuals to seek treatment when their symptoms have increased in severity. Acute environmental events, especially those involving interpersonal conflict or change, may be related to exacerbation in symptomatology. However, the onset of depressive symptoms is usually insidious and long predates the exacerbation. Consequently, these acute precipitants are less likely to provide effective foci for IPT in dysthymia than they are in acute depressions.

Dysthymia, Character Pathology, and IPT

Interpersonal psychotherapy is a brief, focused psychotherapy that does not address character pathology as a treatment target. Yet, when treating dysthymic patients, the IPT therapist is confronted with characterological issues that are impossible to ignore. A major goal of IPT of dysthymia is to help the patient recognize which aspects of what he or she has considered inherent personality or temperament are, in fact, mood related and alterable. An important function of the treatment is to help the patient distinguish state from trait in a condition having a chronicity that tends to merge the two.

An analogy may be made with pharmacotherapy of dysthymia in which patients responsive to antidepressants are aware of perceiving their world from a new perspective. IPT does not propose to change character; but by treating a chronic affective illness that strongly influences identity and outlook, it may indirectly help the patient to reexamine long-standing behaviors and perceptions, diminish chronic difficulties in interpersonal functioning, and improve pervasive poor self-image and low self-esteem (Bronisch and Klerman 1988).

Paucity of Euthymic Memories

Acutely depressed patients can usually be induced to look back to normal premorbid periods, helping them to see depression as a limited episode from which they can recover. However, the patient whose dysthymia had an early onset may be unable to recall euthymia and see depressive symptoms as part of his or her character. This underscores the importance of defining dysthymia for the patient as a chronic but treatable medical illness and of systematically seeking periods of higher social functioning and mood improvement.

Recall is an area that may particularly affect the work of IPT with this population. Studies have suggested that patients' subjective recall of events is often unreliable beyond 6 months, particularly for depressed patients whose current outlook may retrospectively color memories of their past (Beck et al. 1979; Zimmerman et al. 1988). Such cognitive distortions may lead some dysthymic patients to report more continuously persistent symptoms and more impaired interpersonal functioning than they actually suffer. Accordingly, the IPT therapist must be skeptical of blanket descriptions of dysfunction, seeking areas and periods of higher functioning and genuine achievements, which the patient may have forgotten or disregarded in the current dysphoric state, as evidence of potential for recuperation. The acknowledgment of any areas of competence may provide a foundation for developing reality-based self-confidence and self-esteem.

Goals and Tasks of Interpersonal Psychotherapy in the Treatment of Dysthymia

Initial Sessions (Sessions 1–3)

The first one to three sessions of IPT encompass multiple goals, which include the following: 1) establishing the diagnosis of dysthymia, 2) obtaining careful medical and medication histories and an interpersonal inventory; 3) explaining the nature of the mood disorder and the patient role; 4) establishing interpersonal problem areas and linking them to diagnosis in a treatment contract; and 5) pursuing a treatment alliance, providing psychoeducation about dysthymia, and imparting hope.

Establishing the Diagnosis

Patients may not recognize dysthymia as such, unthinkingly accepting their neurovegetative symptoms and hopelessness as part of their core sense of identity. The therapeutic work begins by carefully diagnosing the patient's disorder and then presenting it to him or her as a discrete, treatable disorder. The Hamilton Depression Rating Scale (Ham-D; Hamilton 1960) and the Cornell Dysthymia Rating Scale (Mason et al. 1989) provide symptomatic guidelines.

Psychiatric evaluation includes a history of present illness, a history of previous psychopathology and psychiatric treatment, a family history of psychiatric disorders, and a mental status examination. Particular attention is paid to the interpersonal inventory, assessing the quality, duration, expectations, and outcome of the patient's important past and present relationships. Medical and medication histories are necessary to rule out medical causes of chronic depression (e.g., hypothyroidism, antihypertensive medication) and to convey to the patient that he or she is undergoing a thorough diagnostic evaluation.

The history of previous treatment relationships also deserves careful inquiry. Because of the chronicity of the syndrome, the majority of dysthymic patients will have already undergone one or more therapies that have likely been unsuccessful (Kocsis et al. 1986; Markowitz et al. 1992). Were these psychotherapeutic or psychopharmacological treatments? What issues were discussed, what were the patient's expectations, and does he or she feel that the therapy was beneficial? What does the patient want from therapy now?

Establishing the Problem Area

Most of the dysthymic patients we have treated have had some interpersonal deficits. These deficits have often appeared to be related to their depressed mood. For example, extreme fear of rejection may lead patients to the avoidance of relationships, or fear of abandonment may induce a willingness to accept inequities in the relationships they do have. Because interpersonal deficits have been the least developed area of IPT, it is preferable to choose alternative foci when they exist, working on interpersonal deficits within the context of a role transition, interpersonal dispute, or grief. A more easily attainable success in these focused areas may serve as an impetus for the dysthymic patient to tackle the more threatening and pervasive area of his or her interpersonal deficits. For each problem area the patient can be asked to speculate on the best, worst, and most expectable outcomes. Progress can be measured against these expectations, and the deeply held belief that nothing will change can thereby be challenged.

Legitimizing the Sick Role

One aspect of initiating therapy is legitimizing the patient role. The patient is given the "sick role," as defined by Parsons (1951), which exempts the patient from certain ordinary social obligations and pressures, defines him or her as needing help, and requires his or her cooperation in recovering from the disease state as quickly as possible. Defining the patient as suffering from a discrete psychiatric disorder allows him or her to distinguish symptoms as ego-dystonic rather than as a defective attribute of himself or herself—a crucial differentiation for the lifelong dysthymic patient. The patient's recognition that he or she has an illness can help to render symptoms ego-dystonic rather than accepted, and simultaneously can limit self-blame for "laziness" and other depressive symptoms. The sick role validates a patient's need to decrease work and social pressures, and to increase particular interpersonal contacts and activities.

A depressed person may initially elicit sympathy, reassurance, and support, but those around him or her soon lose patience, tending to become critical and even hostile, and they may withdraw from what they see as morally weak behavior (Klerman et al. 1984). High levels of expressed emotion in a marriage, marital distress, and patients' perceptions of criticism by spouses have all been associated with depressive relapse (Hooley and Teasdale 1989).

At the same time that assuming the sick role may relieve self-criticism and social pressures on the patient, it should not provide an excuse for regressive social withdrawal. Maximizing interpersonal contact is crucial to providing material for IPT and to changing those behaviors, such as social withdrawal, that characterize dysthymia.

Presenting the Formulation

Once convinced of the diagnosis of dysthymia, the therapist presents the constellation of somatic, cognitive, and emotional symptoms as a recognizable, treatable diagnosis. It may be helpful to show the patient the criteria in DSM-III-R as evidence that the symptoms the patient has long taken for granted are in fact a disorder. The therapist lists the elicited signs/symptoms of depression, indicates that they confirm the diagnosis, and then relates them to the crucial problem area(s). The following excerpt from an IPT manual for dysthymia developed by Drs. Markowitz and Klerman gives an example of how an IPT formulation may be presented:

> These symptoms are part of depression, and that depression is related to what has been happening in [the specific interpersonal situation]. Because you've been depressed for so long—all your life—it may be hard to recognize that you have a disorder, that this isn't part of you. Although your situation feels hopeless, enduring, and untreatable, it isn't: that feeling is simply a paradoxical symptom of a highly treatable and common disorder. More than 8% of the population in the United States develop a significant depression in their lifetime, and more than 3% have the kind of long-lasting depression you do. Depression nearly always improves with treatment. Depression affects and is affected by interpersonal relationships. [It is helpful here to point out social withdrawal, losses, and so forth in the patient's own case.] Interpersonal therapy, a brief treatment based on this connection, has been shown to be as effective as medication or any other treatment. We'll try to understand what current stresses and relationships in your life may be contributing to depression.

Obtaining the Patient's Agreement to the Formulation

In addition to explaining the diagnosis of depression, the therapist should weave into his or her recapitulation of the patient's story the interpersonal events relevant to the problem areas he or she proposes therapy should focus on. Therapist and patient should explicitly agree on an interpersonal focus in one or two of the problem areas (i.e., grief, role dispute, role transition, or interpersonal deficits) as the target for the treatment to follow.

Establishing a Therapeutic Alliance

The Epidemiologic Catchment Area study established that dysthymic individuals are frequent users of health and mental health services (Weissman et al. 1988a). It is consequently important to explore previous interpersonal relationships with therapists and other caregivers, including the patient's expectations and the nature of treatment and its outcome. Persons with dysthymia who have already had courses of psychotherapy or pharmacotherapy may describe hopelessness about the outcome of the current treatment based on unrealistic assessments of past treatment. Lack of response to past appropriate treatments should be acknowledged without concession of hopelessness. The IPT therapist can offer confident answers about the treatment and outcome of depression.

As the IPT therapist begins to gather information about the patient's life and to form hypotheses about interpersonal associations with depression, he or she should teach the patient the patient role while establishing a supportive, encouraging alliance. This involves clarity about the nature and limits of the therapeutic relationship and a sense of mutual endeavor. Psychoeducation and the instilling of hope are further aspects of initiating treatment that can help to build trust.

Utilizing Psychoeducation

Psychoeducation should include the nature of depression, symptoms of dysthymia, its likely course, and effectiveness of its treatment. A matter-of-fact, confident tone, backed by reference to appropriate research, can help patients feel that there is a way to structure and deal with their experience. In their manual Drs. Markowitz and Klerman suggest the following approach:

> When you've been depressed for years, as you have been, it's hard to recognize that you have an illness, to see that the disorder isn't you. These symptoms—sleep disturbance, pessimism, fatigue, not wanting to be around people, wishing you were dead—are as much symptoms of depression as your feeling blue is. And you can get control over them, instead of having them control you. I'm going to keep reminding you of this, because I want you to understand what's illness, not you, and that it doesn't have to continue to be that way. As we work on the interpersonal factors that are part of this depression, the symptoms will start to go away.

Instilling Hope

Instilling hope is to some degree an extension of psychoeducation, but it cannot be overemphasized. From the start, the IPT therapist should impart hope:

Dysthymia is a treatable illness and IPT an effective treatment; there always are options, even if they are hard to see when depressed. You're suffering a lot from [name symptoms], but those are symptoms of dysthymia; as treatment proceeds you should begin to feel better. . . . You have options in life that dysthymia has undoubtedly kept you from fully exploring. It's harder to do everything when you're depressed—particularly when you don't even realize that you are depressed. You've been fighting all your life with one hand tied behind your back.

The Middle Sessions (Sessions 4–12)

Initiating the Middle Sessions

The middle phase of therapy begins with agreement on the treatment contract. This stage of IPT has two goals: 1) alleviating depressive symptoms and 2) assisting the patient to explore and rethink the interpersonal problems on which the treatment centers. The "here and now" framework of IPT helps the patient avoid depressive ruminations on the "there and then," including past failures and losses. It mobilizes internal resources by encouraging a sense of mastery of the situation, and external supports by facilitating interpersonal relationships.

The therapist may begin sessions with a statement such as, "Tell me how you have been since we last met." Or, if the focus is an interpersonal dispute, "How have you been doing with [name of person] since we last met?" The patient is likely to respond to these openings in one of two ways: reporting depressive symptoms or discussing interpersonal events. If the patient describes depressive symptoms, the therapist can seek to relate these to contemporary interpersonal events and to the appropriate problem area. Symptoms should be paid careful attention, elicited in detail, and, in a psychoeducational mode, identified as symptoms of dysthymia that are amenable to treatment. If the patient offers an interpersonal issue, the therapist should simply listen and then explore the material, but eventually tie the theme to symptomatic fluctuation.

Understanding the Importance of the Therapeutic Relationship

Because dysthymic patients generally need to rethink their whole approach to relationships, the therapeutic relationship takes on greater importance in IPT for dysthymia than for acute depression. It provides important interpersonal modeling, particularly for subjects with interpersonal deficits. Manifestations of interpersonal deficits within the therapeutic relationship may include a subject's tendency to apologize to the therapist; to present himself or herself as superficially "normal," fearing to reveal a "defective" self; and to avoid the dual risks of expressing anger and of angering the therapist. The therapist should look for and encourage the expression of dissatisfaction about the therapist and therapy, gently confronting and exploring the patient's tendency to idealize and empower the therapist while presenting himself or herself as helpless, ineffectual, and apologetic. The treatment should be framed as a collaboration or joint venture in which the patient's wishes, desires, and goals are paramount. Addressing interpersonal issues in the therapeutic relationship not only strengthens the working alliance but can also provide a springboard for parallel issues in other interpersonal situations.

Determining Applicability of Four Problem Areas

In the sections that follow we modify the application of the four IPT problem areas (Klerman et al. 1984) to the treatment of dysthymic patients based on clinical experience and pilot research to date. Work with a given patient revolves around one (or, at most, two) problem area(s) that has been identified. In the pilot series of nine dysthymic subjects reported above, none were found to have grief as a problem area, two had interpersonal role disputes, three were facing role transitions, and four were experiencing interpersonal deficits. Our discussion is based not only on these pilot cases but on ongoing experience with dysthymic patients in several forms of psychotherapy and combined psychopharmacotherapy, and additional dysthymic patients subsequently treated or in treatment with IPT.

Grief.   Depression has long been associated with object loss. For the purposes of IPT, *grief* is defined as the death of a loved one in a spousal or sexual relationship, one's biological family, or one's circle of friends. Other losses, such as the loss of a job, health, and so on, should be considered role transitions.

Uncomplicated grief is not considered a mental disorder (Lazare 1979); most mourners do not require professional help, particularly if bolstered by interpersonal supports. Because of the chronicity of dysthymic symptoms, acute grief is rarely a focus of IPT. Nonetheless, when the death of a significant other does occur, it provides an excellent focus for exploration of the exquisite sensitivity to loss shown by dysthymic patients, and their difficulty in expressing anger and other ambivalently held feelings. The following case is illustrative:

> A severely dysthymic patient with major interpersonal deficits was experiencing symptom-free periods of increasing duration in response to 10 IPT sessions, at which point her abusive ex-husband died unexpectedly. They had divorced approximately 17 years before, and she had not seen him for more than a year prior to his death. Nevertheless, she responded with anergia, marked psychomotor retardation, and a cornucopia of vague somatic complaints that she completely dissociated from his dying. However, she did summon up her previously acquired mastery of the IPT technique of linking fluctuations in dysthymic symptoms with interpersonal events, and the IPT model for working through grief was implemented, including a reconstruction of her relationship with her ex-husband and her positive and negative feelings toward him. The flare up of depressive symptoms significantly diminished within two sessions.

Interpersonal disputes.   Dysthymia tends to produce limited and unequal relationships. Patients with dysthymia tend toward social isolation, which may be absolute or may confine their relationships to superficiality. When dysthymic individuals succeed in appearing "normal" to others who encounter them, it is usually at the cost of great internal effort and tension, because they inwardly feel inferior, bad, and worth nothing. They are less likely to have intimate relationships, and they are also likely to understate the value of those relationships they do have. When they marry or otherwise risk intimacy, their relationships tend to be masochistic ones. Being dysthymic, they feel unworthy of better relationships and may cling to dysfunctional relationships and roles for fear of losing the little they have.

   In examining an existing relationship, the IPT therapist and patient should consider what each partner wants and expects from the therapy and whether disputes exist and can be negotiated. If the patient and his or her partner have reached an impasse, what options are available to the patient to alter the relationship? Is the relationship genuinely satisfying, or is the patient settling for an unsatisfactory situation based on his or her feelings of inadequacy? Patients may require some prodding to explore what they really desire from relationships, as opposed to what they have been accustomed to receiving or thinking they deserve. What they themselves want is often an unconsidered problem for patients who have predicated their relationships and lives on caregiving and fulfilling the wishes of others as a way of excusing their self-perceived lack of desirability.

A characteristic problem of dysthymic individuals involved in relationships is *suppression of anger* for fear of "rocking the boat" and losing the overvalued partner. Indeed, the patient is often unaware of feeling angry, responding to upsetting situations instead with guilt and self-criticism rather than rage. This "retroflexed rage" often results in a masochistic relationship in which the patient, unwilling to risk setting limits, silently suffers the partner's hurtful behaviors. Such patients frequently have histories of childhood and latter-day traumata (Akiskal 1981: Klein et al. 1988) to which they also respond with guilt rather than anger.

A principle of IPT is that an appropriately outraged, morally justified response to the transgressions of others may be clinically beneficial. IPT should focus on this disequilibrium, helping the patient to explore his or her needs in sessions and to begin to assert them in the relationship. The goal is not simply abreaction and catharsis—which do not in themselves alter interpersonal functioning—but rather the linking of affect to a specific interpersonal situation.

> A 32-year-old single white Roman Catholic photojournalist reported having felt depressed since her early teens, even before her involvement in a teenage trauma for which she felt, undeservedly, guilt. She had a series of unsatisfying relationships with men, who, she felt, took advantage of her; she "stayed with them too long" lest she feel alone and unmarriageable. When she began dating, shortly after therapy started, she foresaw nothing but disaster in her current boyfriend's behavior. She was loath to discuss her feelings and wishes with him for fear of seeming either "too interested" or "too pushy," and losing him. She subsequently discovered that she could alter the relationship in positive directions simply by expressing her reactions to behaviors she found bothersome—which he then promptly ceased. Even anger, which had previously been taboo, she gradually recognized as a useful and increasingly comfortable emotion. The relationship evolved, and her symptoms almost entirely disappeared.

There are unwritten codes for relationships and reasonable expectations partners may have of one another. Because dysthymic individuals are averse to expressing anger, they are at particular risk for being transgressed against. A special type of interpersonal dispute of particular importance to sexual partners concerns *transgressions.* A transgression occurs when a partner breaks the explicit or implicit rules of a relationship; usually this involves a breach of trust or a sexual or financial indiscretion. Sexual infidelity is the most common interpersonal transgression; sexual abuse of children is another.

A crucial therapeutic point is that the victim needs to challenge the transgressor and assert his or her moral right to justice. The therapeutic goal with such patients is not simply catharsis, but mobilization of anger toward the transgressor who has betrayed expectations, perhaps in several respects.[1]

Role transitions. Role transitions are defined as difficulties in coping with life changes that require an alteration in one's social or occupational status or self-view. Examples include the development of an illness, graduation from school, job change, promotion or demotion, moving to a new city, a return to single life in the aftermath of divorce, or prolonged alcohol abstinence following years of dependence. Although dysthymic patients are likely to emphasize the negative aspects of any change, the therapist can help them to recognize actual and potential gains. Any transition is a stress, which can have its negative side but almost always has positive aspects as well.

A novel strategy worth pursuing with patients who lack obvious role disputes or complicated bereavements, and which is preferable to focusing on interpersonal deficits alone, is to consider the diagnosis of dysthymia and its treatment as a *transition.* This is particularly effective in cases where the patient, albeit suffering from dysthymia for the remembered decades of his or her life, has not previously received the diagnosis of dysthymia or realized that it is treatable. This approach charges the IPT treatment with added excitement and may help the patient to feel newly empowered.

Interpersonal deficits. Interpersonal deficits represent the most challenging IPT problem area. Helping the patient to reestablish adaptive coping

---

[1] The case of Ms. B. on p. 251 illustrates transgression in the context of interpersonal disputes.

mechanisms following complicated bereavement, a role dispute, or role transition is less daunting than addressing long-standing and pervasive interpersonal deficits. Patients with interpersonal deficits are the most difficult to treat with IPT, in part because the paucity of relationships limits interpersonal material for therapy. Any of the other three problem areas is a preferable focus; as discussed above, role transition frequently can be invoked instead. Yet most dysthymic patients will have interpersonal deficits.

The interpersonal deficits associated with dysthymia may be mood related, hence vigorous treatment with IPT may alleviate depressive symptoms and simultaneously challenge affectively toned beliefs and behaviors. For dysthymic patients, the deficits typically involve 1) social isolation, 2) a sense of inadequacy, 3) a lack of self-assertion, and 4) a guilty inability to express anger.[2]

Social isolation.   The therapist can attack social isolation by encouraging occupational and extraoccupational activities, especially weekend activities. The question "What did you do over the weekend?" often yields revealing answers. Social activities allow testing and reworking of interpersonal patterns. Dysthymic patients are often slow to recognize or to report pleasurable activities, some of which they may have abandoned years before and forgotten. Hobbies and particularly social activities that bring the patient into contact with others are to be encouraged. Whatever the outcome of such activities, they provide opportunities to examine social behaviors, expectations, and desires. Patients are often surprised to find things have gone better than expected.

Sense of inadequacy.   Too often the patient's efforts have been expended in the pursuit of conformity, to blend in and not be noticed for fear they may be perceived as inadequate, unlovable, or strange. The sense of inadequacy emerges particularly when the patient approaches a relationship that could involve intimacy.

Lack of self-assertion.   Passivity, lack of self-assertion, fear of risk taking, and social embarrassment are often a way of life for the dysthymic individual, with a chronic sense of living at the mercy of his or her mood, and devotion to the needs of others. By expressing needs to others, dysthy-

---

[2] The case of Ms. A. on p. 249 illustrates the role of interpersonal deficits in IPT.

mic patients may learn that they can indeed control their internal and external environments, affecting both the feelings within and the behavior of those around them.

Guilty inability to express anger. Masochistic, avoidant, and dependent schemata may be developed. Assertiveness training, support of expression of anger, and increased tolerance of risk taking are likely to be important goals, directed to the following settings:

1. *Romantic:* Patients may have a fear of dating lest they be rejected. They may have a sense of being boring and uninteresting. These patients are avoidant and seek conformity; many are "wallflowers" who dress conservatively and feel inexperienced in social intercourse. Many lack knowledge of how to demonstrate their interest in or affection toward others.

   A 29-year-old woman with lifelong dysthymia and the sense that she was unlovable and defective had dared hope only for sexual encounters (masochistic), not relationships. In IPT she was encouraged to become involved with a man whom she found attractive and with whom she had long been friendly. She found this relationship sexually and emotionally more satisfying than any previous one.

   Patients frequently are pleased to find that asking and knowing is better than withdrawing and guessing at the motives of others. Taking the risk of being rejected can lead to acceptance, and with it, erosion of the inner sense of defectiveness—of the ineffable depressive "fatal flaw."

2. *Occupational:* Some patients may avoid work responsibility for fear that they may prove inadequate to the stress, attention, and so forth. These patients have difficulties with the social culture of the job milieu, as opposed to paperwork and other asocial aspects of work.

3. *Social:* Some patients may be socially isolated and withdrawn.

A major difference between acute and chronic depression is the chronicity of hopelessness. Patients with good premorbid adjustment who suffer an acute major depression become hopeless but with guidance can usually acknowledge that life has not always seemed that way. Patients with recurrent depressive episodes often benefit from the insight that they have recovered in the past and may do so again. Dysthymic patients, however, often have no euthymic periods to recall. This increases the importance of maintaining the here-and-now interpersonal focus rather than dredging up dispiriting past events.

The Final Sessions (Sessions 13–16):

Termination

In terminating, patients are asked to give up their relationship with their therapist as they move toward recognition of their independent competence to deal with the problem area(s) on which IPT was focused. The therapist announces termination at least three to four sessions before the end and subsequently elicits patients' responses to it. Termination should be recognized as a time of potential sadness, but also as a graduation from the sick role (back) to social competence. In these last sessions the therapist and patient should review key interpersonal issues, consolidate gains made, and appreciate the success of their alliance while lamenting its ending.

Dysthymic patients, who tend to overvalue the importance of others in relationships and to underrate themselves, are often reluctant to end therapy after 4 months. The therapist must help the patient to appreciate both the degree to which they have improved and the patient's own responsibility and credit for that improvement. Markowitz and Klerman, in their manual on IPT of dysthymia, suggest the following summary:

> We've accomplished a lot in a brief time. I want to point out that this wasn't magic: you've gotten out of depression and dramatically changed your relationships because of the things you did, the risks you took. Now that you recognize what you've been dealing with all your life, you know what to do. Continuing to address these issues—expressing your wishes and your anger to your boyfriend when appropriate, risking to ask for the raise you deserve—is likely both to keep you from being depressed and to make you ever more comfortable in those interpersonal situations.

The termination phase of IPT should counter fears of relapse by reviewing the symptoms of depression, summarizing the problem area and how the patient has addressed it, and suggesting that the patient may be able to do the same with his or her newly acquired skills should new problems arise in the future. Patients should leave with the knowledge that they always do have options, even if depression seems to mask these choices, and that by dealing with the interpersonal issues that have given them difficulty in the past they may avert depression in the future.

Booster Sessions

When termination seems clinically contraindicated, alternatives include monthly IPT booster sessions with the same therapist or involvement in a postintervention support group. Given the chronicity of dysthymia and the effectiveness of monthly IPT maintenance for patients with recurrent major depression (Frank et al. 1989, 1990), we consider that this, in fact, may be advisable.

Special Problems in the Application of Interpersonal Psychotherapy for Dysthymia

Treatment Sought for the Acute Precipitant

A common problem the IPT therapist confronts in treating dysthymia involves patients who seek treatment because their depressive symptoms have worsened due to an acute precipitant. These patients determinedly seek relief from the acute distress but do not consider changing their ordinary way of functioning, having an affective disorder so insidious and chronic that they are inured to its pervasive influence.

A defensive self-protectiveness and protests of helplessness, hopelessness, and vulnerability may be evident if changes in chronic maladaptive interpersonal behaviors related to dysthymia are proposed. Behaviors such as social withdrawal and isolation may contribute to the dysthymia, but the dysthymic patient also perceives these behaviors as protecting a fragile self-esteem from exposure to rejection, criticism, abandonment, and so on, which feels potentially much worse than the status quo of dysthymia. Motivation to change may be increased by successfully applying IPT techniques to dispel the distress associated with the acute problem area. However, some dysthymic patients will be inclined to terminate treatment once the acute distress is alleviated, and psychoeducation regarding dysthymia and its treatment should be provided in the initial sessions and reinforced throughout the course of IPT as needed, in order to promote resolution of the chronic affective disorder.

Ms. A. is a 37-year-old white divorced bookkeeper who sought treatment for worsening symptoms at the time that a retrial was scheduled for the neighborhood hoodlum who shot her on a dare as she was walking by the local playground. The previous trial had ended with a hung jury, and Ms. A. presented depressed, angry, and obsessed with obtaining his conviction. She described herself as having been depressed her whole life: "When I look, I can't pick out a whole lot of good days in 37 years." She described the related feeling that her life was never going to change and that she had no control over changing, just surviving, taking no interest or pleasure in anything.

The interpersonal inventory revealed that her parents were depressed, physically and verbally abusive, and inappropriately dependent on her. They had forced her to marry the 23-year-old drug-addicted man who impregnated her when she was 16 years old. He was imprisoned for drug-related manslaughter shortly after their marriage, after which she was supported by welfare. She subsequently obtained her high school Graduate Equivalency Diploma, graduated from college, and got a job as a bookkeeper. Despite her good pay, she disliked her work, but always did what was convenient and practical. Probing her feelings about her ex-husband revealed that she felt he should have been more remorseful about shooting and killing a bystander in a drug war. She was able to make the connection that the kid who shot her reminded her of her ex-husband, and that her explosive feelings about the trial related to long-standing feelings of being abused by those around her whom she should have been able to depend on.

The IPT problem area of role transition was chosen in keeping with her wish to put behind her the court case and all the pain, fear, anger, and helplessness it represented. Understanding the relationship between the trial and her ex-husband, and how her intense feelings during the court case fit into the context of her life, helped her feel better. She was able to derive satisfaction from recognizing that she was both a fighter and a compassionate woman.

The interpersonal inventory also revealed that this appealing woman led an extremely socially isolated existence, having only one friend (who lived out of state) and a depressed daughter. She had a history of only two relationships following her divorce, both with nonmonogamous policemen, the first an abuser of alcohol and the second who was subsequently killed in the line of duty. The emptiness in her life was underscored when she won her case and her assailant was convicted. At first she reported feeling great—she had wanted to be taken seriously and had wanted her assailant to take his crime against her seriously—but then she felt let down, "like there was nobody there for me. There should be someone in my life to go through these things with." Her innate determination and expressed discontent with her isolation suggested that the interpersonal deficits problem area should be addressed, as it appeared powerfully associated with the maintenance of her dysthymia.

With encouragement, she identified her desires in life and identified obstacles that had to be surmounted in order to meet these goals. For example, she presented with marked facial impassivity, possibly because to invite interpersonal attention when she was growing up often was to invite violence. Her lack of expressiveness hindered her goal of initiating new relationships, and she had to be helped to remember to smile and make appropriate eye contact. She overcame her fatigue and her fear of going out alone, joined a health club, bought a party dress, and initiated career counseling in anticipation of a change to a more gratifying and interpersonally involving job. Each moment spent out of bed and in interpersonally productive and engaging activity was an accomplishment that was associated with diminishing of somatic complaints and lessening of her concern that she could not maintain her mood improvement. After 16 IPT sessions, her Ham-D score had decreased from 20 to 4, and her prognosis was considered good for continuing to use IPT principles to maintain euthymia. A follow-up rating 3 months after the last IPT session found her Ham-D score to be 8, with a normal, nondepressed mood.

Changing Long-standing Behaviors That Are Contributing to Dysthymia

In IPT the assumption is made 1) that the development of depression occurs in a social field and 2) that clarifying, reconstructing, and/or changing the social interpersonal context of a patient contributes to recovery. As illustrated in the previous case example, many dysthymic patients seek treatment because their symptoms have worsened in response to an acute stressor. Resolution of acute distress may provide some relief, similar to a partial response to an antidepressant. However, the acute stressor is unrelated to the onset and persistence of the dysthymia. Failure to diagnose and treat the factors in the patient's social field that are central to dysthymia leaves the patient vulnerable to full return of depressive symptoms, similar to a partial responder to antidepressant medication.

Ms. B., a 29-year-old single Hispanic woman, sought treatment for depression that she associated with feeling out of control in her 2-year relationship with a younger man, expressing the fear that "he will desert." His distancing when she moved closer emotionally increased her fears that he had an interest in another woman or did not respect her. Ms. B.'s depressive symptoms varied with the level of his expressed ambivalence. She attempted to intellectualize her feelings and master them by projecting them upon the world, pronouncing during a moment of disillusionment that "the world is at a crisis of mankind being at its worst, turning into objects of consumption; if you don't satisfy someone the way they want you to, they put you in the trash."

Ms. B. was aware of her boyfriend's having lied to his former girlfriend in order to be with her. Despite not trusting him, she entered into a relationship with him. She was disappointed that he refused to live with her, but he did pay for her expenses while she was looking for a job, thereby acknowledging some commitment to and responsibility for her.

Role dispute was initially chosen as the problem area to be focused on, with the aim of helping Ms. B. to renegotiate and resolve the nonreciprocal role expectations in her relationship with her boyfriend and thereby relieve the depressive symptoms that fluctuated with the boyfriend's ambivalence toward her. However, taking the interpersonal inventory revealed that prior to leaving her native country, the patient deferred to her parents on important life decisions because their disapproval of her was the hardest thing for her to bear. She also lived with a man for years in a relationship characterized by the same insecurities and infidelities as the current one, staying on even though she could never love him the same way after discovering infidelities. Analysis of these interpersonal themes indicated an elemental need to depend on someone else for her sustenance, to the extent that she would diminish her functioning and trade away her feelings of competency, self-worth, and personal adequacy.

The therapist proposed that this pattern was more central to maintaining the dysthymia than was the current interpersonal dispute with her boyfriend, which was simply the latest manifestation of this maladaptive interpersonal strategy. The patient agreed to address this chronic contributing factor to her dysthymia. She indicated that her insecurity was the worst flaw in their relationship and felt "challenged to seek inside and cure my deficiency in needing him." A role-transition model was implemented to help her relinquish her long-standing dependency on boyfriends for emotional stability and completeness. Ms. B. observed during her fifth IPT session that she saw her boyfriend in a more balanced way and was more aware of his needs. This made her feel more secure because "a god needs a goddess, but a man needs a woman like me."

She completed 12 IPT sessions, during which time she realized her goals of admission to a Ph.D. program and a professional-level job, in addition to significant diminution of her feelings of desperation regarding men. Her baseline Ham-D of 22 had decreased to 3 at the time of her termination from treatment, despite her boyfriend actually "deserting" her at the time of her seventh IPT session.

Booster Sessions for Dysthymic Patients Who Are in Early Recovery

The data presented in the last section of this chapter indicate that dysthymic patients can respond to IPT treatment within the standard 16-session format designed for acutely depressed patients. However, the option of booster sessions bears careful consideration as a way to maintain gains accrued in acute treatment. Given that dysthymic patients' maladaptive interpersonal modes are deeply ingrained, they may be a population at serious risk for relapse and therefore candidates for maintenance therapy. On the other hand, many dysthymic individuals have dependent personality components and tend to empower others, as in the case of Ms. B. above. In such cases, facilitating independence and a sense of personal competence and self-sufficiency are of primary importance. However, for patients with very impoverished interpersonal resources, as in the case below, scheduled monthly booster sessions may be crucial to maintaining gains and preventing relapse.

Ms. C. is a 35-year-old single white female from an upper-middle-class background who had been depressed her whole life and presented for treatment of increasing feelings of alienation, tension, guilt, and hypersomnia related to her isolating work in the business department of a large corporation. The interpersonal inventory revealed that she was the friendless only child of a sexually abusive alcoholic father and a schizophrenic mother who had multiple hospitalizations throughout the patient's childhood. The parents' pathology was never discussed or overtly acknowledged while she was growing up, and no adult was available to provide Ms. C. with a sense of normal relatedness, to model social skills, or to help her develop social confidence. Ms. C. described her experience of her parents as one of strangeness, disappointment, deception, and lack of nurture, and of feeling responsible for them. For example, her father would conceal that his drinking cost him jobs and would then be unable to pay her private school tuition and unable or unwilling to negotiate scholarship aid. She would unexpectedly have to change schools at the same time that her father was preaching that persons of their class did not attend public schools. He forbade the patient to close the door to her room, intruded on her privacy, and forced her to exhibit herself to him when she was undressing. The patient was completely dissociated from her anger at both parents. The few men with whom she had had relationships were from backgrounds very different from her own. These relationships were characterized by infrequent contact, as she dreaded being intruded on or pressured as she had been by her father. Ms. C. stated that she would like to have a close relationship built on security and trust but did not feel physically attracted to men who could offer her this; put off by their gregariousness and arrogance, she saw them as "neuters" or felt herself to be neuter with them so that sex seemed clumsy and embarrassing. Tall and uncomfortable with her height, and self-conscious about a self-perceived lack of athletic ability, she was currently involved with an unemployed Puerto Rican man 10 years her senior who lived in a basement. Although she was discontented with her boyfriend's passivity and poor planning for the future, which she associated with her father's behavior, and did not want to "move ahead" with him, she feared the loneliness of ending the relationship.

The IPT problem areas of role transitions and interpersonal deficits were selected to help Ms. C. relinquish her maladaptive view of her role in a relationship and develop new relationship behaviors. Strategies were developed to decrease her isolation at work to afford some socializing opportunities. Weeks of agonizing over her fears, role-playing, and identifying the best, worst, and most expectable outcomes predated her even going to the cafeteria for lunch. A work incident in which she was scapegoated made it clear that she did not know how *not* to be the victim. Nevertheless, as she felt more connected to people at work, her hypersomnia decreased and her productivity and energy improved. By Session 16 of her IPT, she felt reasonably good and accepted the termination of treatment, but was sorry to have IPT end, expressing a wish to extend it or to have monthly contact.

Ms. C. articulated that through IPT she had gained awareness of her anger and her inability to express it. She also had become aware of its relation to her isolation, depression, and fatigue, and could understand how that separated her from other people. She further was able to be aware of her father's effect on her expectations surrounding relationships, particularly in terms of intrusiveness and sex, which were the strongest feelings she had. She perceived that she felt best when she felt interpersonally connected but that her anger and concerns about intrusiveness defeated this social goal and made her feel separate from others. She also appreciated learning how reactive her depression was and how she tended to set unrealistically high expectations for herself so that she never felt confident or competent.

Ms. C. made major progress in treating her dysthymia using the role-transition and interpersonal-deficits models, and clearly benefited from this treatment. However, her Ham-D score was still modestly elevated at 13, suggesting incomplete resolution of dysthymic symptoms that could make her vulnerable to full return of depressive symptoms.

In such cases, it may make sense, given the background of extreme interpersonal impoverishment, to renegotiate the length of treatment in order to obtain a more complete response and then use monthly maintenance sessions to prevent relapse.

Recovery From Dysthymia Impeded by Chronic Psychopathology of the Untreated Spouse

Our general experience with dysthymic patients has been that persons with the chronic interpersonal problems associated with dysthymia tend not to be married. However, those individuals that do marry often seem to choose mates with similar chronic psychopathology—that is, they mate assortatively for dysthymia.

The case studies depicted above give a sense of how effortful and threatening it can be for dysthymic patients to change their maladaptive, self-protective behaviors. Instead of responding supportively, untreated dysthymic spouses may feel put off, threatened, or even angered by their spouse becoming more energized and interested in socializing. Consequently, it is important to take the spouse into account when devising an IPT treatment plan. The therapist must first assess the patient's feelings about the marriage to determine if the patient is committed to the relationship. If not, a role-transition model may be selected to help the patient end the relationship in a constructive manner. If the patient is committed to the relationship, the spouse's potential as an ally, rather than as an obstacle, to the IPT treatment should be developed and supported. This can be accomplished by employing strategies to include and mobilize the dysthymic spouse that do not arouse feelings of insecurity, betrayal, and vulnerability. The acceptance of positive change in the patient by his or her dysthymic spouse may be crucial in effecting and sustaining the patient's response to IPT.

Mr. D., a 38-year-old married security guard and avocational writer, reported being depressed his whole life, with an exacerbation of low energy, low libido, and poor self-esteem that he attributed to family strife involving his 12-year-old daughter. He described feeling upset by her emerging sexuality and at his ineffectualness in changing negative traits in her that he likewise perceives in himself (e.g., laziness and lying).

Mr. D. presented as bland, lethargic, and coy. He grinned inappropriately when describing the intense anger, resentment, and vengeful, violent fantasies that followed his frequent perceptions of being slighted by higher-status males. Behaviorally, he adopted a passive-aggressive stance, believing that either you "shut up and take it" or else lose control. He also believed that positive affect is dangerous because "it leaves you vulnerable."

The interpersonal inventory revealed that his father, a career military man, had been physically abusive and had abandoned the family when Mr. D. was 6 years old. The mother, alcoholic, depressed and unable to cope, placed Mr. D. and his younger sister in an orphanage for 2 years, where the siblings were separated and rarely able to see each other. Mr. D. joined the army at 18 years of age and never returned home except as a visitor.

Mr. D. reported having little contact with his relatives and no close friends, although he described some female colleagues and neighbors as potential friends, were it not for his wife's insecurity. He described his wife as overweight, reclusive, and chronically depressed. He stated that she "flies off the handle a lot" and uses him as a "whipping boy" when she is drinking. She "saws sawdust," looking for faults in others to ease her insecurity by forcing him to say, "You're the good one," or "I love you more." He described anger as having some exciting quality and found provoking his wife to be "better than sex."

The IPT role-transition model was selected to facilitate his acceptance of his daughter's maturation, and the interpersonal-deficits model was used to help him decrease his interpersonal inappropriateness and isolation. Mr. D. quickly became energized in the treatment, writing and submitting a story that was accepted for publication in a literary magazine, and made plans to buy a car to decrease boredom and facilitate socializing.

Ms. D. responded to her husband's mobilization with inertia and (unfounded) concern about their finances. One hypothesis was that his passivity assured that he would not leave her. After his commitment to the marriage was explored and verified, techniques and related homework assignments were developed to entice his wife into going out and having a pleasurable experience. Although her initial response would be "no," she would end up having a good time if he did not give up too soon and say that he would go by himself.

Mr. D.'s Ham-D score decreased from 27 to 3 over the course of 16 IPT sessions, but it was felt that he would have a poor prognosis for sustaining and extending these gains if his wife remained untreated and exerted the familiar pull toward lethargy, passivity, and isolation. Ms. D. refused to seek treatment for her own dysthymia. However, the strategies to decrease Mr. D.'s social isolation and inertia included his wife. As a result, she may have experienced a decrease in social isolation with a subsequent diminution of depressive severity. Furthermore, this treatment strategy was oriented toward helping this rejection-sensitive woman feel included, rather than left out, as her husband responded to therapy. Consequently, she agreed to participate in family therapy upon Mr. D.'s completion of IPT treatment.

Preliminary Research

In this section we summarize results from a preliminary trial of IPT for dysthymia in a quasi-experimental comparison with desipramine, a tricyclic antidepressant. The parent compound of desipramine is imipramine, a tricyclic antidepressant that has established efficacy for dysthymia (Kocsis et al. 1988a, 1988b).

Description of Treatment

Characteristics of the patients in the samples involved in this study are given in Table 9–1. Each weekly IPT session lasted 50 minutes. The planned treatment duration was 16 IPT sessions, but four patients terminated prematurely, resulting in an average of 12 sessions per patient. Dr. Mason was the therapist for all IPT cases. Following the classification of problem areas in IPT (Klerman et al. 1984), a primary problem area and a secondary problem area were designated for each patient. As shown in Table 9–2, there were four patients who were judged as having interpersonal deficits, two with interpersonal disputes and three with role transition as their primary problem area.

Desipramine subjects were treated with medication for an average of 14.1 weeks in this study. Clinically indicated doses of desipramine were individually prescribed, based on standardized ratings of response and side effects. The average dose prescribed was 216.67 (SD = 57.28) mg per day.

Design

This comparison study was an uncontrolled clinical trial; no randomization procedures were employed. Patients had to meet DSM-III-R criteria for dysthymia and have a 24-item Ham-D score of 14 or higher to qualify for admission to a study of desipramine treatment of dysthymia. Patients ($n = 9$) were assigned to IPT if they met the above criteria but refused to accept drug treatment, or if they failed to fully respond to desipramine by Week 10 of that study. Nonresponse was defined as a Ham-D score of 12 or greater. Partial response was defined as a Ham-D score of less than 12 but greater than 6, and full recovery was defined as a Ham-D score of less than

Table 9–1.   Demographic and clinical characteristics of the interpersonal psychotherapy and desipramine treatment groups

			IPT sample[a]		
Patient	Age	Sex	Marital status	Duration of depression	Current exacerbation
D01	46	F	Single	Lifelong	6 years
D02	36	F	Divorced	Lifelong	None
D03	42	F	Divorced	Lifelong	1.5 years
D04	29	F	Separated	Lifelong	None
D05	35	F	Single	Lifelong	5 years
D06	42	M	Married	3 years	3 years
D07	36	M	Married	Lifelong	5 years
D08	38	F	Divorced	Lifelong	1 year
D09	29	F	Single	2 years	2 years
			Desipramine sample[b]		
C01	42	F	Single	Lifelong	2.5 years
C02	28	M	Single	16 years	2 years
C03	32	M	Single	15 years	2 years
C04	43	F	Single	26 years	None
C05	32	M	Single	8 years	None
C06	30	F	Single	8 years	None
C07	27	F	Single	12 years	5 years
C08	25	M	Single	Lifelong	6 years
C09	44	F	Single	22 years	None

[a]Mean age = 37.31 years; male:female = 2:7; mean current exacerbation = 3.4 years.
[b]Mean age = 33.7 years; male:female = 4:5; mean current exacerbation = 3.5 years.

7. These patients were continued on desipramine while IPT was added so as to determine whether IPT could promote full recovery in patients not fully responsive to medication.

Comparison of IPT With Desipramine-Treated Sample

To assess the therapeutic efficacy of IPT relative to antidepressant medication, a quasi-experimental comparison was undertaken. From the sample of 25 patients—representing all response categories, with ages between 25 and 49 years—who had completed more than 3 weeks in the desipramine trial, 9 patients were chosen by computer-generated randomization for comparison with the IPT sample. This yielded a sample of 9 desipramine subjects and 9 IPT subjects, whose demographic and clinical characteristics are presented in Table 9–1. Ideally, there would be a group receiving neither drug nor placebo to control for treatment expectancy effects. However, the low rate of placebo response found in dysthymic patients (Barrett 1984; McCullough et al. 1988) indicates that expectancy effects are not a powerful determinant of treatment response in dysthymia. A double-blind clinical trial including the desipramine-treated patients from this study yielded a placebo response rate of less than 13% (Kocsis et al. 1988a, 1988b).

Table 9–2. Interpersonal psychotherapy treatment variables

| | | IPT problem area | | |
Patient	Sequence of IPT[a]	Primary	Secondary	No. of sessions
D01	1	Deficits	Transition	16
D02	1	Deficits	Transition	16
D03	1	Dispute	Deficits	3
D04	1	Transition	None	11
D05	1	Deficits	None	16
D06	2	Deficits	Dispute	16
D07	2	Transition	Deficits	5
D08	2	Transition	Deficits	16
D09	2	Dispute	Transition	9

[a]Sequence of IPT indicates whether patients were referred to IPT as the primary treatment, with no antecedent treatment (1), or as an adjunctive treatment after failing the double-blind desipramine trial (2).

Assessment of Change

Assessment of depressive severity was made before and after treatment on the clinician-rated Hamilton Rating Scale for Depression (Ham-D; Hamilton 1960) and the self-rated Beck Depression Inventory (BDI; Beck 1967). The Global Assessment Scale (GAS; Endicott et al. 1976) was used to measure level of overall functioning. Independent assessors (i.e., research psychiatrists) rated IPT subjects. Ratings of desipramine subjects were done by the treating psychiatrist, as per the study protocol.

Statistical Methods

The hypothesis that efficacy of IPT is comparable to that of desipramine for treatment of dysthymia was tested by comparing the rank order of change scores on the Ham-D, the BDI, and the GAS in IPT and desipramine subjects with the Mann-Whitney U test. This nonparametric procedure was chosen to test the study's hypothesis in order to diminish the influence any extreme score might have in a relatively small sample (Conover 1980). The Mann-Whitney U test was also used to establish equivalence of pre- and posttreatment clinical measures (Ham-D, BDI, GAS) between the two groups. Additionally, Mann-Whitney U tests were used to compare pre- and posttreatment clinical measures of those IPT subjects who were originally desipramine nonresponders with those IPT subjects who were not treated with desipramine prior to IPT. All tests were two-tailed.

Results

Characteristics of the Sample

The drug-treated sample was statistically equivalent to the IPT sample in age and gender. Marital status differed between groups (Chi square = 11.78, df = 4, $P = .02$) as shown in Table 9–1, with desipramine subjects all being single. Ham-D, BDI, and GAS scores at baseline did not vary between groups. Individual and group scores on pretreatment measures are presented in Table 9–3.

The IPT sample was predominantly female (78%). The average age was 37 (range 29–46) years. Patients had long-standing disorder, with current exacerbations averaging 3.4 years. Seven of the patients described themselves as having been depressed "lifelong," similar to the self-assessment of a group of early-onset characterologically depressed patients described by Akiskal (1983). These seven patients could be considered to have "double depression" (Keller and Shapiro 1982).

The desipramine sample was likewise predominantly female (56%). The average age was 33.7 (range 25–44) years. Patients treated with desipramine also had long-standing dysthymia, with current exacerbations averaging 3.5 years.

Table 9–3. Comparison of mean and mean rank ratings for interpersonal psychotherapy and desipramine groups

Between groups	IPT Mean	SD	(MR)	Desipramine Mean	SD	(MR)	U	P
Pre Ham-D	19.33	5.45	(8)	23.89	7.91	(11)	27.0	.231
Pre BDI	21.56	12.08	(8.5)	25.89	9.88	(10.5)	31.5	.426
Pre GAS	60.56	7.68	(11.22)	54.78	5.40	(7.78)	25.0	.160
Post Ham-D	7.22	4.42	(9.78)	10.11	9.49	(9.22)	38.0	.822
Post BDI	8.38	5.76	(8.38)	11.57	14.22	(7.57)	25.0	.727
Post GAS	69.33	9.00	(9.39)	67.78	12.89	(9.61)	39.5	.929
Pre-post Ham-D	−12.11	6.37	(9.72)	−13.78	8.72	(9.28)	38.5	.860
Pre-post BDI	−12.38	10.66	(8.44)	−13.00	4.62	(7.50)	24.5	.685
Pre-post GAS	8.78	10.51	(8.33)	13.00	11.08	(10.67)	30.0	.351

Within groups	IPT Z	P	Desipramine Z	P
Pre-post Ham-D	2.67	.008	2.67	.008
Pre-post BDI	2.38	.028	2.37	.018
Pre-post GAS	2.20	.017	2.38	.017

Note. The Mann-Whitney U test (U) was used for between-group comparisons, and the Wilcoxon signed rank test (Z) was used for within-group comparisons. (MR) = mean rank; Ham-D = Hamilton Depression Rating Scale (Hamilton 1960); BDI = Beck Depression Inventory (Beck 1967); GAS = Global Assessment Scale (Endicott et al. 1976).

Psychotherapy Effects on Outcome Measures

The effects of IPT on the three outcome measures are shown in Table 9–3 and are depicted in Figure 9–1. Based on the Wilcoxon signed rank test, IPT patients displayed statistically significant ($P < .05$) reductions in Ham-D and BDI scores from baseline to termination, with a comparable increase in overall functioning as measured by the GAS.

For five patients IPT was used following an initial drug trial. These five patients had not adequately responded to a mean daily dose of 240 (SD = 41.83) mg per day of desipramine for a mean of 12.80 (SD = 2.28) weeks. However, they were continued on desipramine while receiving IPT to determine whether the addition of IPT would augment response and promote recovery. The other four patients agreed to IPT after refusing assignment to drug treatment.

The two groups did not differ significantly by age, gender, BDI scores, or GAS scores prior to beginning IPT. However, Ham-D scores of the IPT

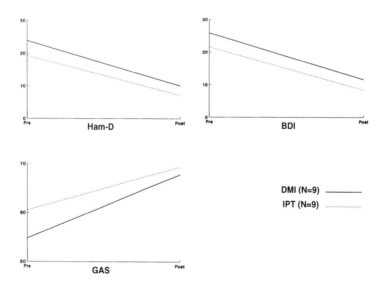

Figure 9–1. Baseline and termination scores on the Hamilton Depression Rating Scale (Ham-D), the Beck Depression Inventory (BDI), and the Global Assessment Scale (GAS) in dysthymic patients treated with interpersonal

group initially receiving DMI (mean = 15.80 ± 4.02) were found, based on the Mann-Whitney U test, to be significantly lower at time of entry into IPT than were the Ham-D scores (mean = 23.75 ± 3.30) of patients treated with IPT alone (U = − 0.5, corrected P = .02). This was primarily a function of one patient (D03) having achieved partial response to 250 mg per day of desipramine over a 6-week period, without further improvement in symptomatology after 10 additional weeks of pharmacotherapy. Addition of IPT was associated in this case with a 7 point (64%) decrease in Ham-D rating (i.e., achievement of full recovery). Similarly, another patient's (D04) Ham-D score had decreased only to 12 after 4 months of treatment with 250 mg per day of desipramine. She obtained a 7 point (58%) decrease in Ham-D rating with the addition of IPT (i.e., achievement of full recovery). Following IPT treatment, Ham-D, BDI, and GAS scores were equivalent in the two IPT groups.

Effects of Desipramine on Outcome Measures

The effects of desipramine without IPT on the three outcome measures are shown in Table 9–3 and Figure 9–1. Based on the Wilcoxon signed rank test, desipramine subjects were found to display significant (P < .01) reductions in Ham-D and BDI scores from baseline to termination, with a comparable increase in overall functioning, as measured by the GAS.

Comparative Efficacy of Treatments

The results from the Mann-Whitney U test indicate that the degree of improvement during IPT was comparable to that of patients treated in the desipramine trial. As shown in Table 9–3, the two treatment groups did not differ on any outcome measure.

Applying study criteria for nonresponse (Ham-D of > 11), partial response (Ham-D of > 6 and < 12) and full recovery (Ham-D of < 7) revealed equivalent proportions of subjects in each outcome category across groups. The IPT sample had two nonresponders, two partial responders, and five fully recovered patients. The desipramine sample had four nonresponders, no partial responders, and five fully recovered patients. Combining partial responders and fully recovered subjects yielded an overall response rate of 78% for IPT and 56% for desipramine. These figures are consistent with a previously reported 60% overall response rate of dysthymic patients to desipramine (Kocsis et al. 1988a).

Discussion

This study had a number of design and methodological limitations: raters were not blind to treatment, treatment assignments were not random, IPT was conducted by the same therapist, and sample size was small. IPT subjects who failed to adequately respond to lengthy trials of therapeutic doses of desipramine were combined with patients receiving IPT alone in order to augment IPT sample size. Ideally, there would be three separate treatment groups (IPT alone, desipramine alone, and IPT with desipramine) and a control group with neither IPT nor desipramine.

Nevertheless, the 78% rate of response to IPT is sufficiently encouraging to warrant more systematic exploration. Accordingly, research is underway to refine a manual to modify IPT for dysthymia and to assess the efficacy of IPT in dysthymia using a more rigorous research design. These data lend preliminary support to the use of IPT for dysthymia, both as a primary treatment for those patients unable or unwilling to take medication, and as a secondary treatment for dysthymic patients who are unresponsive to pharmacotherapy.

References

Akiskal HS: Subaffective disorders: dysthymic, cyclothymic, and bipolar II disorders in the "borderline" realm. Psychiatr Clin North Am 4:25–46, 1981

Akiskal HS: Dysthymic disorder: psychopathology of proposed chronic depressive subtypes. Am J Psychiatry 140:11–20, 1983

Akiskal HS, Rosenthal TL, Haykal RF, et al: Characterological depressions: clinical and sleep EEG findings separating "subaffective dysthymias" from "character spectrum disorders." Arch Gen Psychiatry 37:777–783, 1980

American Psychiatric Association: Diagnostic and Statistical Manual of Mental Disorders, 3rd Edition. Washington, DC, American Psychiatric Association, 1980

American Psychiatric Association: Diagnostic and Statistical Manual of Mental Disorders, 3rd Edition, Revised. Washington, DC, American Psychiatric Association, 1987

Arieti S, Bemporad J: Severe and Mild Depressions. New York, Basic Books, 1978

Barlow DH, DiNardo PA, Vermilyea BB, et al: Co-morbidity and depression among the anxiety disorders. J Nerv Ment Dis 174:63–72, 1986

Barrett JE: Naturalistic change after 2 years in neurotic depressive disorders (RDC categories). Compr Psychiatry 25:404–418, 1984

Beck A: Depression: Clinical, Experimental and Therapeutic Aspects. New York, Harper & Row, 1967

Beck AT, Rush AJ, Shaw BF, et al: Cognitive Therapy of Depression. New York, Guilford, 1979

Becker RE, Heimber RG, Bellack AS: Social Skills Training Treatment for Depression. New York, Pergamon, 1987

Bemporad J: Psychotherapy of the depressive character. J Am Acad Psychoanal 4:347–372, 1976

Bronisch T, Klerman GL: The current status of neurotic depression as a diagnostic category. Psychiatr Dev 4:245–275, 1988

Cassano GB, Perugi G, Maremmani I, et al: Social adjustment in dysthymia, in Dysthymic Disorder. Edited by Burton SW, Akiskal HS. London, Gaskell, 1990, pp 78–85

Conover WJ: Practical Nonparametric Statistics, 2nd Edition. New York, Wiley, 1980

Chodoff P: The depressive personality: a critical review. Arch Gen Psychiatry 25:666–673, 1972

Corney RH: Social work effectiveness in the management of depressed women: a clinical trial. Psychol Med 11:417–423, 1981

de Jong R, Treiber R, Henrich G: Effectiveness of two psychological treatments for inpatients with severe and chronic depressions. Cognitive Therapy and Research 10:645–663, 1986

Elkin I, Shea MT, Watkins JT, et al: National Institute of Mental Health Treatment of Depression Collaborative Research Program: general effectiveness of treatments. Arch Gen Psychiatry 46:971–982, 1989

Endicott J, Spitzer R, Fleiss J, et al: The Global Assessment Scale: a procedure for measuring overall severity of psychiatric disturbance. Arch Gen Psychiatry 33:766–771, 1976

Frank E, Kupfer DJ, Perel JM: Early recurrence in unipolar depression. Arch Gen Psychiatry 46:397–400, 1989

Frank E, Kupfer DJ, Perel JM, et al: Three-year outcomes for maintenance therapies in recurrent depression. Arch Gen Psychiatry 47:1093–1099, 1990

Gonzalez LR, Lewinsohn PM, Clarke GN: Longitudinal follow-up of unipolar depressives: an investigation of predictors of relapse. J Consult Clin Psychol 53:461–469, 1985

Hamilton M: A rating scale for depression. J Neurol Neurosurg Psychiatry 25:56–62, 1960

Harrison W, Rabkin J, Stewart JW, et al: Phenelzine for chronic depression: a study of continuation therapy. J Clin Psychiatry 47:346–349, 1986

Hooley JM, Teasdale JD: Predictors of relapse in unipolar depressives: expressed emotion, marital distress, and perceived criticism. J Abnorm Psychol 98:229–235, 1989

Jacobson E: Depression. New York, International Universities Press, 1971

Keller MB, Shapiro RW: "Double depression": superimposition of acute depressive episodes on chronic depressive disorders. Am J Psychiatry 139:438–442, 1982

Keller MB, Lavori PW, Endicott J, et al: "Double depression": two-year follow-up. Am J Psychiatry 140:689–694, 1983

Klein DN, Taylor EB, Harding K, et al: Double depression and episodic major depression: demographic, clinical, familial, personality, and socioenvironmental characteristics and short-term outcome. Am J Psychiatry 145:1226–1231, 1988

Klerman GL, Weissman MM, Rounsaville BJ, et al: Interpersonal Psychotherapy of Depression. New York, Basic Books, 1984

Kocsis JH, Frances AJ: A critical discussion of DSM-III dysthymic disorder. Am J Psychiatry 144:1534–1542, 1987

Kocsis JH, Voss C, Mann JJ, et al: Chronic depression: demographic and clinical characteristics. Psychopharmacol Bull 22:192–195, 1986

Kocsis JH, Frances AJ, Voss C, et al: Imipramine and social-vocational adjustment in chronic depression. Am J Psychiatry 145:997–999, 1988a

Kocsis JH, Frances AJ, Voss C, et al: Imipramine treatment for chronic depression. Arch Gen Psychiatry 45:253–257, 1988b

Kocsis JH, Markowitz JC, Prien RF: Comorbidity of dysthymic disorder, in Comorbidity in Anxiety and Mood Disorders. Edited by Maser JD, Cloninger CR. Washington, DC, American Psychiatric Press, 1990, pp 317–328

Koenigsberg HW, Kaplan RD, Gilmore MM, et al: The relationship between syndrome and personality disorder in DSM-III experience with 2,462 patients. Am J Psychiatry 142:207–212, 1985

Kovacs M, Feinberg TL, Crouse-Novak MA, et al: Depressive disorders in childhood, I: a longitudinal prospective study of characteristics and recovery. Arch Gen Psychiatry 41:229–237, 1984

Lazare A (ed): Outpatient Psychiatry. London, Williams & Wilkins, 1979

Markowitz JC, Moran ME, Kocsis JH, et al: Prevalence and comorbidity of dysthymic disorder. J Affective Disord 24:63–71, 1992

Mason BJ, Kocsis JH, Frances AJ: Cornell Dysthymia Rating Scale, in New Research and Abstracts, 142nd annual meeting of the American Psychiatric Association, San Francisco, CA, May 1989, NR231, p 134

McCullough JP: Psychotherapy for dysthymia: a naturalistic study of ten patients. J Nerv Ment Dis 179:734–740, 1991

McCullough JP, Kasnetz MD, Braith JA, et al: Longitudinal study of an untreated sample of predominantly late onset characterological dysthymia. J Nerv Ment Dis 176:658–667, 1988

Parsons T: Illness and the role of the physician: a sociological perspective. Am J Orthopsychiatry 21:452–460, 1951

Paykel ES, Rowen PR, Parker RR, et al: Response to phenelzine and amitriptyline in subtypes of outpatient depression. Arch Gen Psychiatry 39:1041–1049, 1982

Rounsaville BJ, Sholomkas D, Prusoff BA: Chronic mood disorders in depressed outpatients. J Affective Disord 2(2):73–88, 1980

Stewart JW, Quitkin FM, McGrath PJ, et al: Social functioning in chronic depression: effect of 6 weeks of antidepressant treatment. Psychiatry Res 25:213–222, 1988

Ward NG, Bloom VL, Friedel RO: The effectiveness of tricyclic antidepressants in chronic depression. J Clin Psychiatry 40:49–52, 1979

Weissman MM, Akiskal HS: The role of psychotherapy in chronic depressions: a proposal. Compr Psychiatry 25:23–31, 1984

Weissman MM, Bothwell S: Assessment of social adjustment by patient self-report. Arch Gen Psychiatry 33:1111–1115, 1976

Weissman MM, Leaf PJ, Bruce ML, et al: The epidemiology of dysthymia in five communities: rates, risks, comorbidity, and treatment. Am J Psychiatry 145:815–819, 1988a

Weissman MM, Leaf PJ, Tischler GL, et al: Affective disorders in five United States communities. Psychol Med 18:141–153, 1988b

Wells KB, Stewart A, Hays RD, et al: The functioning and well-being of depressed patients: results from the Medical Outcomes Study. JAMA 262:914–919, 1989

Zimmerman M, Pfohl B, Coryell W, et al: Diagnosing personality disorder in depressed patients: a comparison of patient and informant interviews. Arch Gen Psychiatry 45:733–737, 1988

C H A P T E R   1 0

Applications of Interpersonal Psychotherapy to Depression in Primary Care Practice

Herbert C. Schulberg, Ph.D.
C. Paul Scott, M.D.
Michael J. Madonia, M.S.W.
Stanley D. Imber, Ph.D.

In more than 80 epidemiological studies conducted over the past two decades, investigators consistently have found that depressive disorders are highly prevalent among patients treated by primary care physicians. Structured interview schedules were administered in 11 of these studies, and from their findings Katon and Schulberg (1992) concluded that 4.8% to 8.6% of ambulatory medical patients meet diagnostic criteria for a current major depression. The point prevalence of dysthymia approximates 2.1% to 3.7%, of minor depression 3.4% to 4.7%, and of intermittent depression 5.0%. The total point prevalence of diagnosable affective disorders in primary care practice, thus, ranges from 15% to 22%. At least as many ambulatory medical patients report mood and neurovegetative symptoms at a distressing but subclinical level of severity.

Preparation of this chapter was supported by Grant MH-45815 from the National Institute of Mental Health, Bethesda, Maryland. We express appreciation to the clinicians serving as IPT therapists in our study: Patricia Cluss, Ph.D., Judy Grumet, Ph.D., Robert Howland, M.D., Barry Judd, M.D., Ana Rivera-Tovar, Ph.D., and Mark Webb, M.D.

265

In addition to depression's high prevalence in the ambulatory medical sector, it also has been found that a) comorbid physical illnesses intensify the depression's severity (Coulehan et al. 1990; Wells et al. 1989); 2) persons with affective illness utilize the health care system at significantly higher rates than persons without psychiatric illness (Katon et al. 1990); and 3) treatments for depression are readily available but underutilized or utilized inappropriately by generalist physicians (Callies and Popkin 1987; Gullick and King 1979).

Recognizing these epidemiological, clinical, and service delivery issues, various providers and researchers have focused on the question of which treatment could be used to most effectively resolve the depression experienced by ambulatory medical patients (Blacker and Clare 1987; Goldberg 1988; Katon 1987). Concern also has been expressed as to whether interpersonal psychotherapy (IPT) retains its demonstrated effectiveness (Klerman et al. 1984) when delivered in medical settings rather than psychiatric ones.

In light of these uncertainties, we first consider emerging national guidelines for treating depression in primary medical care and the clinical ambiguities still to be addressed in future investigations. We then describe the characteristics of major depression experienced by medical patients in terms of the disorder's severity and comorbidity, as well as treatment practices and constraints associated with the unique sociocultural and medical rituals of primary care facilities. Case examples germane to each of IPT's four problem areas are provided to illustrate the psychotherapeutic management of a mood disorder presenting in the medical setting, where comorbid physical illness often affects the patient's chief complaint and course of depression.

Depression Treatment Guidelines

A significant gap is evident between the growing body of scientific knowledge about how to assess and treat depression, and the continuing failure of primary care physicians to apply this knowledge in routine medical practice. This disparity led the United States Public Health Service's Agency for Health Care Policy and Research (AHCPR) in 1990 to include affective disorders among the seven medical conditions initially selected for guideline development (Rush et al. 1992). Through this effort, the federal government is formulating treatment guidelines and options that are designed to assist primary care practitioners and their patients with decisions about appropriate care for depression in specific clinical circumstances. Within the framework of these AHCPR practice guidelines, care of depression is deemed appropriate when the psychiatric, physical, and social benefits of treatment appreciably outweigh the expected negative outcomes. Conversely, the care is judged inappropriate when the risks appreciably exceed the anticipated benefits.

The AHCPR Depression Panel responsible for establishing guidelines for the diagnosis and treatment of depression will present its findings and recommendations to the federal government in 1993. Among the topics is the role of IPT and other psychosocial treatments in resolving depression during the acute, continuing, and maintenance phases of therapy. Treatment during the acute phase aims at removing symptoms of depression and typically lasts 2 to 4 months. Continuation treatment seeks to prevent a relapse of symptoms and usually is of 6 to 9 months' duration. Maintenance treatment seeks to prevent or reduce the frequency of further episodes (recurrences) and can extend for 2 to 3 years (or even longer given recent findings by Frank et al. [1990]).

The AHCPR panel is analyzing randomized controlled clinical trials for findings about outcome of acute episodes. Pending publication of this comprehensive review, it would appear from several major studies that there is a 45% to 55% probability of very significant improvement or remission among patients treated with time-limited psychotherapy alone (Elkin et al. 1989; Murphy et al. 1984; Rush et al. 1977). There is little evidence of direct and immediate harm or complications during such acute phase treatment with IPT or cognitive therapy. If the effectiveness of psychotherapy is substantiated by the AHCPR review, this may well be the treatment of choice for primary care patients experiencing a mild or moderate depression, and for those whose psychosocial problems are chronic in nature or are markedly troublesome during the acute mood episode. Other reports indicate that if the depression is not recurrent, there is a 50% to 75% probability of staying well by continuing treatment with psychotherapy alone (e.g., Blackburn et al. 1981) and a minimal chance of significant harm during this extended phase of treatment. If the AHCPR review supports this conclusion as well, psychotherapy alone may be clinically useful for the sizable segment of primary care patients who cannot be medicated for health reasons, who refuse to take additional drugs, who will not comply with prescribed dosages because of intolerable side effects, or who are unresponsive to drug treatments. With regard to psychotherapy's effectiveness during the maintenance phase of treatment, monthly IPT sessions successfully delay recurrence among persons experiencing multiple depressive episodes (Frank et al. 1989) but when provided alone at this frequency are less effective than full dosage antidepressant medication (Frank et al. 1990).

Because evidence regarding the effectiveness of psychotherapy and pharmacotherapy is derived from studies conducted with depressed patients at psychiatric facilities, Schulberg et al. (1991b) have questioned whether these tertiary care findings pertain to depressed primary care patients as well. The question's cogency is supported by earlier reports that major depression in primary care patients may be less severe, of briefer duration, and more affected by physical comorbidity than it is in psychiatric patients (Blacker and Clare 1987). The AHCPR Depression Panel recognizes this clinical uncertainty but likely will conclude that, absent data to the contrary, treatment outcome patterns derived in psychiatric settings form a reasonable basis for selecting treatments in ambulatory medical practice.

This critical assumption requires scientific validation. Randomized controlled trials (RCTs) are appropriate for this purpose but have rarely been implemented. Despite their methodological rigor, the costs and practical complexities of RCTs are formidable. Certainly, no investigator has yet conducted an RCT to determine the efficacy of IPT in treating a depressed medical population. Given this lack of relevant information, University of Pittsburgh researchers are investigating the clinical course of depressed primary care patients who have been randomized for treatment to either IPT alone, nortriptyline alone, or a physician's "usual care" (Schulberg et al. 1991b). Study findings will address the question of IPT's effectiveness when extended into a clinical population rarely treated with this psychotherapy, as well as the broader issue of whether treatment standards are validly generalized across different sectors of the health delivery system.

Evaluating the Effectiveness
of Interpersonal Psychotherapy
in Primary Care Patients

The effectiveness of IPT in treating currently depressed primary care patients remains scientifically unproven. Nevertheless, IPT or other forms of psychotherapy are a treatment option for individuals seeking help for depression, including those persons who are unwilling or unable to take an antidepressant medication. The effectiveness of pharmacotherapy in primary care practice similarly is scientifically uncertain. It may be prescribed for those primary care patients seeking medication and/or those resisting psychotherapy because they view depression as a biological rather than a psychological disorder. Given a continued demand for both types of treatment, findings from a clinical trial investigating the effectiveness of each will permit physicians and their patients to make choices based upon scientific evidence as well as personal preference.

A crucial conceptual decision in designing a meaningful clinical trial is the intervention with which the effectiveness of psychotherapy or pharmacotherapy is to be compared. In addition to its implications for sample size, the selected yardstick must be clinically relevant to physicians reviewing the study's findings if current practice is to be modified. We therefore consider the outcome produced by an internist or family practitioner's "usual care" the proper reference condition. The nature of "usual care" for depression differs among physicians; it may include psychotherapy, pharmacotherapy, or no treatment at all. This intervention nevertheless consistently expresses the physician's composite clinical judgment about the patient as a total person—that is, the relative importance of various biopsychosocial factors in the patient's syndrome and, most importantly, whether depression-specific interventions are indicated. By comparing the outcome experienced by patients receiving psychotherapy or pharmacotherapy with outcomes experienced by patients receiving a physician's "usual care," we can determine whether treatments provided within the guidelines already validated with psychiatric patients are superior to the "usual care" provided primary care patients by their own physicians.

We have hypothesized that psychotherapeutic and pharmacological treatments for depression delivered within treatment manual standards are significantly more effective than a physician's "usual care." This hypothesis is being tested in an RCT (funded by the National Institute of Mental Health) designed to balance internal and external validity (i.e., scientific rigor with features maximizing the generalizability of outcome findings) (Schulberg et al. 1991a). To achieve this balance, our protocol incorporates key methodological decisions about characteristics of the research setting, the clinicians who are providing treatment, and the population of eligible depressed medical patients. We believe that, collectively, these decisions advance existing frameworks for studying the effectiveness of IPT and other depression-specific treatments in primary care practice.

Research Setting

Depressed ambulatory medical patients who can be treated within the primary care setting are best managed there because many do not comply with a referral to a specialist facility (Byrd and Moskowitz 1987). Given this reality, research on treatment effectiveness with a medical population should be performed in the medical setting if outcome data are to be ecologically valid. Our study, therefore, is being conducted in a general internal medicine clinic and two family health centers typifying large urban fee-for-service primary care practices with patient populations from lower socioeconomic classes. Whereas pharmacotherapy of depression is an established treatment in the medical setting, IPT is not. Administrative and clinical accommodations by the health center and by the researcher are needed if psychotherapy is to be delivered in conformance with both routine medical facility practice and IPT treatment manual requirements. Given our desire to maximize the generalizability of our study findings while maintaining the specificity of IPT, we describe later in this chapter how IPT sessions are conducted in the health center and how they resemble or differ from psychotherapy sessions in a mental health center.

Clinicians

In selecting clinicians to deliver protocol treatments, we again have been strongly influenced by the wish to generalize findings about treatment effectiveness to practitioners at other health centers. Earlier reports indicated that primary care physicians routinely prescribe antidepressants

(Beardsley et al. 1988; Haggerty et al. 1986), so we are utilizing internists and family practitioners rather than psychiatrists as the study's pharmacotherapists. We were readily able to recruit and train such primary care physicians in treatment manual procedures for prescribing nortriptyline (Fawcett et al. 1987). Audiotaped monitoring of the physicians' interactions with patients indicated that compliance remains high on such pharmacotherapy procedures as identifying and focusing on target symptoms, maintaining dosage schedules, and avoiding psychodynamic themes.

While primary care physicians can serve as pharmacotherapists, it is unclear whether they are professionally skilled and/or motivated to serve as psychotherapists in routine medical practice. Even if the RCT could successfully recruit and train physicians in IPT procedures, the feasibility of extending their psychotherapeutic role beyond the research protocol into daily activities is uncertain. We therefore have selected psychiatrists and psychologists to deliver IPT, and they do so within the treatment manual specifications established by Klerman et al. (1984).

Patients

An RCT investigating treatments for major depression in medical patients must enroll subjects who meet DSM-III-R criteria (American Psychiatric Association 1987) for this disorder, and who also are clinically eligible on additional inclusionary/exclusionary criteria for randomization to any of the study's three treatment conditions. By choosing pertinent clinical criteria and by systematically assessing potential subjects to determine their eligibility, the investigator increases the study's internal validity. A consequence of this "purifying" strategy, however, is that RCT subjects often constitute but a small proportion of the patient population experiencing the disorder. Thus, the quest for scientific rigor in the RCT typically is achieved at the price of diminished generalizability.

Given our desire to test IPT's effectiveness with depressed ambulatory medical patients and to generate valid findings applicable beyond the participating study sites, what, then, has been our recruitment experience during the RCT's initial 6 months?

Depressed primary care patients may be recruited for an RCT in any of several ways. The first is to assess and randomize those patients identified by their primary care physicians as depressed. The resulting subgroup would include patients whom physicians clearly judge as needing treatment, but it would exclude the majority of potentially eligible depressed patients, because physicians fail to diagnose this disorder properly in the course of routine practice (Blacker and Clare 1987). A second recruitment strategy is to advertise for eligible subjects among patients at the participating health center study sites, a technique commonly used in clinical research. The resulting patient cohort likely would be motivated to comply with protocol procedures. However, the cohort would not include depressed patients failing to recognize their symptoms as a mood disorder nor those unable or unwilling to initiate help-seeking behavior. A third recruitment strategy, that which we chose to utilize, is to assess all health center patients waiting to meet their physicians for a regular medical visit. While this strategy inevitably stimulates refusals from persons unwilling to consider the possibility that they are depressed or unwilling to participate in a research project, approaching all health center patients minimizes selection bias while maximizing the pool of clinically eligible patients who are willing to accept a randomized treatment assignment.

Major Depression in Primary Care Practice

The nature of major depression in primary care practice creates complex diagnostic and treatment decisions for internists and family practitioners as well as psychiatrists. Cameron (1990), Cohen-Cole and Stoudemire (1987), Katon and Sullivan (1990), and others have emphasized the following factors:

1. A functional depression may mimic a recognized medical disorder.
2. Depressive signs may indicate a true underlying medical disorder.
3. Depressive symptoms may occur as a functional reaction to the impairment created by a medical disorder.
4. A functional depression may occur simultaneously with an unrelated medical disorder.

Before considering some of these depression–medical illness subtypes, it should be noted that various researchers (e.g., Abbey et al. 1990; Williamson and Yates 1989) have studied whether severity of depressive symptoms can differentiate affective and organic disorders. Cameron (1990) concluded from such analyses that depressed patients typically experience more severe mood and neurovegetative symptomatology. However, much of the earlier research suffers from logical circularity because the diagnosis of depression typically considers, at least in part, the presence of more intense symptoms. Cameron suggested, therefore, that depression be diagnosed on the basis of clinical symptoms different from those that are likely to characterize a medical illness.

Accurately assessing symptom severity and determining whether a medical patient has a coexisting depressive syndrome have significant implications for choice of treatment. As was noted previously, medical illness and depression have additive effects. Because persons experiencing both disorders experience greater morbidity and mortality (Fava et al. 1988), interventions are indicated for the depression as well as the medical illness.

Somatic Concomitants of Depressive Disorder

In their prior review of how functional depression can mimic a recognized medical disorder, Schulberg et al. (1987) emphasized that major depressive disorder is a complex psychobiological syndrome involving mood disturbance, neurovegetative signs, and/or distorted cognitive schemata. From the physiological perspective, major depressive disorder involves multilevel impairment of brain neurotransmitters, hormonal systems, circadian rhythm, and rapid eye movement (REM) sleep (Katon 1982). However, this disorder can also be a severe reaction to overwhelmingly stressful life events and interpersonal losses. From a phenomenological perspective, the symptoms include a sad mood; loss of interest, motivation, and pleasure; increased guilt; impaired concentration; changes in appetite, weight, and sleep; and thoughts of death or suicide.

Some patients experience disturbing life events or losses but fail to report a depressed mood. When this happens, physicians may fail to consider the possibility of an underlying depression. Many patients will express their distress by somatic symptoms such as headache, nonspecific pain, gastrointestinal complaints, dizziness, fatigue, respiratory difficulties, and many others. Somatic manifestations of depression may serve to bind anxiety and relieve dysphoria in personally and culturally acceptable idioms (Katon 1982) or may be a function of rigid defense mechanisms (Stoudemire et al. 1985). Patients who express their depression through somatic equivalents persist in this symptom expression from episode to episode even though the type of physical symptom may change across episodes. Early family patterns of illness behavior (for example, increased attention, or serious or frightening illness in childhood) may also predispose an individual to somatic rather than affective depression. Physical symptoms can also generate the secondary gain of disability and dependence in a more acceptable form. Somatic symptoms, however, continue to affect the patient's social and vocational adjustment and the homeostasis of the family.

Sociocultural as well as psychodynamic factors can also influence and reinforce somatic expressions of depression. Some Western and non-Western cultures lack proper terms for describing emotional states or pose strong sanctions against perceiving depression as an emotional state. When a patient's beliefs and practices about disease are not derived from modern science, physicians may fail to recognize depression expressed in the unique idiom of the patient's culture of origin.

The question arises as to whether medical patients present distinctive physical signs/symptoms that can facilitate the diagnosis of depression. It is known that physical symptoms associated with depression in patients seeking medical care include musculoskeletal, neurological, gastrointestinal, and cardiopulmonary types. In addition, fatigue, chronic pain, and sleep discontinuity are commonly reported by depressed primary care patients. Nevertheless, no specific somatic symptoms, by themselves, are indicative of an underlying depression. In diagnosing depression when it presents as somatic symptomatology, the clinician needs to be attentive to the presence of concomitant depressive symptoms and to the patient's psychosocial context.

Depressive Concomitants of Medical Illness

Just as depressive symptoms can mimic a medical disorder, organic illnesses can assume the form of a mood disorder. Katon (1982) considered the biological and psychological processes that could produce the affective clinical presentation and concluded that it is unclear whether this form of somatopsychic illness results from pathological central nervous system monoamine changes stimulated by the medical disease, or whether it is a response to the stress of coping with such disease. A combination of both could be involved.

The possible medical conditions presenting with depressive symptoms are extensive and pertain to most bodily systems (Stoudemire and Fogel 1991). Among the organic illnesses that most commonly cause depressive signs are hypothyroidism, hyperadrenalism, hypoglycemia, systemic infections, autoimmune deficiency syndrome, multiple sclerosis, temporal lobe and psychomotor epilepsies, essential hypertension, rheumatoid arthritis, pernicious anemia, diabetes mellitus, nutritional deficiencies, cardiovascular disease, and cancer (especially pancreatic and brain tumors). A wide range of neurological diseases and structural brain damage can also produce distinct affective symptoms (Tucker and Price 1987). In addition to organic conditions that may potentiate a depression, various drugs ranging from birth control pills to antihypertensives can produce depressive signs and symptoms (Zelnik 1987).

These findings suggest that physicians and psychotherapists must be vigilant in distinguishing functional depression from medical illness with depressive symptomatology, regardless of its etiology and mechanisms. When the patient lacks a family history of depression, underlying medical illnesses should be considered. Furthermore, women and older patients presenting with dysphoria or vegetative symptoms of depressions (e.g., sleep changes, weight changes, appetite changes) should be evaluated for endocrine disorders. As a general principle, any physical symptomatology should be thoroughly evaluated before initiating psychosocial or psychobiological treatments. Further medical assessments also are warranted if the physical symptoms worsen or new ones appear during the course of treatment.

Depression: Medical-Psychiatric Comorbidity in a Randomized Controlled Trial

Given this range of potential interactions between major depression and organic illnesses (as well as between major depression and other DSM-III-R disorders), what is the effect of these interactions on the selection of subjects for an RCT focusing on treatments for depression? As we noted previously, only a small proportion of patients with a given disorder typically qualify for an RCT because this research design seeks to "purify" the pool of subject participants. Thus, our study requires that patients with affective symptomatology meet DSM-III-R criteria for a current major depression as well as a severity level dictating active treatment rather than "watchful waiting." Diagnostic and severity indices (plus others, such as ability to be managed as an outpatient) and absence of psychotic features or serious suicidal ideation apply to an RCT studying psychotherapy of depression. However, in a protocol including pharmacotherapy, medical contraindications must be considered as well when determining patient eligibility for randomization to any of the treatment alternatives. Consequently, our RCT excludes primary care patients with medical problems precluding assignment to nortriptyline (e.g., malignant ventricular arrhythmia or urinary retention), even though they would be eligible for IPT.

Epidemiological studies administering structured interview schedules found that 4.8% to 8.6% of primary care patients experience a current major depression (Katon and Schulberg 1992). However, such cases were not further assessed psychiatrically and medically to determine whether depression-specific treatment was indicated. In the face of repeated reports that affective disorder often is untreated by primary care physicians (e.g., Ormel et al. 1991), it is striking that almost 40% of our study's primary care patients meeting Diagnostic Interview Schedule (DIS; Robins et al. 1981) criteria for a current major depression and participating in a psychiatric assessment were found to be clinically ineligible for a randomized treatment assignment. Of this excluded group, approximately 75% failed to display sufficient depressive severity or had diagnoses such as history of bipolar illness. The remaining 25% of excluded depressed patients had medical conditions precluding the use of antidepressant medication prior to ascertaining whether the physical illness had been properly treated (e.g., thyroid dysfunction or organic mood disorder). These findings again emphasize the need to carefully assess affectively disturbed primary care patients, as well as the unique complexities confronting generalist physicians when deciding whether to treat the depression immediately or observe its course prior to intervening.

An RCT requires that patients meet rigorous eligibility criteria and that they consent to a randomized treatment choice. Thus, primary care patients adhering to particular "health beliefs" about the etiology of major depression and its proper care may refuse informed consent so as to preclude a treatment assignment antithetical to their beliefs. Less than 10% of our psychiatrically assessed, protocol-eligible patients have exercised this option. Nevertheless, our study likely omits patients wishing to avoid IPT because they consider major depression biological in nature as well as patients wishing to avoid nortriptyline because they believe that medication cannot resolve stressful interpersonal relationships that are producing depression.

Within this framework for recruiting depressed primary care patients, what are the characteristics of the initial 60 subjects entering our clinical trial? Analyses are still to be performed of the participants' medical condition, but data regarding their psychiatric status are quite revealing. Rather than displaying the lowered levels of symptom severity reported previously, our patients are at least as affectively distressed and dysfunctional as psychiatric patients with major depression. When assessed for clinical eligibility, they had mean scores of 36 on the Center for Epidemiologic Studies Depression Scale (Radloff 1977), 27 on the 17-item Hamilton Rating Scale for Depression (Hamilton 1967), and 49 on the Global Assessment Scale (Endicott et al. 1976).

Equally pertinent to the nature and treatability of major depression in primary care practice are findings about the prevalence of DSM-III-R comorbidity among these initial 60 patients. In addition to the current major depression, 82% had a lifetime history of at least one other Axis I disorder. When administered selected sections of the DIS, 38% met Escobar et al.'s (1987) modified criteria for somatization and 45% had experienced panic disorder, 62% a generalized anxiety disorder, 12% alcohol dependency, and 15% some type of drug dependency.

Findings about Axis II comorbidity are equally compelling with regard to their implications for treating major depression in primary care patients. Based on the Structured Clinical Interview for DSM-III-R Personality Assessment (Spitzer et al. 1989), 86% of study subjects met criteria for at least one Axis II disorder. More specifically, 38% were classified in Cluster A (i.e., paranoid, schizotypal, and schizoid); 29% in Cluster B (i.e., borderline, histrionic, and narcissistic); and 67% in Cluster C (i.e., avoidant, obsessive-compulsive, dependent, and passive-aggressive). Thus, the depressed patients enrolled in our clinical trial display extensive psychiatric comorbidity in addition to the medical comorbidity for which they are being treated at the primary care clinics. The impact of these associated illnesses on psychotherapy and pharmacotherapy's effectiveness in resolving a major depression will be examined in later stages of our study.

Interpersonal Psychotherapy in Primary Care Facilities

When a primary care patient is diagnosed as having a current major depression, the physician must decide whether to treat the disorder with psychotherapy or pharmacotherapy. Intense psychosocial problems are thought to favor a psychotherapeutic intervention, whereas severe neurovegetative symptoms are thought best treated pharmacologically. However, scientific evidence regarding which depressed patients benefit from which treatment remains uncertain. Major recent studies of acute- and maintenance-phase therapies with depressed psychiatric patients were unable to distinguish predictors of differential response to psychotherapy and pharmacotherapy (Frank et al. 1990; Sotsky et al. 1991). No such study has been conducted in primary care settings. It is not surprising, therefore, that treatment of depression in primary care practice often is determined by a patient's clinical symptoms and health beliefs interacting with 1) the physician's health beliefs and his or her personal comfort in counseling the patient or prescribing antidepressant medication, and 2) the costs, financing mechanisms, and availability of alternative interventions outside of the health center.

Given this complex interplay in selecting a treatment, Schulberg and Scott (1991) urged physicians to assess more carefully the psychosocial stressors underlying many of the episodic depressions presenting in their medical patients, and to more frequently select a time-limited psychotherapy specifically geared to interpersonal issues. The psychotherapy should respect the patient's somatic presenting complaints while still dealing with the psychosocial context in which these complaints arose or are experienced. The treatment also should convey an optimism to the patient that particular relationship problems associated with the depression will be addressed and resolved shortly, while others must await future consideration. Furthermore, termination must be addressed from treatment's onset, because the therapeutic contract, for clinical and administrative reasons, is of a time-limited nature. Interpersonal psychotherapy meets these requirements, and we next describe how patients in our clinical trial are being treated with this modality.

Conducting IPT in Health Centers

Because health centers aim to diagnose and treat physical illness, their staff hierarchy, organizational rituals and symbols, and daily clinical procedures are structured accordingly. For example, physicians play a dominant role in the patient's management, medical symbols such as white coats abound, and procedures are performed that reinforce the patient's sense of being treated for a physical disorder. Indeed, some examinations and test procedures may be conducted to reassure a worried patient without any expectation that additional clinical data will be obtained. Given a sociocultural environment that focuses upon organic morbidity, can the psychosocial aspects of depression be treated within it?

Our experiences thus far are positive and reflect the growing availability of time-limited psychotherapy in health maintenance organizations (HMOs) and managed health care facilities. In our clinical trial, patients randomized to IPT are willing to make weekly appointments with the treating psychiatrist or psychologist at the health center and keep approximately 80% of these appointments. It is feasible to monitor the depressive state through regular administration of the Beck Depression Inventory and to detect possible clinical deterioration. The IPT therapist readily contacts the patient's health center physician when necessary, and harmful splitting tactics are infrequently employed by the IPT patient.

These features of IPT conform with the IPT treatment manual standards (see Klerman et al. 1984) and are consistent with its practice in any caregiving setting. However, we also strive to ensure that IPT conforms with the clinical and sociocultural characteristics of a primary care center, because we deem it important that the patient continue perceiving himself or herself as a health center patient. Therefore, we permit vital signs to be taken and blood pressure to be read when the patient arrives at the center. The patient then is led by a nurse to the psychotherapy room, which contains not only chairs but also an examining table and standard medical instruments. When medical crises necessitate a patient's hospitalization, the IPT therapist visits the ward when possible and conducts sessions in the inpatient environment so as to minimally disrupt the continuity of treatment. When a patient's social crises threaten to disrupt the psychotherapy, IPT is maintained with assistance from local human service agencies linked to the health center.

In contrast to these experiences, we also have observed that routine health center practices can complicate rather than facilitate the psychotherapist-patient relationship. For example, health center receptionists occasionally have commented about a therapist's personal life circumstances in the patient's presence even though such remarks clearly cross the doctor-patient boundaries enforced by mental health center personnel. Concerns about privacy and confidentiality have also led therapists to limit the kind of information that is entered in the patient's medical record given the diverse and sometimes uncertain access to it in the course of health center operations.

Interpersonal Problem Areas

In IPT, four interpersonal problem areas are identified as producing, or being associated with, depressive disorders: grief reactions, role transitions, interpersonal role disputes, and interpersonal deficits. These problem areas generally are distinct and readily identified through careful interviewing of the patient. However, they are not mutually exclusive, and patients often will present with simultaneous difficulties in two or three problem areas. Furthermore, the targeted problem areas may shift as therapy progresses. With depressed psychiatric patients, difficulties in role transitions and interpersonal disputes predominate and, indeed, often occur simultaneously.

It is our impression that depressed ambulatory medical patients more frequently experience unresolved grief that has been extensively somatized, or the combination of grief and role transition difficulties associated with chronic physical morbidity. In the remainder of this section, we describe these four problem areas in IPT and illustrate each with the case of a primary care patient.

Grief Reaction

Acute symptoms of grief reactions tend to resolve spontaneously within 4 to 6 months of the loss of a loved one as the bereaved person gradually distances himself or herself from emotions and experiences associated with that person. When this process fails to occur within the expected sequence and duration, however, abnormal grief of the delayed or distorted type should be considered. An abnormal grief reaction may be readily diagnosed when the patient's symptoms have a clear temporal relationship to the loss of a loved one. Often, though, the relationship is more subtle or indirect and requires careful probing by the therapist. With depressed primary care patients, the unresolved grief often presents as intense anxiety about serious personal illness or illness in a significant other. The patient may then display depressive symptoms but lack any awareness of their relationship to the past unresolved grief.

The IPT treatment of grief-related depression has two goals: 1) facilitating the delayed mourning process and 2) helping the patient establish interests and relationships that can substitute for the relationship with the lost loved one.

Ms. D., a 28-year-old single mother of three children, was a nurse by profession. She was repeatedly evaluated at the health center for symptoms of chronic intermittent abdominal pain, indigestion, fatigue, headache, and shortness of breath. She underwent many tests including endoscopy and abdominal ultrasound, but her epigastric discomfort could not be adequately explained. She finally took a leave of absence from work, returning to her physician with the above complaints plus "difficulty getting up in the morning." He referred the patient for a psychiatric evaluation, which revealed a 2-year progressive history of depressed mood, hypersomnia, anhedonia, and weight gain (of 40 pounds).

Upon closer questioning, it appeared that Ms. D.'s depressive symptoms dated back to the time when Jim, her second husband and the father of her youngest child, separated from the family. She described her sorrow at the loss of a father figure for her children, particularly since Bill, her first husband (and father of her two older children), had died several years earlier. Though reluctant to talk about the past, Ms. D. gave additional history indicating that her father had abandoned the family when she was a child, leading her to form a close, protective relationship with her mother and older sisters but without a male figure in the household. Ms. D.

reported that she had moved to Pittsburgh to be near her mother and sisters, while her first husband remained in St. Louis. Bill was killed in a fight a year later. During the year they were separated, Bill continued supporting Ms. D. and his children, frequently admonishing her to return home so they could be a family once again. Ms. D. was shocked to learn of Bill's unexpected death and guilt-ridden over ways she might have prevented it. Although she tried hard not to think of him, in recent months intrusive and disturbing memories of Bill had returned.

Ms. D. readily acknowledged the temporal connection between her losses and symptoms and agreed to IPT therapy centering around unresolved grief. Nevertheless, she experienced much difficulty talking about Bill. Dr. G., the therapist, gently but persistently urged her to review Bill's and her life together, assuring Ms. D. that she could control and resolve the painful memories. Ms. D. then did so with a burst of bitter tears, anguish, and sorrow. Midway through treatment, Ms. D. decided that she must travel to St. Louis, visit Bill's grave, and speak to his family for the first time since his death. Several difficult, intense psychotherapy sessions prepared the way for this visit. Ms. D. returned shaken but less guilty and more hopeful than previously. Following this experience, rapid progress in the resolution of Ms. D.'s depressive symptoms led to her terminating psychotherapy after 14 sessions. Ms. D. was seen in three monthly follow-ups. At the last visit, she was markedly improved, back at work, sleeping well, actively attending to her children's needs, and only occasionally experiencing abdominal discomfort when eating certain foods.

Role Transitions

Psychologists and psychiatrists have long focused on the manner in which people cope with new roles and the impaired social functioning that results from the inability to manage a transition involving altered status. When the new role (of an objectively negative or positive nature) is too difficult to manage, a clinical depression often results. Klerman et al. (1984) propose that depressions induced by role transitions stem from 1) the loss of familiar social supports, 2) problematic management of the accompanying affect, 3) demands for a repertoire of new social skills, and 4) cognitive disturbances produced by diminished self-esteem.

Depressed primary care patients experience the same role-transition problems as do depressed psychiatric patients—for example, coping with a job change, accepting a change in parental or marital status, retiring, and so on. However, medical patients also commonly confront severe role problems produced by the disabling effects of a chronic physical illness. Such illness can create major limitations in the person's social roles as a parent, spouse, or co-worker and require that he or she fundamentally revise the manner in which these roles are to be played. Depressive illness results when the person cannot accept the limitations produced by the physical morbidity—for example, dependency, loss of long-standing social relationships, the need to develop new social skills, altered social status and group identification, and so on. The functional limitations produced by normal aging processes may also generate depressive illness in medical patients. Acceptance of these limitations and coping with their consequences can be unusually debilitating when there is a need to alter long-standing social roles and patterns.

In clarifying the patient's reaction to a physical limitation, it is useful to distinguish the feelings associated with the lost role (which may resemble a grief reaction) from difficulty in performing a new social role. For example, not all newly diagnosed diabetic patients facing significant dietary restrictions or insulin dependence experience an affective disorder. For those who do, it is vital to understand the patient's cognitive beliefs about this illness, the subjective reactions to having a chronic condition, the patient's feelings of dependency and loss of control associated with needed medical procedures, and the ways in which the procedures affect the person's daily ability to function as student, spouse, wage earner, parent, and so on. The goal of IPT in treating role transition–related depression is to shift the patient's emphasis from feelings of loss and inadequacy to an appreciation of future opportunities for recovered self-esteem and rewarding social relationships.

Ms. B. is a 62-year-old divorced mother of four grown children who was being actively treated at the family health center for chronic obstructive pulmonary disease, moderately severe degenerative arthritis, recurrent heme-positive stools, and generalized tiredness. Three months earlier, a routine thyroid test level had been mildly elevated (12), and she was being treated with levothyroxine sodium, 0.075 mg, with no apparent symptomatic improvement. Ms. B. had undergone three colonoscopies, with no source found for her gastrointestinal bleeding, and she worried that her right leg weakness might lead to paralysis and helplessness. Her nonspecific complaints of tiredness, anhedonia, greater shortness of breath, and increased arthritic pains were increasingly accompanied by insomnia (difficulty falling asleep [DFA], early morning awakening [EMA]), withdrawal from family, and hopelessness. She was not suicidal, other than vague passive ideation, and was not psychotic or organically impaired. In a psychiatric consultation obtained by the family practitioner it was determined that Ms. B. was in the midst of a major depression for which IPT could be effective.

It became apparent in the initial sessions that Ms. B's growing physical disabilities left her resenting a lifetime role of responsibility for family members and others, which was not reciprocated by them. She recited a litany of such complaints. She recalled that her mother, now dead for several years, had been insensitive, always criticized her, and was locked in repetitive angry clashes with Ms. B.'s father. Both Ms. B.'s father and husband were verbally abusive toward her. Thus, she "hated men," including the several male physicians and the psychologist whom she had seen over the years, and wondered if she would be able to work with Dr. Y., her male IPT therapist. In this relationship, though, Ms. B. felt "listened to," and ended up feeling positively toward Dr. Y. Compounding Ms. B.'s feelings of excessive burden, early in therapy the patient's daughter left her husband and returned to live with Ms. B., bringing a 12 year-old granddaughter along as well. Ms. B. bemoaned this development, complaining that even though her daughter had been offered other lodging and had money to pay for it, she instead chose to impose on Ms. B.

The patient's appearance underscored her complaints. She was obese, sad, and plodding, looking a decade older than her stated age. Ms. B. spoke deliberately and bitterly, and was quickly moved to tears when speaking of her own mother's insensitivity. Dr. Y. observed that at a stage of life when Ms. B. might be anticipating increased dependency, she still was required to care for members of her family. He proposed that therapy focus on how Ms. B. could alter her relationships with others so that they better reflected the roles that she presently wished to play.

Ms. B. readily agreed, and, despite initial difficulties, the course of therapy was surprisingly smooth. At first, Ms. B. attempted to engage Dr. Y. in talk about her numerous somatic complaints. Dr. Y. recognized the trap in these discussions, which would again leave Ms. B. feeling unsatisfied and uncared for. Instead, he redirected her attention to underlying feelings of sadness, fear, and the unmet needs that these somatic complaints masked. Ms. B. was soon won over to this perspective. Recognizing that Dr. Y. sincerely wished to understand her, Ms. B. quickly dropped the somatic preoccupation, discussing instead with intense feeling the unfair impositions from people in her current personal and work life.

As Ms. B. and Dr. Y. discussed her options for achieving a new age-appropriate role with others, the sad mood began to noticeably improve. Ms. B. suggested to her daughter that she could help financially by paying rent; later they agreed that the daughter was ready to move into a place of her own. At work, Ms. B. delegated more tasks to co-workers and subordinates, and was commended by her boss for devoted work efforts. Ms. B. became reinvolved with her religious community and, at the end of her 16 scheduled visits, gave Dr. Y. a special Bible as a token of thanks and connection. Ms. B. was seen to smile for the first time by nurses who had known her for years. These clinical gains were maintained at the 1- and 2-month follow-up visits. Ms. B.'s medical complaints also decreased substantially as she developed comfort in less demanding roles. She walked daily, was breathing better and sleeping well, and had not visited her family practitioner in 10 weeks at last contact.

Interpersonal Role Disputes

Situations in which the patient and a "significant other" hold widely discrepant expectations about their relationship have been characterized by Klerman et al. (1984) as interpersonal disputes. Commonly reported by medical patients, such disputes become the focus of psychotherapeutic attention only when judged by the physician as significant in the depression's etiology or persistence. Typical maladaptive behaviors that maintain the dispute are the patient's poor communication patterns, any truly irreconcilable differences, and/or the patient's sense of helplessness and hopelessness intrinsic to the depression.

The interpersonal disputes upon which IPT focuses with depressed primary care patients may well resemble those presented by depressed psychiatric patients—for example, physically abusive behavior by the spouse, altered but unsatisfactory roles upon the birth of a child, and so on. In the primary care setting, however, the therapist also should carefully elucidate how physical illness has affected the patient's relationship with a significant other. Chronic illnesses like colitis or arthritis can profoundly disturb long-established marital roles and shift the prior equilibrium in conflicting directions. IPT treatment goals in the event of an interpersonal dispute are to 1) help the patient identify the conflict; 2) guide the patient toward an awareness of choices and the formulation of alternative actions; and 3) encourage the patient to modify expectations of the significant other so that they are more realistic and achievable.

Ms. C., a 25-year-old mother of two young children, presented at the health center with a long history of depression. She complained of insomnia, weight loss of 15 pounds, irritability, fatigue, anhedonia, and persistent suicidal ideation. She had been followed by her family practitioner for routine gynecological care (i.e., examinations and birth control) and was known to be depressed for at least 2 years. Initially, her family physician prescribed nortriptyline. Ms. C. was unable to tolerate the side effects of lethargy and dizziness and was switched to fluoxetine (Prozac), resulting in fair symptomatic improvement. She soon, however, reported disturbing nightmares of a murder she had witnessed. When her agitation and fear increased, the Prozac was discontinued. No other depression-specific treatment was attempted. Ms. C. angrily refused referral to a local mental health center. After continued distress, however, Ms. C. did agree to schedule weekly psychotherapy sessions within the health center itself.

Ms. C.'s family and social histories were complex and chaotic. She was one of two children from the second of her mother's three marriages. Male adult figures were transient in her household and often abusive (physically and sexually) toward Ms. C. and her step-sisters. Ms. C.'s mother was also quite volatile and abusive, so that the patient felt "lucky to be alive today." She managed, nevertheless, to complete high school and worked for a time before marrying. However, the marital relationship deteriorated after two children were born, ending in many angry, though nonviolent, fights. All of Ms. C.'s relationships were intense and often revolved around drug use or promiscuous sexual encounters. She herself barely escaped being killed several times and was in trouble with the law on occasion. Dr. L., the IPT therapist, identified interpersonal conflict as the central issue, clearly recognizing the dramatic character pathology complicating treatment of the diagnosed major depression.

For many weeks, Ms. C. was alternatively testy and seductive. She provoked Dr. L. in conversation and dress, trying to break down his professional reserve in a way that would surely have replicated the prior troubling relationships about which she complained so bitterly. When Dr. L. did not accept these overtures and instead persisted in exploring Ms. C.'s complaints, she would lash out angrily and pointedly inquire into the details of his marriage and sexual life. Ms. C. did attend sessions faithfully, at times to Dr. L.'s secret chagrin, as he saw no apparent improvement in her depressive symptoms or provocative manner. It was not until the last three scheduled sessions that change became evident. Ms. C. reported setting firm limits with her boyfriend who had previously used her car and money irresponsibly. She directly addressed the manner wherein seductive behavior had led her into harmful relationships, and she evidenced more respect for Dr. L. and apologized if she had offended him.

Ms. C. indicated a readiness to terminate at 16 visits with a clear feeling of enhanced self-respect even though depressive symptoms had not yet fully remitted. Medical problems never became a focus of the therapy, and Ms. C.'s mild somatic complaints persisted. Nevertheless, it was striking that this patient with severe character pathology and significant depression, who failed on antidepressants and adamantly refused referral to a mental health center, was able to engage in focused psychotherapy and benefit from it when treated at the health center.

Interpersonal Deficits

Exploration of the clinical depression may reveal that the patient has a history of social isolation marked by inadequate or unsustaining interpersonal relationships. Such persons may never have established intimate relationships as adults; indeed, disrupted childhood relationships frequently are evident as well. The diagnosis of depression accompanied by interpersonal deficits should seek to distinguish whether the patient is 1) socially isolated because of long-standing or temporary deficiencies in interpersonal skills, 2) socially unfulfilled despite an adequate number and range of social relationships, or 3) socially withdrawn because of a persisting depression that has not been adequately treated. The third case is evident in primary care patients who have made poor adjustments to a chronic physical illness and whose relationships with others have become progressively withdrawn and limited. This pattern can also be seen in patients with AIDS or communicable diseases that lead them to avoid social contacts. The goal of IPT with depressed patients displaying interpersonal deficits is to reduce their social isolation.

> Ms. A. is a 30-year-old single mother of a somewhat hyperactive 11-year-old boy. She visited the health center with complaints of sadness, frequent crying episodes, loss of appetite, sleep disturbance (DFA, difficulty staying asleep [DSA], EMA), loneliness, and mild suicidal ideation. At times, Ms A. felt that life was not worth living. She would frequently lash out angrily at her son, with guilty feelings afterward. Given these disturbing moods and behaviors, Ms. A.'s primary care physician referred her to the health center's psychologist for psychotherapy.
>
> Ms. A. presented as a Peter Pan–like thin, wiry, boyish-looking woman with short hair and a striking childlike demeanor. She deferred readily to any authority figure, disclaimed any personal competence, and accepted without question even obviously misleading statements such as when a friend told her that it was impossible to get AIDS from initial sexual intercourse. Ms. A. misused words and expressions in a childish and

unself-conscious way. For example, in discussing her ex-boyfriend's alcoholism, she stated that "he does drink to Bolivia." Ms. A.'s relationships with her mother and son were also characterized by a profound inability to assert herself. She attributed her loneliness and depression to the recent loss of a long-standing boyfriend, a man who drank and was verbally abusive. While drunk, he had caused a traffic accident that resulted in his becoming paraplegic. Ms. A. tried to visit him in the hospital and maintain their relationship but was ushered out by his family. Though she wanted desperately to return to him, she felt unable to negotiate any reconciliation with his mother. Ms. A.'s own mother and son took turns bullying her, and she was similarly unable to assertively speak her mind.

Ms. A. and her psychotherapist, Dr. M., identified interpersonal deficits as the focal problem and contracted for 16 weekly sessions plus 4 monthly follow-ups. Initially, Ms. A. found the work of psychotherapy daunting. There were several late cancellations and no-shows, often related to characteristic battles with mother and son. When Ms. A. did attend sessions, she seemed genuinely puzzled by Dr. M.'s gentle but persistent attention to her inadequate, childlike responses to those around her. Ms. A. felt this was the way she had been raised and was expected to behave even presently, and could not imagine herself otherwise. However, as her temper outbursts increasingly were perceived as the natural result of suppressed rage from repeated attacks on her, Ms. A. had a glimmer of understanding.

She met and began dating a new man, also a problem drinker but otherwise more willing to encourage her assertiveness in dealing with her son and later with her mother. Dr. M. repeatedly focused on the more complex social skills required to succeed in the adult world. Toward the end of therapy, Ms. A. felt substantially more in charge of her relationships and was training for a career as a paralegal.

An additional outcome of this psychotherapy was Ms. A.'s general health care behavior. She had been visiting her family practitioner regularly for nonspecific gynecological symptoms and episodic lower abdominal discomfort. When discussing this with Dr. M., Ms. A. assumed her typical childlike attitude, evincing puzzlement that the physician could not definitively diagnose and treat her problems. Nevertheless, Ms. A. passively persisted in medical visits. As she became more comfortable with adult ways of talking to authority figures, however, Ms. A. more precisely defined her symptoms, and her family physician could then properly diagnose and treat them. With the resolution of these problems, Ms. A.'s visits to her family physician ceased until she next appeared several months later with typical symptoms of a viral upper respiratory infection.

Summary

Depressed primary medical care patients require effective treatment for this disorder so as to alleviate distress and reduce excessive utilization of health care services. In this chapter we reviewed various complexities facing the physician in distinguishing affective and somatic illnesses in a medical population, and in determining whether and how to intervene. IPT's ability to reduce depressive symptomatology has been demonstrated with psychiatric patients, and guidelines developed by the Depression Panel of the U.S. Public Health Service's Agency for Health Care Policy and Research will likely recommend the use of IPT with depressed primary care patients as well.

References

Abbey S, Kennedy S, Kaplan A, et al: Self-report symptoms that predict major depression in patients with prominent physical symptoms. Int J Psychiatry Med 20:247–258, 1990

American Psychiatric Association: Diagnostic and Statistical Manual of Mental Disorders, 3rd Edition, Revised. Washington, DC, American Psychiatric Association, 1987

Beardsley R, Gardocki G, Larson D, et al: Prescribing of psychotropic medication by primary care physicians and psychiatrists. Arch Gen Psychiatry 45:1117–1119, 1988

Blackburn I, Bishop S, Glen A, et al: The efficacy of cognitive behavior therapy in depression: a treatment trial using cognitive therapy and pharmacotherapy, each alone and in combination. Br J Psychiatry 139:181–189, 1981

Blacker C, Clare A: Depressive disorder in primary care. Br J Psychiatry 150:737–751, 1987

Byrd J, Moskowitz M: Outpatient consultation: interaction between the general internist and the specialist. J Gen Intern Med 2:93–98, 1987

Cameron OG: Guidelines for diagnosis and treatment of depression in patients with medical illness. J Clin Psychiatry 51 (No 7, Suppl):49–54, 1990

Callies A, Popkin M: Antidepressant treatment of medical/surgical inpatients by non-psychiatric physicians. Arch Gen Psychiatry 44:158–160, 1987

Cohen-Cole S, Stoudemire A: Major depression and physical illness. Psychiatr Clin North Am 10:1–16, 1987

Coulehan J, Schulberg H, Block M, et al: Medical comorbidity of major depressive disorder in a primary medical practice. Arch Intern Med 150:2363–2367, 1990

Elkin I, Shea T, Watkins J, et al: National Institute of Mental Health Treatment of Depression Collaborative Research Program: general effectiveness of treatments. Arch Gen Psychiatry 46:971–982, 1989

Endicott J, Spitzer RL, Fleiss J, et al: The Global Assessment Scale: a procedure for measuring overall severity of psychiatric disturbance. Arch Gen Psychiatry 33:766–771, 1976

Escobar J, Burnam A, Karno M, et al: Somatization in the community. Arch Gen Psychiatry 44:713–718, 1987

Fava G, Sonino N, Wise T: Management of depression in medical patients. Psychother Psychosom 49:81–102, 1988

Fawcett J, Epstein P, Fiester S, et al: Clinical management–imipramine/placebo administration manual. Psychopharmacol Bull 23:309–324, 1987

Frank E, Kupfer D, Perel J: Early recurrence in unipolar depression. Arch Gen Psychiatry 46:397–400, 1989

Frank E, Kupfer D, Perel J, et al: Three-year outcomes for maintenance therapies in recurrent depression. Arch Gen Psychiatry 47:1093–1099, 1990

Goldberg R: Depression in primary care: DSM-III diagnoses and other depressive symptoms. J Gen Intern Med 3:491–497, 1988

Gullick E, King L: Appropriateness of drugs prescribed by primary care physicians for depressed outpatients. J Affective Disord 1:55–58, 1979

Haggerty J, Evans D, McCartney C, et al: Psychotropic prescribing patterns of nonpsychiatric residents in a general hospital in 1973 and 1982. Hosp Community Psychiatry 37:357–361, 1986

Hamilton M: Development of a rating scale for primary depressive illness. British Journal of Social and Clinical Psychology 6:278296, 1967

Katon W: Depression: somatic symptoms and medical disorders in primary care. Compr Psychiatry 23:274–287, 1982

Katon W: The epidemiology of depression in medical care. Int J Psychiatry Med 17:93–112, 1987

Katon W, Schulberg H: Epidemiology of depression in primary care. Gen Hosp Psychiatry 14:237–247, 1992

Katon W, Sullivan MD: Depression and chronic mental illness. J Clin Psychiatry 51 (No 6, Suppl):3–11, 1990

Katon W, Von Korff M, Lin E, et al: Distressed high utilizers of medical care: DSM-III-R diagnoses and treatment needs. Gen Hosp Psychiatry 12:355–362, 1990

Klerman G, Weissman M, Rounsaville B, et al: Interpersonal Psychotherapy of Depression. New York, Basic Books, 1984

Murphy G, Simons A, Wetzel R, et al: Cognitive therapy and pharmacotherapy. Arch Gen Psychiatry 41:33–41, 1984

Ormel J, Koeter M, van den Brink W, et al: Recognition, management, and course of anxiety and depression in general practice. Arch Gen Psychiatry 48:700–706, 1991

Radloff LS: The CES-D Scale:a self-report depression scale for research in the general population. Applied Psychological Measurement 1:385–401, 1977

Robins LN, Helzer JE, Croughan J, et al: National Institute of Mental Health Diagnostic Interview Schedule: its history, characteristics, and validity. Arch Gen Psychiatry 38:381–389, 1981

Rush A, Beck A, Kovacs M, et al: Comparative efficacy of cognitive therapy and pharmaco-therapy in the treatment of depressed patients. Cognitive Therapy and Research 1:17–37, 1977

Rush A, Trivedi M, Schriger D, et al: The development of clinical practice guidelines for the diagnosis and treatment of depression. Gen Hosp Psychiatry 14:230–236, 1992

Schulberg H, Scott C: Depression in primary care: treating depression with interpersonal psychotherapy, in Managed Health Care: The Optimal Use of Time and Resources. Edited by Austad C, Berman W. Washington, DC, American Psychological Association, 1991, pp 153–170

Schulberg H, McClelland M, Burns B: Depression and physical illness: the prevalence, causation, and diagnosis of comorbidity. Clinical Psychology Review 7:145–167, 1987

Schulberg H, Coulehan J, Block M, et al: Investigating primary care treatments for depression through culturally compatible clinical trials. Paper presented at the Fifth Annual NIMH International Research Conference on the Classification, Recognition, and Treatment of Mental Disorders in General Medical Settings, Bethesda, MD, September 1991a

Schulberg H, Coulehan J, Block M, et al: Strategies for evaluating treatments for major depression in primary care patients. Gen Hosp Psychiatry 13:9–18, 1991b

Sotsky S, Glass D, Shea T, et al: Patient predictors of response to psychotherapy and pharmacotherapy: findings from the NIMH Treatment of Depression Collaborative Research Program. Arch Gen Psychiatry 148:997–1008, 1991

Spitzer RL, Williams J, Gibbon M, et al: Structured Clinical Interview for DSM-III-R Personality Disorders. New York, New York Psychiatric Institute, September 1989

Stoudemire A, Fogel B (eds): Medical Psychiatric Practice, Vol 1. Washington, DC, American Psychiatric Press, 1991

Stoudemire A, Kahn M, Brown J, et al: Masked depression in a combined medical-psychiatric unit. Psychosomatics 26:221–228, 1985

Tucker G, Price T: Depression and neurologic disease, in Presentations of Depression. Edited by Cameron O. New York, Wiley, 1987, pp 237–250

Wells K, Stewart A, Hays R, et al: The functioning and well-being of depressed patients: results from the Medical Outcomes Study. JAMA 262:914–919, 1989

Williamson P, Yates W: The initial presentation of depression in family practice and psychiatric outpatients. Gen Hosp Psychiatry 11:189–193, 1989

Zelnik T: Depressive effects of drugs, in Presentations of Depression. Edited by Cameron O. New York, Wiley, 1987, pp 355–402

Interpersonal Psychotherapy for Other Psychiatric Disorders

CHAPTER 11

Interpersonal Counseling for Stress and Distress in Primary Care Settings

Myrna M. Weissman, Ph.D.
Gerald L. Klerman, M.D.

Interpersonal counseling (IPC) is a brief treatment (six 30-minute sessions) focused on the patient's current psychosocial functioning and administered by health care professionals, usually a nurse practitioner. It is designed for nonpsychiatric patients who are in distress and have symptoms due to current stresses in their lives but who do not have serious concurrent psychiatric disorders or medical conditions. Attention is given to recent changes in the person's life events; sources of stress in the family, home, workplace, and friendship patterns; and ongoing difficulties in interpersonal relations. In IPC it is assumed that such events provide the interpersonal context in which bodily and emotional symptoms related to anxiety, depression, and distress occur. Although designed to be used in a primary care facility, IPC may be suitable in other types of medical settings.

Interpersonal counseling derives directly from interpersonal psychotherapy (IPT; Klerman et al. 1984). It differs from IPT in that it is briefer in number and duration of sessions. Because it can be administered by a

Permission has been granted to reprint portions of the following article: G. L. Klerman, S. Budman, D. Berwick, et al.: "Efficacy of a Brief Psychosocial Intervention for Symptoms of Stress and Distress Among Patients in Primary Care." *Medical Care* 25:1078–1088, 1987. Copyright 1987.

non–mental health professional, the actual scripts of each session are out-lined, and homework has been added to accelerate the process. The IPT manual was used as a general guide in developing the IPC manual (Weiss-man and Klerman 1988).

The purpose of IPC is to reduce stress, enhance social functioning, and reduce inappropriate health care utilization. This is accomplished by iden-tifying the current stressors in the patient's life that lead to distress and by helping the patient to consider more effective strategies for dealing with the stress.

The development of IPC is based on research documenting the high frequencies of anxiety, depression, and functional bodily complaints in patients in primary care settings (Goldberg 1972, 1979; Hankin and Otay 1979; Hoeper et al. 1979; Jencks 1985; Ormel et al. 1991). Some of these patients have diagnosable psychiatric symptoms that do not meet estab-lished criteria for psychiatric disorders, and the diagnostic status of these patients remains a source of controversy. They are variously described as "the worried well," or as having "minor affective disorder," "anxiety and depression," "problems of living," "stress reactions," and "transient situa-tional disturbances" (Schubert et al. 1979; Uhlenhuth et al. 1983). Not only are suitable diagnostic criteria lacking, but considerable disagreement ex-ists over the legitimacy of the utilization of health care services by this population. Some critics propose that these individuals are not medically ill but experience the "exigencies" of everyday life (Illich 1976). Other critics, concerned about the increasing cost of health services, question the efficacy of extending expensive health care services to individuals with distressing emotional symptoms and psychosocial problems without phys-ical pathology or serious psychiatric illness.

Uncertainty exists as to the appropriate treatment of patients with these common conditions of psychological distress. Often, these patients receive psychoactive drugs, particularly benzodiazepines (Uhlenhuth et al. 1983), a practice that has led to the criticism that ours is an "overmedicated society." Greater use of nonpharmacological techniques, such as psycho-therapy and counseling, has been proposed, but the efficacy of psychoso-cial treatments alone or in combination with drugs for such patients has not been firmly established by controlled trials (Budman 1981; Budman and Clifford 1979; Catalan et al. 1984a, 1984b; World Health Organization 1989).

Psychologically distressed patients use a disproportionate share of ambulatory services and hospitalizations. Some research suggests that psychological treatment for patients with emotional and psychosocial problems associated with bodily complaints and a physical illness can reduce the use of laboratory tests, radiological examinations, and hospitalization (Jones and Vischi 1979; Mumford et al. 1984; Schlesinger et al. 1983). However, the results from such studies of "medical offset" are not conclusive (Budman et al. 1982). Not only does the type of treatment remain in dispute, but also the appropriate locus of care for these patients. Are they best treated in primary care settings? Should they be referred to mental health specialists?

To address some of these questions, a mental health research program was initiated at the Harvard Community Health Plan (HCHP), a large health maintenance organization (HMO) in the greater Boston area. Primary care for adults at HCHP is provided by teams of internists and nurse practitioners. Informal surveys of practitioners and studies of utilization have indicated that "problems of living" and symptoms of anxiety and depression are among the main reasons for individual primary care visits. These clinical problems contribute heavily to high utilization of ambulatory services at HCHP, as in other similar settings.

Over a 6-month period IPC was developed through an interactive and iterative process in which the research team met on a weekly basis with the nurse practitioners to review previous clinical experience, discuss case examples, observe videotapes, and listen to tape recordings. The treatment manual (Weissman and Klerman 1988), which derives from IPT, describes session-by-session instructions as to the purpose and methods for IPC, including "scripts" to ensure comparability of procedures among the nurse counselors. The conduct of IPC occurs in three phases:

1. In the *assessment phase* (which requires one or two sessions) are included a review of symptoms, assessment of the chronology of the symptoms in relation to recent life events and stress, and an interpersonal inventory. Based on these sources of information, the subject's distress, as in IPT, is "reformulated" into one of four problem areas: a) unresolved grief; b) role transitions; c) role disputes; and d) interpersonal deficits (i.e., loneliness and social isolation).

2. In the *middle phase*, IPC encourages the patient's capacity for coping with the problem area. ·

3. In the *termination phase* (usually Sessions 5 and 6), the patient is encouraged to use improved modes of coping with these problems, facilitating independence rather than continued reliance on the counseling relationship.

As a means of minimizing dependency and discouraging unnecessary utilization, patients who felt sufficiently improved following any session were not urged to continue in the IPC sessions. Thus, many treatment sessions ended with fewer than six visits.

The nine internal medicine nurse practitioners who served as counselors for the development of IPC were supervised weekly in small groups by two senior psychotherapists (i.e., a psychiatrist and a psychiatric nurse).

Interpersonal counseling, like IPT, is based on the premise that symptoms of psychological distress, regardless of biological vulnerability or personality, occur in a psychosocial and interpersonal context. Thus, the focus of IPC is mainly on the patient in current life situations, with the therapist engaging the patient in a self-evaluation in relation to the current situation. The patient is viewed as a person in distress who is experiencing symptoms, not as a patient with a specific psychiatric diagnosis.

Referral to Interpersonal Counseling

The basis of the referral to IPC was a primarily negative physical examination and high levels of subjective symptoms of distress as evidenced in the examination and/or a general screening questionnaire such as the General Health Questionnaire (GHQ; Goldberg 1979). The GHQ is a symptom inventory in which respondents are asked if they have been experiencing each of a variety of feelings or behaviors "less than usual," "the same as usual," "more than usual," or "much more than usual" in the previous few weeks. For negative symptoms (such as feeling "constantly under strain"), responses in either of the last two categories earn a score of 1. For positive feelings (such as feeling "full of energy"), responses of "less than usual" or "much less than usual" earn a score of 1. The GHQ score is the simple sum of item scores over the 30 items, and cutoff scores have been established. Widely used in research in general medical settings, the GHQ was the primary measure of symptoms in our development of IPC, although other scales may do equally as well.

To rule out serious psychiatric illness, a clinical interview by the physician can be used. A structured interview such as the Diagnostic Interview Schedule (DIS; Robins et al. 1981), the Schedule for Affective Disorders and Schizophrenia (SADS) (Endicott and Spitzer 1978), or the Structured Clinical Interview for DSM-III-R (SCID) (Spitzer et al. 1992; Williams et al. 1992) can be completed by the nurse and reviewed by the physician.

The Structure of Interpersonal Counseling

Visit 1: Initiating IPC

The first visit is used to establish rapport with the patient. During this session, the previous physical and psychiatric examination and laboratory studies that ruled out a major illness as an explanation of the symptoms are reviewed. The patient is informed of the negative physical findings. The possible relationship between symptoms of distress and current life stress, and the patient's current interpersonal and social situation is discussed, and the patient is offered an opportunity to receive help for his or her problems. Because much has to be accomplished in the first visit, this is the longest session, usually lasting 1 hour. A second visit may be necessary, especially if the full results of the physical or psychiatric examination are not yet available. All subsequent visits are 30 minutes or less, unless some undue problem arises.

In order to begin a discussion of the patient's symptoms of distress, the nurse reviews the results of the GHQ directly with the patient. This is done, item by item, for positive responses so that the patient has an opportunity to respond and also feels that some attention is being given to his or her distress. Patients with definitive physical disorders who meet the diagnostic criteria for current alcoholism, major depression, bipolar disorder, or antisocial disorder, who are psychotic or suicidal, or who have any other serious mental disorder are referred to appropriate services consistent with current clinical procedures. Patients with minor depressive symptoms or past psychiatric disorders can be included.

The nurse proceeds to discuss with the patient the negative physical findings. The possible relationship between symptoms and concerns and stress in the patient's life is stated explicitly:

> Your symptoms [state symptoms, e.g., headaches, sleep problems, fatigue, etc.] don't seem to have a physical basis. The tests are negative. How are you feeling now? Just because there is no physical basis doesn't mean that the symptoms are not real and that you are not feeling well—that is, your headache, fatigue, [etc.] are real. Stress in your life can also cause these symptoms. Let's try to review what has been going on in your life.

The nurse begins to ask the patient about recent changes in life circumstances, mood, and social functioning. Specific scripts are suggested to elicit this information.

At the end of Visit 1, the patient is given a scale assessing life events to complete as homework. This can be explained as follows: "I'd like you to complete these and bring them to our next visit. They may help us to identify what the recent stresses have been in your life."

Patient reactions to this type of exploration can be of at least one of three types:

1. The patient may insist that he or she has an undetected physical illness.
2. The patient may remain focused on the distress—for example, the sleep disturbance or fatigue—and deny any possible connection to life stress.
3. The patient may acknowledge with varying degrees some current life stress.

The first response is the most difficult one to deal with. In any case, if the patient denies an association, coercion or lecturing is avoided. If the patient's denial persists, it may be necessary to offer the opportunity for review of the results from the physical examination. As in usual clinical practice, it may be reassuring to the patient to get a second opinion from the physician. However, at this point, the nurse is advised to go gently, not to get into an argument, and to follow the patient's lead, never denying the reality of the symptoms and the real discomfort they produce. A second visit is offered. For the reluctant patient who denies current problems, you might say the following: "I can understand that these [state patient's symptoms] are uncomfortable. I'd like to try to understand over the next few weeks what may be causing them. Let's see how you are doing next week."

In some cases it may be appropriate to enter into a negotiation with the patient about his or her perceptions. You may state the following: "We both agree that you have problems with [state symptoms, e.g., sleep, energy], but we have different ideas about what is producing them. Can we, working together, see how things go for you and see what we find out over the next few weeks?"

Visit 2: Determining the Specific Problem Area(s)

The purpose of this visit is to establish directly with the patient the specific current stress area(s) in the patient's life that may be contributing to the symptoms and that will form the focus of the remaining visits.

The results of a scale assessing life events are reviewed item by item, and the one or two areas that seem to be most troubling (e.g., threat of loss of job, problems with children, marital friction) are focused on. If the patient forgets to bring in the form, this may be mentioned briefly but in a *noncritical* fashion, saying, for example, "Patients frequently forget to complete these and find it difficult to think about problems, etc." The items or areas can be reviewed during the course of the session. It is important to *listen*, letting the patient describe the answers in his or her own terms. Let the patient unburden himself or herself. However, the patient is not allowed to dominate the interaction by irrelevant preoccupations.

A systematic outline in which all salient historical points and examination results are listed can be useful to help focus a brief treatment. These points do not have to be applied in a mechanical order, but by the end of this process the area(s) should have been adequately covered. The goal is to find a focus of problems and to help the patient make sense of his or her symptoms and their onset in relationship to life circumstances. In order to achieve the above, the following areas are reviewed:

- History of present symptoms
- History of current life circumstances
- History of current close interpersonal relationships
- History of recent changes in any of the above

The nurse's task is to help the patient discover the key person(s) with whom the patient is having difficulties, what the trouble is about, and whether alternatives are open to the patient to make the relationship(s) more satisfactory.

By the end of Visit 2, the nurse (and possibly the patient) will have a sense of the major problem area(s). The problem area(s) should be stated explicitly to the patient and should derive from what the patient has been describing. It should be made explicit that the purpose of the next visits is to help with the problem(s) in question.

Visits 3–5: Working With the Specific Problem Area(s)

The purpose of Visits 3, 4, and 5 is to help the patient deal more positively with the specific problem area(s) as outlined. This is achieved by 1) continued clarification of the problem, 2) allowing the patient to unburden himself or herself to a concerned person, and 3) pointing out aspects of the situation the patient may have overlooked and suggesting steps that might help the patient better cope with the problem.

The conceptualization of the problem area(s) follows directly from IPT, with the exception that "interpersonal deficits" from IPT are described as "loneliness" and "social isolation" in the IPC manual. The problem areas include 1) grief; 2) interpersonal disputes with spouse, lover, children, other family member, friend, co-worker, and so forth; 3) transitions (i.e., new job, leaving family, going away to school, divorce, economic change, other changes in family, relocation to new home, city, or state), and 4) loneliness and social isolation.

The problems are obviously not mutually exclusive. The patient may present with problems in several areas, or there may be no one clear-cut problem. In a brief treatment, however, it is useful to choose one or two areas to work on. For patients with wide-ranging problems, the nurse may be guided in his or her choice by focusing on the stress precipitating the current symptom. The specific details for handling each problem area as described in the IPC manual follow from IPT. The use of homework is a departure from IPT and is described below.

Homework

Grief.   In order to accelerate the grieving process, the assignment might be to look over old photographs or see old friends. For example, the nurse might say: "It is often helpful to review old memories. Do you have any albums? Or do you have any old friends that you haven't seen since [name of the deceased] died? Before our next session, I'd like you to go over the albums or meet with your old friends and review your past times together. Let me know how this review was for you next time we meet."

In order to encourage the patient to become active in new social activities, the task of going to a new organization or calling up an aquaintance may be assigned: "I'd like you to do something you don't normally do, for example, call a friend or go out to dinner with a friend. Let's see how that goes. I'd like to hear about it the next time we get together."

The next sessions are used to learn about the assigned homework, how it went, and how the patient felt, beginning each session with, "How did it go last week?"

Interpersonal disputes.   Homework assignments that may be useful for interpersonal disputes, especially those with significant others, often involve expressing one's wishes more directly. All assignments, of course, must relate to the nature of the dispute and the parties involved. (For example, expressing one's wishes more directly to a tyrannical supervisor at work may not be productive.) In most cases, the dispute is between intimate family members, and the patient has not been able to express wishes directly because the wishes have been unclear or not considered legitimate by the patient.

The patient's expectations in the relationship, and how realistic they are, are discussed. As these issues become more clear, the homework assignment might include the following:

> Over the next week could you try to talk to [name family member or friend]. Let him know calmly how you feel about [identify the issue]. What would you like and how would you like it? Try to get to his point of view and why he feels the way he does. Try to understand where you agree and where you disagree, and how you both can give in to reach a better solution. If there are positives in the situation, express them directly.

While this type of negotiation will take on a different flavor with nonintimate persons who are in authority positions, the principles of negotiation can be the same. For the employee/employer relationship, you might say:

Over the next week could you ask to speak to your supervisor? You might acknowledge that things at work haven't been going as well as they could. Explain your point of view. Ask for hers. Find out what she would like to improve in the situation and try to see where you agree and disagree and how you can work out a better solution. If you like your job and really wish to improve the situation, say so directly.

Role transitions. The homework tasks for role transition are similar to those of grief with the emphasis on establishing new relationships. To help the patient make the transition, it is sometimes useful to seek transitional objects. The patient may be encouraged to bring old pictures or a piece of furniture from his or her former place or life into the new role. As homework, the patient may be encouraged at the different sessions to find transitional objects, to review old memories, and to make new contacts: "Over the next week try to look over some pictures, etc., from your old life and/or call your old friends and review your past times together. Let's talk about how this went the next time we meet."

To encourage the patient to become active in new social activities, the therapist may say, for example, "I'd like you to call up one of the new neighbors and/or work associates, etc., and go out together."

Loneliness and social isolation. In the IPT manual these problems are called *interpersonal deficits*. In the training of nurses or any counselors with nonpsychiatric training, the terminology is made more straightforward. Social isolation is chosen as the focus of treatment when a patient presents with a history of social impoverishment involving inadequate or unsustaining interpersonal relationships and when he or she has general pervasive feelings of loneliness and social isolation not specifically related to some recent transition.

In the *socially isolated group*, patients may lack relationships with either intimates or friends, or at work; they may have long-standing or temporary deficiencies in social skills or have an adequate number of interpersonal relationships but seem unable to enjoy them. Such individuals may have chronically low self-esteem despite apparent interpersonal or occupational success, or they may complain angrily about chronic exhaustion that results from repeatedly taking on more than they can manage.

Finally, there is a *chronically distressed group* of patients who may have lingering depressive symptoms that were untreated or inadequately treated in the past. Although some of the patients' acute symptoms may have resolved, persistent multiple symptoms of low intensity continue to cause distress, particularly in interpersonal situations.

The goal and strategies of dealing with the interpersonal-deficits problem area are described in the IPT manual. If the patient has no current meaningful relationships, the focus is on finding examples of relationships in the past that may have been meaningful and on forming new relationships. Homework for this problem area includes assignments to make contact with old friends or possible new ones and to seek out social situations (e.g., clubs, church, sports, other groups):

> Over the next week I'd like you to find at least one new activity with people that you haven't done before such as [give examples based on patient's age, interests, and social group]. Let's see how it goes, what problems, if any, come up, and how you can handle them differently next time. Let's see how you felt.

In helping the patient to apply the learning taking place in treatment to outside situations, it is useful to have the patient report efforts, successful or unsuccessful, to increase his or her interactions with others. A detailed review of these attempts may reveal easily correctable deficits in the patient's communication skills. In helping the patient to overcome his or her hesitations in approaching others, the nurse may invite the patient to role-play difficult situations with her, as, for example, "Let's pretend that you are going into a room full of strangers at a party. What could you do to meet people?" If the patient has been able to talk openly about an issue, the nurse might encourage this by saying, "You have been able to be very open in our talk. Is there anyone else [friends or family] you can try to be like this with? Let's imagine you are with [friend's name] and you want to start an intimate conversation. Let's pretend now that I'm this person. How would you start?" It should be emphasized that the brief treatment of interpersonal impairment is a most difficult task. Goal setting should be limited to "starting" to work on these issues, not necessarily resolving them.

Visit 6: Termination

Many patients will terminate before the full six sessions, and no effort should be made to encourage continuation if the patient feels that his or her distress has resolved. For patients who continue the full six sessions, mention again should be made of the time-limited treatment contract at Week 5. In the last session, the nurse reviews the developments over the past 6 weeks and the patient's current state, and explicitly discusses the end of IPC. For most patients, this will be the last visit. At the patient's discretion, an additional visit (see below) can be held in 2 weeks or a telephone contact can be arranged as needed. The explicit discussion of termination is a major focus in Visit 6.

Most patients and many health care providers have some discomfort with termination. Even though the patient will not be terminating the usual clinic contacts with the nurse, the IPC contacts specifically around issues of patient stress and coping will end after this visit.

If the treatment has been useful, the patient faces the task of establishing a sense of competence to deal with further problems without the aid of the sessions. It must be emphasized to the patient that the goal of the treatment is to assist the patient with mastery of life work, love, friendship, and so forth, on the outside. The nurse/patient relationship is to enhance the patient's health and competence outside of therapy and is not a substitute for friendship that is lacking on the outside.

The nurse should bring up the topic of termination and elicit the patient's reactions to this if the patient has not already volunteered this information. Many patients are unaware of having any feelings about the end of treatment, or they may be hesitant to acknowledge that they have come to value the relationship with the nurse. If these patients find themselves missing the treatment or experiencing slight worsening as termination approaches, they may interpret their feelings as a relapse. To prevent this misunderstanding, such patients should be told that at the end of treatment it is usual for patients to have some feelings—apprehension, sadness, and so forth—about ending the treatment but that the appearance of these feelings does not portend a return of distress.

As in IPT, to aid the patient's perception of his or her own competence to cope with new problems, the nurse calls attention to the patient's independent successes, friends, family, church, and the supports that are available on the outside, and emphasizes the extent to which the patient has handled his or her own difficulties. In this last visit, the nurse may bolster the patient's sense of being capable to handle future problems by reviewing with the patient his or her anticipation of areas of future difficulty and guiding the patient through an exploration of how various contingencies could be handled. Of particular importance in this regard is the patient's being able to assess early warning signals of distress. Situations of potential stress should be identified, and ways and resources for coping should be discussed (e.g., the patient's family and friends and their availability discussed). The problems of termination have been described in detail in the IPT manual.

Visit 7: Optional Extra Termination Visit

The purpose of this optional extra termination visit is to complete the termination of IPC for the patient who expresses a need to have this extra visit. This visit is held 2 weeks after the sixth visit and may be held over the telephone.

This optional visit is essentially a recapitulation of the previous one. A review of accomplishments at self-mastery and resources (e.g., friends, family, church, work) is undertaken. The termination of the 30-minute sessions is made explicit to the patient: "This will be the last time we will get together for these 30-minute sessions." If the patient is hesitant, the nurse might again say the following:

> Many patients have some uneasiness about ending these sessions if they have found them helpful. We have found that a treatment-free period is also helpful. During this next period, you should continue to use and seek out new friends or family with whom you can confide. You should continue to work on the gains you have made in taking charge of your own life. Let's see how you are doing over the next 8 weeks before making any decisions about further treatment. You can, of course, call me or the plan if you need to, and, of course, your regular clinic care will continue as usual.

Special Problems

The types of problems encountered in ITP and procedures for dealing with them have been described in earlier chapters of this book. Some problems that are unique to IPC if conducted in a primary care facility or an HMO are described below.

Differentiating Between IPC and Continuing Clinical Responsibility

Interpersonal counseling is a brief, focused treatment with specific goals and a well-defined termination point. However, all persons in a health care facility are entitled to continuing clinical care for all medical conditions. Usual clinical care continues unchanged while the patient is receiving IPC, and when IPC ends (e.g., if a patient develops a fever during the course of IPC or after it ends), he or she would seek treatment for the condition in the usual fashion. Moreover, if the patient abruptly terminates IPC or refuses to participate, the clinical care would continue as is customary.

Referral of Patients When an Illness Emerges During the Course of IPC

Although patients are screened before beginning IPC and are included if they are without serious physical psychiatric illness, medical or psychiatric problems may emerge or become unmasked during the course of the six IPC sessions. The overriding consideration is always the patient's well-being. Any life-threatening situation and all physical illness should be referred to the appropriate sources consistent with customary practice and good clinical care. The patient can also complete the IPC course if this is possible.

If non–life-threatening psychiatric symptoms or mild alcohol abuse becomes unmasked, then a referral can be delayed until the IPC course has been completed and the referral can be discussed as part of the termination phase of IPC. The rationale behind this delay is that the ensuing visits may help clarify the extent and nature of the problem. In some instances the problem may resolve, and when there is no resolution, the additional time for clarification may help in the initiation of appropriate referral.

Efficacy of Interpersonal Counseling: The Harvard Community Health Plan Study

Design

The site for the efficacy study of IPC was the Harvard Community Health Plan (HCHP), the largest HMO in New England. New enrollees are routinely encouraged to choose a primary care team consisting of an internist and a nurse practitioner to arrange an "initial health assessment" visit, which includes a baseline medical history, physical examination, and screening tests. Follow-up consultations with a specialist, including mental health personnel, are available as needed upon referral from the primary care clinician. Each year approximately 7% of HCHP members are evaluated or treated in the mental health specialty component at one of the HCHP centers (see Klerman et al. 1987 for description of efficacy study).

There were two phases of the study. In the first phase, 2,791 consecutive new enrollees were mailed questionnaires soon after joining the HCHP. The purpose was to generate a large sample for an ongoing naturalistic survey of the distribution of symptoms of stress and distress and for prospective analysis of patterns of utilization. This questionnaire included items concerning the enrollee's sociodemographic background, eight questions from the current health subscale of the GHQ (Goldberg 1979), and questions about levels of previous utilization of general health and mental health services, self-perception of social functioning questions from the Social Adjustment Scale (SAS; Weissman and Bothwell 1976), and expectations for health care.

Previous reports have recommended a cutoff score of 5 or more on the GHQ as an index of psychosocial morbidity. To select a group of patients with slightly higher symptom severity, a cutoff point of 6 or above was chosen as the criterion for entry into the second phase of the study. The second phase consisted of the IPC intervention trial. In this phase, 5,339 consecutive new enrollees were sent the GHQ by mail, and 2,868 (52%) returned completed GHQs. Those with scores of 6 or higher were selected for assignment to an experimental group that was offered IPC, or to a comparison group that was followed naturalistically. Subjects selected for IPC treatment were contacted by telephone and invited to make an appointment promptly with one of the study's nurse practitioners. During this telephone contact, reference was made to items of concern raised by the subject's response to the GHQ, and the subject was offered an appointment to address these and other health issues of concern in an initial health assessment.

In the course of the intervention study, the original intent to randomize subjects strictly was modified in order to provide a steady stream of subjects for the IPC treatment. Randomization, though methodologically desirable, would have left too much idle capacity in the treatment condition. Instead of randomizing the subjects, a comparison group was formed consisting of subjects with high GHQ scores during the month of June 1984. During the months of October 1983 through May 1984, all enrollees with high scores were thus assigned to the experimental condition.

A total of 127 patients were contacted and asked to participate in the intervention phase of the research study. Seventy-nine (62%) of those contacted agreed to make an initial appointment. Fifteen subjects (12%) made an initial appointment but either cancelled or failed to keep it, and a total of 64 subjects actually entered the treatment phase. For purposes of outcome assessment, these 64 patients were compared with a subgroup of 64 untreated subjects with similar evaluations in GHQ scores during June 1984, matched to treated subjects on gender.

Assessments Prior to Treatment Assignment

Prior to assignment to treatment, symptoms of stress and distress, general health status, and social adjustment status were assessed by the questionnaire administered to all enrollees. Medical status was evaluated by the routine initial health assessment. Patients with serious medical problems were excluded from the trial.

Enrollees who agreed to participate in the treatment intervention were also evaluated using the National Institute of Mental Health Diagnostic Interview Schedule (DIS; Robins et al. 1981), which provides for assessment of major DSM-III psychiatric diagnoses. These interviews usually took place within a week or two after the initial health assessment. The DIS findings were not available to the nurse clinicians at the time of the first visit. If, however, the DIS revealed significant psychotic functioning, serious suicidal ideation, current heavy use of alcohol, or other drug abuse, this information was provided to the nurse practitioner and her supervisor. As a result of this assessment, two patients were referred for immediate psychiatric care. Patients in the comparison group did not receive the DIS.

At the end of the last IPC session, the 30-item version of the GHQ was readministered. Enrollees in the comparison group were mailed a second GHQ 3 months from the date of the first GHQ, an interval that approximated the average time between entry and postintervention GHQs in the IPC group.

Characteristics of the Sample

As expected, the sample consisted mainly of young adults (mean age = 28 years). The two groups did not differ on any variable except initial GHQ score, with the IPC group having higher scores. The distribution of scores in the GHQ in a large initial sample in the HMO was almost identical to that reported in previous studies of primary care populations. The large majority of enrollees (approximately 80%) scored below the cutoff point of 4 that was recommended as representing "normal."

Based upon the results of the initial health assessment, most of the enrollees who were selected for the trial group and the comparison group were judged in good physical health. Many of the subjects had some past psychiatric diagnoses based on DIS. The most common diagnoses were major depression, dysthymia, phobias, and psychosexual dysfunction.

Results

The average number of completed IPC sessions was 3.4. Thirty percent of subjects had only a single session; 22% completed the entire course of six sessions. There was no significant relationship between number of sessions and symptom reduction. The GHQ was readministered at completion of treatment, with 73% of IPC subjects and 67% of comparison subjects returning completed postintervention questionnaires. By use of previously established norms of scores of 4 or below as indicating "normality," 83% of the IPC group reached this criterion, compared with 63% of the comparison group. This difference in proportions is highly significant statistically ($P = .01$). The mean GHQ score among IPC subjects fell from 14.2 at entry to 3.8 after intervention. In the same interval, the mean GHQ score among comparison subjects fell from 11.0 to 6.9.

The main determinants of the final GHQ score were initial level and treatment groups. The treatment effect remained even after statistical adjustment for the initial higher GHQ score of the IPC subjects. Thus, regression to the mean did not account for the observed effect. The statistical model accounted for 20% of the variance in the final score, and two-thirds of the outcome variance could be attributed to the IPC intervention.

Utilization of medical care.   Sufficient data were available for 56 (88%) of the IPC subjects and 52 (81%) of the comparison subjects to permit analysis of the rate of utilization of health care services in the HMO for the 12 months following entry into the study. Mean annualized rates for the following five utilization variables were assessed: 1) scheduled visits to clinicians other than mental health clinicians, 2) unscheduled nonmental health visits, 3) visits with mental health clinicians (not including IPC visits), 4) hospitalizations, and 5) the total of all ambulatory care visits. IPC subjects showed higher rates of use of all ambulatory care, especially in mental health, but simple statistical comparisons of mean rates were not possible because of the highly skewed distributions of rates among individuals. Nonparametric tests (i.e., the Mann-Whitney U test) comparing the two groups failed to reach statistically significant difference levels; thus, the apparently higher rates among IPC subjects suggest a trend but do not firmly demonstrate it.

Clinical Observations

Few subjects in the intervention study experienced serious medical or psychiatric problems. There were no psychotic episodes. One patient experienced severe back pain throughout the study; there were no other instances of major medical illness. Two subjects out of 64 expressed thoughts of suicide during the course of their sessions. One of these patients (with an initial GHQ score of 11) successfully completed six IPC sessions and expressed positive feelings about the intervention. The other patient completed two sessions with her nurse therapist before being referred to the mental health department for further treatment, and returned for two further sessions a short time later. Her GHQ score fell from 13 at entry to 1 at her final session.

Interpersonal psychotherapy proved feasible in the primary care environment. It was easily learned by experienced nurse practitioners in a short training program of 8 to 12 hours. The brevity of the sessions and the short duration of treatment rendered IPC compatible with usual professional practices in a primary care unit. No significant negative effects of treatment were observed, and nurses were able, with weekly supervision, to counsel several patients whose levels of psychiatric distress would normally have resulted in direct referral to specialty mental health care.

In comparison with a group of untreated subjects with initial elevations in GHQ scores, those patients receiving the IPC intervention showed greater reduction in symptom scores over an average interval of 3 months. Many patients who had undergone IPC reported significant relief of symptoms after only one or two sessions.

Selection biases could partially explain the difference in change scores between treated and comparison subjects, because the former group consisted only of subjects who agreed to an initial appointment with the nurse practitioners, whereas the latter consisted of an unselected group of patients with comparable elevations in GHQ scores at enrollment. In fact, of the 182 subjects initially judged eligible for IPC, 10 did not speak English, and 45 were otherwise technically unavailable for assignment to treatment. Such subjects would also not have been included in the comparison group. Overall, 127 subjects were realistically available for IPC treatment, 79 (62%) agreed to treatment, and 64 (50%) actually attended an initial session, thus gaining entry into the IPC-treated group in this analysis. It is possible that the treatment effect found in this study is attributed to the selection bias introduced by the process of agreement to treatment; only further, fully randomized designs can avoid this potential bias.

Our findings conform to those of other investigators, such as Shepherd et al. (1979) and Corney (1984), who evaluated psychosocial interventions within primary care settings. One prior controlled prospective trial evaluating a form of brief therapy in family practices was not able to demonstrate a positive effect on health status (Brodaty and Andrews 1983), but the patients in that study were, on the average, considerably more impaired than those in the sample reported here.

This pilot study provides preliminary evidence that early detection and outreach to distressed adults followed by brief treatment with IPC can, in the short term, reduce symptoms of distress as measured by the GHQ. The main effect seems to occur in symptoms related to mood, especially in those forms of mild and moderate depression that are commonly seen in medical patients. Such outreach to distressed individuals may also result in reduction in utilization of health care services.

Alternately, it is possible that IPC patients, having been introduced to psychological reframing of physical symptoms, will more often seek and receive mental health care afterward. If IPC acts as such an entry into mental health care, then experimental subjects may demonstrate increased, not decreased, use of health services. Early entry into mental health services may delay or prevent less appropriate later use of primary care for physical symptoms. Previous studies of "offset" effects of mental health services, as noted before, are inconclusive (Budman et al. 1982; Schlesinger et al. 1983).

The current study raises questions about the appropriate timing of psychological interventions in primary care settings. The approach used here (i.e., screening of all adults at the time of enrollment) proved feasible but inefficient for several reasons. First, although mild levels of distress are common, only a few of those subjects screened report marked levels of symptoms. These few subjects are of special interest in intervention studies because the vast majority of subjects with milder elevations of GHQ scores probably have transient and self-limited problems for which interventions are not needed. Second, mild or moderately distressed people contacted through outreach may lack sufficient motivation to initiate or continue in counseling. It is possibly significant that subjects who refused treatment in this outreach study had lower mean GHQ scores than those who agreed to treatment. Third, at least some of the individuals needing help will seek and find it themselves outside the primary care setting or other health care facility, and prompt outreach may interrupt or delay these self-motivated efforts.

Based upon the observations in this study, we developed a model of the "career" of the patient in primary health care. We hypothesize that patients progress through time from enrollment to the first visit for symptomatic health care, to a pattern of multiple visits for a variety of acute, and subsequently chronic, physical symptoms, and, for some, eventually to overt psychiatric illness. Whether or not such a sequence exists in primary care settings remains to be demonstrated, but the model offers a conceptually appealing rationale for potential opportunities for intervention. In theory, it would be desirable to intervene at a stage in the career late enough that an individual can be known with some certainty to be manifesting dysfunctional utilization patterns and when he or she may be motivated to seek help, but early enough that the sequence of events can be interrupted. Further empirical studies with randomized designs can help resolve the issue of timing of psychosocial intervention in primary care.

The nature of interventions appropriate to the primary care setting also warrants further study. Four major considerations are involved in planning psychosocial intervention: 1) scheduling of treatment, including the choice between intermittent and continuous treatment schedules; 2) the duration of individual treatment encounters; 3) the theoretical rationale for intervention, especially the choice between approaches centering on specific behaviors and those focusing on symptom relief; and 4) the professional discipline and training of the counselor-therapist.

Summary and Conclusions

Interpersonal counseling is a brief form of therapy focused on specific symptoms and problem-solving strategies using an interpersonal model of the therapeutic process. This therapy is delivered by experienced primary care nurse practitioners without extensive specialized training in mental health care to patients with mild and moderate distress in general health care systems. Modification of duration, timing, or type of treatment or the training of the therapist may improve the efficiency and feasibility of the treatment. It may be that intermittent sessions would be more effective than a scheduled sequence; encounters of 1 hour might be better than 30-minute sessions; or perhaps nonprofessionals attached to health care units would be as effective as health professionals, and less expensive. These issues remain to be resolved through appropriate prospective trials.

An additional issue not directly addressed by the current study is the choice of thresholds for referral of patients to specialized mental health treatment. Even if options like IPC exist within primary care units, some patients are so ill, or so insistent, that prompt specialty referral is necessary. Studies indicate that primary care physicians are uncomfortable treating patients who are overtly psychotic, demented, suicidal, severely depressed, alcoholic, or addicted to drugs. Our experience with IPC suggests that treatment for patients with these conditions may nonetheless be done safely and effectively by some nonmental health professionals. Rational thresholds for referral should be developed, but these remain to be defined by future investigations.

The purpose of this study was to demonstrate the feasibility of IPC administered by nurse practitioners in a primary care setting and to begin testing the efficacy of IPC. The pilot nature of this study must be emphasized. Further testing should include a broader range of outcome measures, including clinician symptom rating, and long-term follow-up to assess whether the short-term reduction in symptoms with IPC is sustained over time, and whether associated changes occur in general health care and mental health care utilization. Additional comparison groups to control for the effects of attention should be included.

IPC is being tested by Jan Mossey, Ph.D., at the Medical College of Pennsylvania in Philadelphia. In Dr. Mossey's study, IPC is administered by nurse clinical specialists in a randomized clinical trial with medically ill hospitalized older patients who have dysthymia or elevated levels of depressive symptoms. IPC will be continued through outpatient aftercare. The purpose is to see if IPC reduces complications and rehospitalization, and limits use of nonpsychotropic medication and visits to physicians for medical reasons.

Although definitive evaluation of IPC awaits these results, and its effect on utilization is not yet determined, the short-term reduction in symptoms suggests that this approach to outreach and early intervention may be an effective alternative to current practices. If so, then IPC may be a useful addition to the repertoire of psychosocial intervention skills that can be incorporated into routine primary care.

The IPC manual as it stands has been developed by us for one pilot study, although modifications probably are being made by Dr. Mossey for her study noted above. Users of the IPC manual would need to make some modification to fit their particular site and/or protocol. It should also be noted that Dr. Schulberg at the University of Pittsburgh is using IPC in a primary care facility (see Chapter 7).

References

Brodaty H, Andrews G: Brief psychotherapy in family practice: a controlled prospective intervention trial. Br J Psychiatry 143:11–19, 1983

Budman SH: Looking toward the future, in Forms of Brief Therapy. Edited by Budman SH. New York, Guilford, 1981, pp 461–467

Budman SH, Clifford M: Short-term group therapy for couples in a health maintenance organization. Professional Psychology 10:419–429, 1979

Budman SH, Demby A, Randall M: Psychotherapeutic outcome and reduction in medical utilization: a cautionary tale. Professional Psychology 13:200–207, 1982

Catalan J, Gath D, Bond A, et al: The effects of nonprescribing of anxiolytics in general practice, II. factors associated with outcome. Br J Psychiatry 144:603–610, 1984a

Catalan J, Gath D, Edmonds G, et al: The effects of nonprescribing of anxiolytics in general practice, I: controlled evaluation of psychiatric and social outcome. Br J Psychiatry 144:593–602, 1984b

Corney RH: The effectiveness of attached social workers in the management of depressed female patients in general practice. Psychol Med Monograph Supplement 6, 1984

Endicott J, Spitzer R: A diagnostic interview: the Schedule for Affective Disorders and Schizophrenia. Arch Gen Psychiatry 35:837–844, 1978

Goldberg DP: The Detection of Psychiatric Illness by Questionnaire. Institute of Psychiatry Maudsley Monogr No 21. London, Oxford University Press, 1972

Goldberg DP: Detection of and assessment of emotional disorders in primary care. International Journal of Mental Health 8:30–48, 1979

Hankin J, Otay JS: Mental disorder and primary medical care: an analytic review of the literature (DHEW Publ No ADM-78-661). Washington, DC, National Institute of Mental Health, 1979

Hoeper EW, Nycz GR, Cleary PH, et al: Estimated prevalence of RDC mental disorder in primary medical care. International Journal of Mental Health 8:6–15, 1979

Illich I: Medical Nemesis: The Expropriation of Health. New York, Pantheon, 1976

Jencks SF: Recognition of mental distress and diagnosis of mental disorder in primary care. JAMA 253:1903–1907, 1985

Jones KR, Vischi TR: Impact of alcohol, drug abuse, and mental health treatment on medical care utilization. Med Care 17(suppl):1–82, 1979

Klerman GL, Weissman MM, Rounsaville BJ, et al: Interpersonal Psychotherapy for Depression. New York, Basic Books, 1984

Klerman GL, Budman S, Berwick D, et al: Efficacy of a brief psychosocial intervention for symptoms of stress and distress among patients in primary care. Med Care 25:1078–1088, 1987

Mumford E, Schlesinger HJ, Glass GV, et al: A new look at evidence about reduced cost of medical utilization following mental health treatment. Am J Psychiatry 141:1145–1158, 1984

Ormel J, Maarten WJ, Koeter MA, et al: Recognition, management, and course of anxiety and depression in general practice. Arch Gen Psychiatry 48:700–706, 1991

Robins LN, Helzer JE, Croughan J, et al: National Institute of Mental Health Diagnostic Interview Schedule: its history, characteristics, and validity. Arch Gen Psychiatry 38:381–389, 1981

Schlesinger HJ, Mumford E, Glass GV, et al: Mental health treatment and medical care utilization in a fee-for-service system: outpatient mental health treatment following the onset of a chronic disease. Am J Public Health 73:422–429, 1983

Schubert DSP, Gabinet L, Friedson W, et al: The identification of psychiatric morbidity by internists and subsequent selection for psychiatric referrals. Int J Psychiatry Med 9:317–327, 1979

Shepherd M, Harwin BG, Depla C, et al: Social work and the primary care of mental disorder. Psychol Med 9:661–669, 1979

Spitzer RL, Williams JBW, Gibbon M, et al: The Structured Clinical Interview for DSM-III-R (SCID), I: history, rationale, and description. Arch Gen Psychiatry 49:624–629, 1992

Uhlenhuth EH, Balter MB, Mellinger GD, et al: Symptom checklist syndromes in the general population: correlation with psychotherapeutic drug use. Arch Gen Psychiatry 40:1167–1173, 1983

Weissman MM, Bothwell S: Assessment of social adjustment by patient self-report. Arch Gen Psychiatry 33:1111–1115, 1976

Weissman MM, Klerman GL: Interpersonal Counseling (IPC) for Stress and Distress in Primary Care Settings. New York, New York State Psychiatric Institute, 1988

Williams JBW, Gibbon M, First MB, et al: The Structured Clinical Interview for DSM-III-R (SCID), II: multisite test-retest reliability. Arch Gen Psychiatry 49:630–636, 1992

World Health Organization: Psychosocial interventions in primary health care settings in Europe. Report (EUR/ICP/PSF 020, #5695B) on a WHO consultation, Sofia, Bulgaria, 1989

CHAPTER 12

Interpersonal Psychotherapy for Patients Who Abuse Drugs

Bruce J. Rounsaville, M.D.
Kathleen Carroll, Ph.D.

Starting in 1977 our research group has adapted interpersonal psychotherapy (IPT) for use in controlled clinical trials evaluating psychotherapy and pharmacotherapy for opioid-addicted individuals and persons who abuse cocaine. In this chapter we describe 1) the rationale for using individual psychotherapy in general and IPT in particular for these two groups of patients, 2) the adaptations we have made in IPT to meet the specific clinical needs of drug-abusing patients, 3) the design and results of two clinical trials evaluating the efficacy of IPT with opioid-addicted patients and cocaine-abusing patients, and 4) recommendations for enhancing the efficacy of IPT with drug-abusing patients.

Rationale for Interpersonal Psychotherapy With Drug-Abusing Patients

Is Psychotherapy Necessary in the Treatment of Drug Abuse?

What are the alternatives to psychotherapy? Of course, many, if not most, individuals who use psychoactive substances either do not become abusers

This work was supported by National Institute on Drug Abuse Grants 1-018-DA06963 and 1-RO1-DA04299.

of these substances or eventually stop or limit their substance use without formal treatment (Brunswick 1979; O'Donnell et al. 1976; Robins 1979; Robins and Davis 1974). Most people who seek treatment only do so after numerous unsuccessful attempts to stop or reduce drug use on their own (Robins 1979). For those who seek treatment, the alternatives to some form of psychotherapy are either structural (e.g., sequestration from access to drugs in a residential setting) or pharmacological. Removal from the setting in which drug use takes place is a useful and sometimes necessary part of drug treatment but is seldom sufficient, as is shown by the high relapse rates typically seen from residential detoxification programs or incarceration during the year following patients' return to their community (Hubbard et al. 1984; O'Donnell 1969; Simpson et al. 1982; Valliant 1966).

The most powerful and commonly used pharmacological approaches to drug abuse are maintenance on an agonist that has a similar action to the abused drug (e.g., methadone for opioid-addicted patients, nicotine gum for persons who smoke tobacco), use of an antagonist that blocks the effect of the abused drug (e.g, naltrexone for opioid-addicted patients), and the use of an aversive agent that provides a powerful negative reinforcement if the drug is used (e.g., disulfiram for alcoholic persons). While all of these agents are widely used, they are seldom used without the provision of adjunctive psychotherapy. This is because methadone dispensing alone has been shown to have unacceptably high rates of continued use of opioids and other drugs (Senay 1989), naltrexone maintenance alone is plagued by high rates of premature dropout (Kleber and Kosten 1984), and disulfiram use without adjunctive psychotherapy has not been shown to be superior to placebo (Fuller et al. 1986). Even when the principal treatment is seen as pharmacological, psychotherapeutic interventions are needed to complement the pharmacotherapy by 1) enhancing the motivation to stop drug use by taking the prescribed medications, 2) providing guidance for use of prescribed medications and management of side effects, 3) maintaining motivation to continue taking the prescribed medication after the patient achieves an initial period of abstinence, 4) providing relationship elements to prevent premature termination, and 5) helping the patient to develop the skills to adjust to a life without drug use. These elements that psychotherapy can offer to complement pharmacological approaches are likely to be needed even if "perfect" pharmacotherapies are available. However, the repertoire of pharmacotherapies available for treatment of drug abuse is limited to a handful, with the most effective agents limited in their utility to treatment of opioid abuse (Jaffe and Kleber 1989; O'Brien and Woody 1989; Senay 1989). The development of effective pharmacotherapies for abuse of cocaine, marijuana, hallucinogens, sedative-hypnotics, and stimulants is still in its infancy (Kleber 1989; Kosten 1989).

The Place of IPT in Treatment of Drug Abuse

Given the general need for psychotherapy as a component of treatment for persons who abuse drugs, we adapted IPT for use in two specific contexts: 1) as an adjunctive treatment to be used with opioid-addicted individuals being maintained on methadone, and 2) as a treatment to be used alone and in combination with promising pharmacotherapies for ambulatory cocaine-abusing patients.

Ambulatory Psychotherapy in Opioid-Addicted Patients Being Maintained on Methadone

Before the advent of methadone maintenance, psychotherapy alone as treatment for ambulatory opioid-addicted patients was widely thought to be ineffective. Brill (1977) has summarized the problems in psychotherapy treatment with addicted individuals, including failure of the addicted person to become engaged in treatment, early dropout, relapse to illicit drug use, and other types of impulsive behaviors. In the early 1970s, it was shown clinically that psychotherapy offered in a general psychiatric clinic failed to engage even a significant minority of opioid-addicted patients who initially sought help. However, stabilization with methadone maintenance confers several benefits, including facilitation of nonpharmacological intervention. Because of the maintenance with methadone, retention in treatment may be improved, craving for illicit drugs may be eliminated, the need to engage in illegal behavior may be removed, and the addicted person may be able to engage in psychotherapy because he or she is freed from the preeminent need to obtain a constant supply of drugs. As an additional consideration, evidence has accumulated that a majority of opioid-addicted patients presenting to treatment have significant coexistent psychopathology that may require more intensive treatment than is typically offered in a simple methadone-dispensing program (Ross et al.

1988; Rounsaville et al. 1982a, 1982b, 1991; Weiss et al. 1986). Thus, in the late 1970s, the success of many aspects of methadone maintenance afforded us with the opportunity to evaluate psychotherapy for ambulatory opioid-addicted patients in a new and more promising context than previous work that evaluated psychotherapy alone.

Ambulatory Psychotherapy for Patients Who Abuse Cocaine

Widespread use of cocaine in the United States is a comparatively recent phenomenon, with large numbers of cocaine-abusing persons seeking treatment only since the early 1980s (Adams et al. 1986; Colliver 1987). To meet their needs, service providers have generally adapted methods that have been standard for treating persons who abuse other substances, including opioids and alcohol. Given the need for treatments of demonstrated efficacy, our group has conducted a series of studies of promising pharmacotherapeutic (Gawin and Kleber 1986; Gawin et al. 1989) and psychotherapeutic (Carroll et al. 1992) strategies. For patients who abuse cocaine, several clinicians have contended that psychotherapy alone may be sufficient (Kleber and Gawin 1984; Rawson et al. 1986; Washton et al. 1986). The absence of a medically dangerous physical withdrawal syndrome from cocaine suggests that ambulatory psychotherapy is more likely to be adequate than it is for opioid-, sedative-, or alcohol-dependent individuals, for whom a period of medical intervention such as detoxification is often an essential prerequisite for treatment.

Why Adapt IPT for Use With Patients Who Abuse Drugs?

We chose IPT for as a potentially effective treatment for opioid-addicted individuals and cocaine-abusing persons because many of its features fit well with clinical problems presented by drug-abusing patients and with widely available systems of care. Devised by Klerman and associates for treatment of depression (Klerman et al. 1984), IPT is based on the concept that psychiatric disorders, including depression and drug abuse, are intimately related to disturbances in interpersonal functioning that may be associated with the genesis and/or perpetuation of the disorder. This type of psychotherapy has four definitive characteristics: 1) it attempts to immediately address the presenting symptom picture (i.e., depression, drug abuse), 2) it focuses on the patient's difficulties in current interpersonal functioning, 3) it is brief and the emphasis is on therapists taking an active, focused stance, and 4) it uses a traditional exploratory/supportive therapeutic stance that is familiar to traditionally trained psychotherapists.

Interpersonal therapy has been described in a training manual (Klerman et al. 1984) and has been shown to be effective in several clinical trials with depressed patients who do not abuse drugs. Several of these features fit well in the treatment of drug-abusing patients. Intervening with the presenting symptom is essential for engaging the patient into treatment and demonstrating the treatment's relevance. Focus on interpersonal problems is highly relevant for drug-abusing patients, who have been shown to have many social and interpersonal impairments associated with their drug abuse (McLellan et al. 1981; Rounsaville et al. 1982a, 1982b). The brevity and focused nature of the treatment is likely to enhance its cost effectiveness in the context of limited treatment resources for these patients. Also, the traditional stance of IPT and its description in a training manual are likely to facilitate training of therapists in its use. Finally, the efficacy of IPT with depressed patients is promising because of the high rates of depression reported in drug-abusing individuals (Rounsaville et al. 1983, 1991).

Adapting Interpersonal Psychotherapy for Treatment of Drug Abuse

In this section we describe the revisions in the topical content and strategy of IPT that were made to meet the specific needs of drug-abusing patients. The overall rationale for IPT, the therapist's stance, and the phases of treatment are unchanged from those described elsewhere for treatment of depressed patients (Klerman et al. 1984). The focus on depressive symptoms has been changed to a focus on reducing or eliminating drug use, and the handling of current interpersonal problem areas has been adapted to the kinds of issues presented by drug-abusing patients.

Just as the two primary goals of interpersonal psychotherapy of depression are symptom reduction and improved social functioning, the major aims in treating drug-abusing patients are 1) to help the patient reduce or cease drug use, and 2) to help the patient develop more productive strategies for dealing with social and interpersonal problems associated with the onset and perpetuation of drug use. The techniques for achieving the two kinds of goals differ and are described below.

Strategies to Help the Patient Stop Drug Use

Achieving cessation of drug use involves helping the drug-abusing patient reach three subgoals: 1) acceptance of the need to stop; 2) management of impulsiveness; and 3) recognition of the context of drug use and of supply.

Acceptance of the Need to Stop

Persons who occasionally use drugs usually do not seek treatment. The vast majority of people coming to our attention for treatment are those for whom drug use has become an important part of their lives. They usually approach treatment with ambivalence even though they may seek treatment from an internal conviction that they have lost control of the use and pay too heavy a price for it, both financially and personally. However, there is still a feeling that they can control their substance use. They do not want to give up the positive effects and euphoria produced, and instead are seeking treatment chiefly because of external pressure from family members or the law. Moreover, drug-abusing patients are often convinced that the drug use is essential to certain activities, such as maintaining energy level at work, developing creative ideas, being comfortable in social situations, and so on. In this vein, Cummings (1979) asserts that many persons who compulsively use drugs seek treatment primarily with the hope of reducing dosage sufficiently that drug use will become enjoyable and possible again.

Psychotherapy early on must address this ambivalence if the client is to remain in treatment. In effect, the therapist must puncture the patient's idealized, romantic view of drugs or of himself or herself as a drug user. This is done by placing clear emphasis on the the deleterious effects of drugs for the abusing patient. The therapist is careful in taking the history to elicit from the patient the various costs that his or her drug use has entailed. By enumerating these costs repeatedly and comparing them with the perceived benefits of continued drug use, the balance may be persuasive in clarifying to the abusing patient just how self-destructive his or her drug use has been. At times, joint interviews with family members or significant others may be necessary to make these points more clearly.

Management of Impulsiveness

In his description of the "impulsive personality," Shapiro (1965) suggests that the essential feature of persons with this character structure is the lack of cognitive structures that may prevent antisocial or impulsive behavior from being carried out once the impulse is felt. For delay of gratification there must be an awareness that there is a future in which alternative gratification is available. The ability to forgo short-term gains in favor of meeting long-term goals, the presence of lasting and stable relationships, and recognition of adverse consequences are factors that typically prevent the ordinary individual from becoming engaged in impulsive behaviors. The therapist can use several strategies to help the addicted patient temporize his or her behavior.

First, the therapist may attempt to help the drug-abusing patient re-create the train of thought that precedes the use of drugs. By doing this the abusing patient may become aware that many of the thoughts that precede drug use are irrational and overblown, such as "I'll die if I don't have some drugs," or, "I deserve it because of the work that I did." Recognition of the irrational nature of such thoughts may be helpful in the addicted individual's cognitive renunciation of drug use. Also, revealing the thoughts that precede the drug use may help the addicted patient recognize the needs that the drug use fills and help him or her focus on alternative sources of gratification. The careful verbal reconstruction of the train of thought that led to drug use may also be useful simply because the behavior is ordinarily highly impulsive and experienced in a nonverbal way. The articulation alone may help prevent drug use because now there are thoughts that may intervene between the impulse and the use of drugs.

An important technique used by Alcoholics Anonymous (AA) is to provide a continuously available social support group that the alcoholic person can call upon when he or she feels the urge to drink. Similar organizations now exist for cocaine- and opioid-abusing persons. Alternatively, it may be useful to identify a spouse, friend, other family member, and so forth, with whom contact can be sought when the patient feels the urge to use drugs. An important aspect of the self-help group approach is the formation of a dependent relationship on the group that can in part substitute for the dependent relationship on the drug that is being renounced. In the early stage of psychotherapy for drug-abusing patients, the therapist may find it useful to offer support and direction to a greater extent than is typical of traditional psychotherapy. The therapist may make between-session visits or phone calls an option to the patient who is having difficulty in managing his or her impulsive, peremptory desires to use drugs. An important aspect of fostering a substitute dependency on the therapist is the temporary nature of this aspect of the psychotherapy. As patients gain better control of their compulsive drug use, therapists should gradually emphasize the patients' independence and ability to manage themselves on their own.

Recognition of the Context of Drug Use and of Supply

In taking a history of the pattern of drug use, it may become apparent that it takes place in association with particular settings, including physical states and social settings, or during certain affect states. Association with particular individuals, arguments with family members, coming from work to an empty house, and weekend parties are typical situations that may precede drug use. The therapist may help the drug-abusing patient explore ways to simply avoid these situations, such as cutting off contact with dealers and drug-abusing friends, increasing contact with non–drug-abusing friends, and destroying drug paraphernalia. Many persons who use drugs find that they must change routes taken to and from work because these lead to familiar streets or freeway exits that have been associated with buying drugs.

Strategies for Improving Interpersonal Functioning

A key concept for an interpersonal approach to drug abuse is that drug use plays a role in the individual's attempts to cope with problems in social relationships. The abusing individual has chosen to use drugs in an attempt to solve problems in living. Drug use has come to serve important functions in his or her life. These functions may have been those that were initially sought, such as compensation for frustration resulting from failed relationships in work or marriage, or those that have become manifest only after abusing drugs, such as enabling a weak family member to play a key role in family dynamics following the discovery of the patient's drug use. The interpersonal therapist, as a step in helping the patient manage his or her life without resorting to drug use, must determine the functions that drug use plays and help the patient find other ways to perform these functions. Unless the patient can meet these needs in other ways, he or she will be highly vulnerable to relapse, even if the patient has long been free of withdrawal symptoms.

As part of the psychiatric history performed in the initial sessions, the therapist explores the patient's drug history as a means of uncovering the functions of drug use in the patient's psychological and interpersonal life. This includes the course of substance abuse beginning with first use of legal and illegal drugs (including alcohol and cigarettes), the pattern of abuse, the types of drugs used, the sequence of abuse periods and drug-free periods, the means of supporting compulsive use, the nature of previous interactions with treatment programs, and any legal problems or illegal activities associated with drug use. There is special emphasis on interpersonal events and mental states around periods when the patient has relapsed back to drug use after abstinence, for such events may reveal the patient's particular vulnerabilities and provide a foundation for further work on symptom control.

In exploring the patient's drug use, the therapist pays close attention to the meanings of such use in the interaction between the drug use and the patient's relationships with others. The following questions are particularly relevant:

- How did drug use begin?
- Did the patient use drugs early on or recently? primarily alone or in a group?
- How are others in the abusing patient's life affected by his or her drug use?
- How has the patient's drug use influenced other family members? Are family members hurt or exploited by the drug use? Do they contribute to the drug use whether overtly or covertly?
- How does the drug influence the patient's perception of sexual behavior? behavior with casual friends? behavior with strangers and other people?
- Does conflict or, alternatively, greater intimacy with others occur before drug use or after drug use?
- What behaviors are necessary to obtain drugs and to finance drug use?
- What deceptions are necessary?

- Is the money obtained legally or illegally? If money is obtained illegally, what kind of behavior is necessary—violence, deception, theft?
- What risks are taken?

From responses to questions such as these, the therapist can form a picture of the psychological and interpersonal context of the patient's drug use.

To perform IPT for depression, the therapist attempts to focus interventions toward resolving interpersonal problems of four types: interpersonal role disputes, role transitions, grief, and interpersonal deficits. In our experience, the constellation of issues subsumed under each of these problem types is also found in persons who abuse drugs, and the strategies devised for managing these issues in depressed patients can be adapted to the treatment of abusing patients. In approaching interpersonal problems in depressed patients and drug-abusing patients, a key similarity is that interpersonal problems are seen as a determinant of the symptomatic behavior. However, while depression may result from the sense of loss at being unable to resolve interpersonal problems, drug abuse represents a dysfunctional attempt to cope with it. Thus, when attempting to help the abusing patient resolve problems in one of the four areas, the therapist must not only address the patient's problem but also find a replacement for the function that drugs have played in the past.

The four interpersonal problem areas are described below as they relate to drug abuse. Each problem area is associated with a defined set of psychotherapeutic strategies. In taking the psychiatric history it is useful to determine the problem type that best characterizes each patient. Although any given patient may have multiple problems, in a brief therapy the therapist should choose to focus only on those issues that are most closely associated with the perpetuation of drug abuse.

Interpersonal role disputes

Description. *Interpersonal role disputes* refers to a situation in which the patient and at least one significant other have nonreciprocal expectations about the roles they should play in their relationship. The disputes are seen as related to overt or unspoken rules that govern several dimensions of the relationship, including intimacy, dominance, communication, and boundaries. Drug use can be initiated or continued as a dysfunctional attempt to resolve a wide range of disputes. For example, drugs may be used to modulate intimacy in a marriage. Closeness may be a problem if the patient fears being engulfed or overwhelmed by the partner. Too much distance may be a problem if it leads to an overwhelming sense of loneliness or emptiness. Attempts to resolve fears of intimacy or abandonment may involve excessive efforts to achieve either end of the spectrum or else a frequent vacillation between intimacy and distance. Drugs may fit into this scheme in a number of ways. Drugs may give to drug-abusing partners a safe focus of shared activity. Alternatively, they may help the abusing patient obtain a needed distance from a partner both by necessitating time away from home and by allowing the patient to establish a drug-induced distance from the other person even while they are together. Also, the patient may use the drugs to ease the dysphoria after repeated stereotypical, ritualistic arguments.

Drug use can function in the balance of power within a marriage or family. A person who abuses drugs may use his or her disorder as a way of declaring himself or herself incompetent and thereby avoid the tensions of competing for dominance with a significant other. Conversely, the drug-abusing person may use the drug to enhance his or her power in a relationship by relying on the direct energizing effect of the drug or through threats to resume drug use if his or her demands are not met. Drug use can also serve a function in communication such that a family member may make his or her needs known in this form of nonverbal signaling rather than through more direct and explicit verbal communication. A very common pattern is for one partner to use drugs to compensate for satisfactions that are seen as irretrievably lost from a relationship in which disputes have reached an impasse.

Therapist's strategy.   When drug use is related to the patient's role disputes, the goal of treatment is to help the patient to clearly identify the dispute and to begin to resolve it through renegotiation of the relationship with the significant other. The therapist attempts to explore the differences in expectations and values between the patient and the significant other, to place the patient's current problems into the context of other important relationships in his or her life, to help the patient identify options for change, and to assist the patient as he or she resolves the dispute by fostering clearer and more honest communication. An important aspect of this work with drug-abusing patients is helping them to identify the hollowness of the gratification derived from drug abuse in comparison with that derived from meaningful intimate relationships. Compulsive drug abuse often begins as an attempt to console oneself over a breakdown in a relationship that the patient has not been able to resolve or even admit.

Role Transition

Description. As a normal part of development throughout the life cycle, everyone is faced with the periodic necessity of giving up old roles and taking on new ones. This process is seldom smooth and leads to psychiatric symptoms when the individual is unable to accept the demands of a new role or is unable to move out of a role that is no longer appropriate. Role transitions can be normative and expectable, or non-normative. Examples of normative role transitions include moving out of the parental home, obtaining a first job or changing jobs, getting married, initiating parenthood, or entering retirement.

Drugs are often used in coping with difficult role transitions to reverse dysphoric affects associated with the role change. Drug use can be used to combat the pain of non-normative role transitions such as breakup of a marriage, or loss of a job. As another example, highly visible sports stars may find that the drug-induced euphoria helps relieve the tension related to being in the limelight and being outside a context in which familiar values hold. Alternatively, use of drugs may be a covert attempt at reversing the role transition by paving the way for removal from the limelight.

Another way that drugs can function in the management of role transitions is by providing an alternative social network and life-style that is seen as being easier to enter than that which is conventionally available to the patient. Thus, if a poor but ambitious high school student sees college or other opportunities for career enhancement as closed to him or her, he or she may opt to enter the drug-using subculture. For such patients drug use and involvement in a drug-using deviant subculture may be a major organizing feature of their lives. Drug use may become an occupation, because many serious users (unless independently funded) offset drug cost by actively dealing or at least taking a "cut" in obtaining drugs for others. It can also become a leisure time recreational activity (so that empty hours pass unnoticed when the user is high or pass rapidly because the time is filled with the frantic effort to obtain drugs), and a source of friendship through interactions with a drug-using peer group. For some persons who abuse drugs, giving up the drug use means a loss of more than just giving up a pharmacological agent. It means a profound change of life-style. The pharmacological nature of the particular drug may be less important than the metapharmacological meaning of the drug in the patient's self-perception and microculture. Patients need to give up the satisfactions derived in this way to find a socially appropriate alternative to drug use. They must also find non–drug-using friends, tolerate interaction with others when not high, find alternative ways of filling leisure time, and explore their external bases of self-esteem.

Therapist's strategy.   When drugs perform a function in managing role transition difficulties, the therapist's goal is to help guide the patient through the phase without the patient's relying on drugs. There are three fundamental parts to this work:

1. To help the patient recognize the need to give up the old role and to mourn those aspects that are lost
2. To help the patient develop a more realistic and positive acceptance of the demands of the new role
3. To aid in the development of social skills needed to perform the new role

The therapist engages the patient in a systematic review of positive and negative aspects of the old role (e.g., high school student living with family) and of positive and negative aspects of the new one (e.g., worker living away from home). In this process the therapist is alert for evidence that the patient is idealizing the desirable aspects of what is lost and exaggerating the difficulties in performing in the new role. Frequently, managing a role transition involves the fear of losing one's identity, and the therapist may aid the patient in the transitional process by helping him or her to focus on ways of expressing this identity in new circumstances.

Interpersonal Deficits

Description.   Many persons who abuse drugs have a history of severe impoverishment of social relations with a failure to become engaged in adult intimate relationships or even in sustaining friendships. Such patients may lack the necessary social skills, or they may have long-standing, pervasive, maladaptive ways of reacting to relationships that prohibit their development. Such patients may be quite socially isolated or involved with others in such a superficial fashion that the relationships are chronically unfulfilling.

Drug use can perform two important functions in individuals with interpersonal deficits. First, the direct pharmacological effects of the drugs can help to compensate for the sense of failure in social functioning. If the patient does not develop sustaining intimate relationships, become involved in meaningful hobbies or leisure time interests, or experience satisfaction in some occupational pursuit, the drug-induced state offers euphoria, escape, and relief of depression and anxieties that might result from a sense of failure or inner emptiness associated with social isolation and frustration. Second, some abusing patients feel that drugs provide them with desirable personality characteristics that they feel do not or cannot exist in them when they are not under the influence of drugs. For instance, patients often describe themselves as more sociable, friendly, and empathic when high. Paradoxically, by the time they reach the stage of chronic heavy use, they tend to be withdrawn, irritable, and self-absorbed, and often are alone more frequently.

Likewise, while some abusing patients use drugs to overcome sexual inhibition or to enhance the sexual experience, chronic use may lead to the opposite effects. Many chronic patients feel that they require drugs for "normal" sexual functioning or are unable to function sexually with or without drugs. This then becomes another important psychotherapeutic focus.

Therapist's strategy.   If drug effects are used to reduce feelings of depression or failure resulting from social problems, the therapist's strategy is to help the drug-abusing patient focus on the appropriate interpersonal problem areas and devise more successful strategies for handling them. If drugs are used to provide the patient with a feeling of having new social skills, such as interest in others, vibrancy, and so on, the therapist may use a confronting approach. The therapist may explain that use of drugs cannot create social skills that are not already present but rather that drug use may help to reduce the anxiety that may have prevented the patient from exhibiting personality characteristics that he or she, in fact, possesses while straight. The therapist may then attempt to help the patient recognize that the use of drugs is unnecessary for successful role behavior.

In helping the patient reduce his or her social isolation, the therapist can review past relationships in detail with the aim of helping to discover the attitudes and behaviors that have led the patient to past failures. The ways that the patient relates to the therapist may be focused on in the therapy with the aim of discovering dysfunctional attitudes and of imparting social skills within the context of a protected relationship.

Grief

Description.   Although it is common and normal for individuals to experience symptoms of depression in response to the death of a significant other, the grieving state is usually time-limited, and serious symptoms are resolved within 1 year or sooner. However, some individuals suffer from prolonged grief reactions in which dysphoric symptoms do not remit, and others who are ostensibly functioning well may have hidden or distorted grief reactions with pathological changes in mood or behavior that may not be consciously linked to the loss.

Drug use may begin or become exacerbated in the context of prolonged or distorted grief reactions as the patient uses the pharmacological effects of the drug or the involvement in the drug world as a way of avoiding painful affects associated with the loss.

Therapist's strategy.   In managing patients with prolonged or distorted grief reactions, it is often difficult to link the drug use and other symptoms to the death of a loved one. Careful review of important life events, attention to the detailed elaboration of the sequence of events, and the use of clues such as anniversary reactions can be helpful in recognizing the role of grief in the patient's symptomatic behavior. Once recognized, the therapist's aims are to help the patient go through a more healthy mourning process and to help him or her find ways of filling the space left by the loss. The central concept related to pathological grief is that the patient has not been able to give it up because of powerful distorted ideas related to the memories of the person. For example, the patient may feel responsible for the death of a father because he harbored murderous fantasies about him.

To help the patient more adequately mourn, the therapist engages him in a detailed review of the lost relationship, the events surrounding the death, and subsequent reactions to the death. Through this process the therapist usually has the opportunity to correct distorted interpretations of events and to help the patient put the death into a more realistic context. The supportive relationship with the therapist makes this process more bearable. When the patient can tolerate the feelings related to the loss, the need to use cocaine is reduced.

Preventing the Patient From Sabotaging Treatment

For a variety of reasons, persons who abuse drugs are not always willing or able to cooperate with treatment. In most cases, focusing on the therapeutic relationship itself is not an important part of IPT, and the patient's positive feelings for the therapist and positive expectations of treatment are not systematically explored unless they interfere with progress (e.g., a patient with such high expectations of being helped by the omnipotent therapist that he makes no independent effort to solve problems himself). However, the therapist should monitor the treatment for signs that the patient is developing negative or countertherapeutic feelings about the therapist or treatment. These may take the form of relatively subtle verbal or nonverbal messages or may be expressed in problematic behavior such as lateness, missed appointments, silence, excessive discussion of tangential material, or direct uncooperativeness, among others.

When countertherapeutic attitudes and behaviors arise, the therapist has two goals: 1) to stop or mitigate the behavior and 2) to use the behavior as a clue to obtaining a better understanding of the individual motivations that have led to the behavior in treatment and to related problems outside of treatment. There are two general levels for approaching these goals: the practical and the exploratory.

At the *practical* level, the therapist is simply interested in stopping the behavior. For example, if a patient frequently changes topics, the therapist may simply refocus the discussion. The therapist may choose to leave the issue at this level, especially if the intervention solves the problem. At the *exploratory* level, the therapist follows the general principle that countertherapeutic behavior arises when the patient comes up against the very motivations and feelings that stop him or her from solving his or her problems in the first place. Because of this relationship of countertherapeutic behavior to the patient's targeted problems, the manifestations of such behavior are often a valuable sign that can provide a key to the therapy rather than be a nuisance.

As a general sequence, the therapist usually tries to manage countertherapeutic behavior at a practical level first before exploring its meaning. Hence, with lateness, for example, the initial approach is simply to call attention to the behavior and to ensure that trivial misunderstandings are cleared up or that realistic problems are not responsible. For instance, the patient may expect that coming late to an appointment is not a problem because other types of doctors ordinarily have a large backup in the waiting room and long waits are commonplace. In this case it should be explained that the allotted time is kept open for him or her and that the therapist has no conflicting appointments. The patient may also be reminded that missed sessions or lateness means less time to work on problems.

If the behavior persists despite practical interventions, the therapist should help the patient to understand the functions that the countertherapeutic behavior serves. The assumption here is that countertherapeutic behavior is intentional and represents a way of dealing with interpersonal relationships in and out of therapy. In order to discover the purpose of the behavior, attention is paid to the contexts in which it arises and the results of the behavior both within and outside of therapy. It is assumed that the results are intended. If the patient is always late in both contexts, the therapist may ask what reaction this produces between therapist and patient, or in those whom they have kept waiting? What might be the function of generating these reactions? For example, the patient may use lateness as a way of indirectly expressing hostility to authority figures, to gain attention, or to reinforce a sense of his or her life being out of control. If the patient has been punctual up to a particular point in treatment, what new issues preceded the onset of lateness? By focusing on when the countertherapeutic behavior began, the therapist can be alert to which issues pose special difficulties for the patient.

The most important countertherapeutic behaviors that are specific to the treatment of substance-abusing patients are 1) continued drug use without achieving abstinence and 2) relapse to drug use if a period of abstinence is achieved. In the case of a patient who continues heavy drug use despite outpatient psychotherapy and/or pharmacotherapy, the therapist must consider the risks and benefits of continuing a prolonged treatment that does not appear to be succeeding. The important thrust of the message that the IPT therapist gives the abusing patient is that he or she, the patient, is responsible for and capable of controlling his or her drug abuse, and that continued use causes painful consequences that the patient recognizes are serious. For some patients this message does not penetrate, while others seem to understand it but do not appear able to curtail or even substantially reduce drug use to a less self-destructive level. If treatment has not begun to show effects by 4 to 6 weeks, or in a shorter time if drug abuse is severe, the therapist should consider inpatient treatment, which more forcefully disrupts drug-using behavior by eliminating access to drugs.

Relapse

Relapse is the rule and not the exception in treating all substance-use disorders, and dealing with its occurrence is a fundamental part of treatment. Of particular importance is preventing the relapse from terminating the treatment. Patients who relapse may not return to treatment either out of anger that the therapist's promises have not been kept or out of shame that they have failed the therapist (and themselves) by failing to be a "good," successful patient. In order to prevent termination stemming from a patient's relapse, it is important to discuss the possibility in the early phase of treatment, emphasizing that, although undesirable, relapse can become "grist for the mill." Should relapse occur, it can allow the patient and therapist to examine factors related to it more directly with the goal of achieving more lasting abstinence.

In discussing the patient's relapse, the therapist avoids a disapproving or punitive manner and reiterates the fact that avoiding drug use is the patient's decision. It is vital to help the patient avoid the conclusion that a relapse is a cause for giving up attempts to fight drug abuse because it indicates the hopelessness of this cause. On the other hand, it is usually unproductive to conduct treatment when the patient is acutely intoxicated or "crashing," and the therapist should refuse to meet with the patient when the patient is in this state. Frequently, a patient's relapse is not full blown but represents an experimental "flirting" with drug use again with the thought that controlled use will be possible after a period of abstinence.

In such instances the patient should be made aware that this is a very serious matter, in that return to controlled use only is highly unlikely.

Cocaine Use in the Context of Role Transition

M.J. is a 34-year-old black man who has used cocaine for the past year. His cocaine use began shortly after he left his wife and children and moved into an apartment with another divorced man. Coming from a working-class background, he had built a successful small business from scratch through determined, methodical effort. His marriage to a plain, dutiful, matronly woman had been supportive but not passionate. At the age of 33 the patient had some pride in his achievements but lacked involvement or excitement in his job and marriage. He had married and begun work directly after graduating from high school and felt that he had never had a chance to "live."

Leading the single life for the first time, he spent many late evenings at bars or playing cards with other unattached men. These activities were usually accompanied by drinking, for which the patient had a low tolerance, and he found that cocaine use allowed him to remain alert after drinking heavily. He became involved with an attractive, exciting divorced woman who had been admired and popular in the patient's high school. She was willful, temperamental, and tended to abuse drugs herself, but appeared in some respects an appealing contrast to the patient's ex-wife.

In the context of keeping up ties with single friends and dating his new girlfriend, the patient became increasingly involved with cocaine, using large amounts at least three times weekly. The expense of this use led him to take money from his business and borrow heavily from friends and relatives. His cocaine abuse also led to the breakup of the relationship with his new girlfriend, who had kept her level of cocaine use comparatively under control. His moods had become progressively labile in relation to the overwhelming life events and his cycle of cocaine use, in which its use was followed by sleep loss, fatigue and oversleeping, and then cocaine use. His depressive symptoms were sufficient to warrant a DSM-III diagnosis (American Psychiatric Association 1980) of major depression. He had made several attempts to curtail cocaine use on his own before seeking treatment, and the duration of heavy use had been 6 months at that time.

Because of the patient's depressive symptoms, he was placed on desipramine, to which he responded with improved mood over the course of 10 days. During the first week after starting treatment the patient used cocaine once heavily, and during the second week he used cocaine on one occasion. During the subsequent year he did not return to cocaine use. The focus of psychotherapy was to help the patient reassess the current position in his life course and to choose a future direction. By weighing the satisfactions and dissatisfactions of married and single life, the patient became more aware of his own conservative values and obsessional personality style. He recognized that he, in fact, felt most comfortable and satisfied when in stable relationships and when he was able to judge his successes and failures in a familiar context. He recognized the hollowness and unsustaining quality of satisfactions derived from his version of the single life with its emphasis on excitement and superficial relationships. Because of this, he had little difficulty in avoiding the contexts in which he typically used cocaine (i.e., in bars and with groups of drug-using male friends). He increased his involvement in his business and with his family. In early weeks the therapist was very active in helping the patient plan his schedule around activities that did not involve cocaine use. He also was highly confrontive regarding the ways that cocaine had been destructive in the patient's life. The therapist also engaged the patient in role-playing about how he would react to being offered cocaine, seeing others use cocaine, and so on. Renunciation of cocaine use became progressively easier as the patient's mood improved and he reestablished relationships with family and non–drug-using friends.

Individual psychotherapy sessions were held for 4 months followed by biweekly contact over the course of 1 year. During this time the patient considered returning to his marriage and briefly began to date his ex-wife. Again feeling that the marriage would not be satisfying, he began to date more appropriate women, eventually becoming more seriously involved with a stable but more emotionally giving woman. Guilt over the breakup of his marriage was lessened when his ex-wife began dating other men. He revitalized his business and used much of this energy and time in the early course of treatment in this process. However, recognizing that his excessive involvement with the business and inability to reward himself had resulted in the loss of interest in it, he restructured his role in a way that allowed him more leisure time. On discharge from treatment he appeared to have built a more fulfilling life structure that did not require drug use.

In this case, cocaine abuse had become an enduring side effect of the patient's attempt to dramatically revitalize his life by adopting a "youthful" life-style to which he was unsuited. His ability to stop cocaine use was aided by his recognizing the problem before he had lost all that he had worked for, and by his high level of premorbid functioning. The therapy was aimed at helping to determine what his needs and goals were and to help him develop a more realistic strategy for fulfilling them.

Efficacy Studies of Interpersonal Psychotherapy With Patients Who Abuse Drugs

IPT for Opioid-Addicted Patients Who Are Being Maintained on Methadone

IPT was evaluated as an adjunctive treatment for a full-service methadone clinic in New Haven, Connecticut (Rounsaville et al. 1983) as part of a collaborative research project in which a parallel study (Woody et al. 1983) evaluated two other psychotherapies, cognitive-behavior therapy and supportive-expressive therapy, as treatment for methadone-maintained veterans in Philadelphia, Pennsylvania. These two studies included important design features such as random assignment to treatment conditions, specification of treatments in manuals, extensive training of therapists and monitoring of therapy implementation, use of well-trained therapists who were committed to the type of approach they administered, multidimensional ratings of outcome by raters who were blind to the study treatment received, and adequate sample sizes.

For the New Haven study evaluating the efficacy of IPT, 72 opiate-addicted subjects were selected who had been maintained on methadone for a minimum of 3 months and who were found to have a current psychiatric disorder (e.g., depression) based on the Research Diagnostic Criteria (Spitzer et al. 1978). The subjects were randomly assigned to one of two treatment conditions, both of which lasted 6 months: 1) IPT, consisting of 1 hour per week of individual psychotherapy with a psychiatrist or psychologist (a form of treatment that has been shown to be efficacious with ambulatory depressed patients in previous clinical trials); and 2) low contact, consisting of one 20-minute meeting per month in which symptoms and social functioning were reviewed.

Thirty-seven subjects were assigned to IPT and 35 to the low-contact group. Both groups received treatment as usual in a full-service methadone maintenance program that was an administratively separate component from the research program. The methadone program included a weekly 90-minute session of group counseling. Outcome measures included: 1) programmatic measures such as treatment dropout, illicit drug use, etc.; 2) psychological symptoms, including those of depression; 3) personality measures; 4) ratings of social functioning; and 5) change in targeted problem areas measured through a goal-attainment scaling method. Ratings were made by clinical evaluators who were independent of the treatment team and blind to the treatment condition that the addicted patient was receiving.

The first major finding was the difficulty in recruiting and engaging subjects in the study. Despite high rates of psychopathology such as depression among treated opiate-addicted patients, less than 5% of the methadone clinic population participated in the study at any given time. In addition to the low recruitment rate, there was a high dropout rate, with only 38% completing 6 months of treatment in the IPT condition and 54% completing treatment in the low-contact condition. The second major finding was the similarity of outcomes in addicted subjects receiving the two study treatments. Out of 12 major outcome measures, significant differences between IPT and low-contact groups were detected on only two scales, with one measure favoring IPT and the other favoring low contact. However, in many of the outcome areas, subjects in both treatment conditions were shown to have attained significant clinical improvement during the 6-month period. The lack of difference in treatment outcomes did not change when the samples were divided into those with high and those with low levels of depressive symptoms.

In the Philadelphia study evaluating two other forms of psychotherapy, Woody and colleagues (1983) randomly assigned 110 subjects entering a Philadelphia methadone maintenance program to a 6-month course of one of three treatments: 1) drug counseling alone, 2) drug counseling plus supportive-expressive psychotherapy, or 3) drug counseling plus cognitive-behavior therapy. While the supportive-expressive psychotherapy and cognitive-behavior therapy groups did not differ significantly from each other on most measures of outcome, subjects who received either form of professional psychotherapy evidenced greater improvement in more outcome domains than the subjects who received drug counseling alone. Furthermore, gains made by the subjects who received professional psychotherapy were sustained over a 12-month follow-up, whereas subjects receiving drug counseling alone evidenced some attrition of gains. Differential responsiveness to treatment by both presence and type of the addicted subject's psychopathology was found: addicted subjects with low levels of psychopathology tended to show significant improvement regardless of treatment received, but addicted subjects with higher levels of psychopathology were likely to improve only if they received professional psychotherapy (Woody et al. 1984). Addicted subjects with antisocial personality disorder tended not to benefit from treatment, whereas those with concurrent depressive disorders showed improvements in all areas assessed (Woody et al. 1985).

Although the two studies were similar in many design features, their outcomes were different. The Philadelphia study suggested that ancillary professional psychotherapy is likely to provide additional benefit to methadone-maintained clients with high levels of psychiatric symptoms. The New Haven study, on the other hand, suggested that individual professional psychotherapy does not add further to the benefits obtained in a full-service methadone program. One possible explanation is that the types of psychotherapy offered in the Philadelphia study were superior. However, an evaluation of audiotaped sessions from the two studies showed IPT to be highly similar to the supportive-expressive treatment.

Several differences in the administrative aspects of the two studies may have accounted for the comparative lack of psychotherapy efficacy found in the New Haven study. First, and most important, the subjects in the control condition were receiving intensive treatment in the New Haven methadone clinic, which requires that all clients attend at least one 90-minute group psychotherapy session per week in addition to daily contact with the methadone clinic, monitoring of urine, and meetings with a program counselor on an as-needed basis. It is noteworthy that both treatment groups experienced some clinical improvement over the first 6 months of the study.

Second, the timing of recruitment in the New Haven study may have been a limiting feature. Clients were taken into the psychotherapy study only after they had been on the methadone program for a minimum of 6 weeks. Data derived from the New Haven clinic (Rounsaville et al. 1985) indicate that the number of addicted subjects with high levels of depressive symptoms falls after 6 weeks in the methadone program, and this factor may have removed some of the subjects' motivation to become engaged in the psychotherapy.

Third, the participation in the psychotherapy program was likely viewed as a separate treatment that was not integrated into the general methadone program and the client's overall treatment plan. This feeling was further created by the delayed onset and the physical separation of psychotherapists' offices from the methadone program. In this regard, Kaufman and Blaine (1974) reported that addicted patients on methadone maintenance were far more likely to keep psychotherapy appointments when the therapist's office was on the same floor as the clinic than if it was necessary for them to take an elevator to a different floor. In the Philadelphia study, therapists' offices were in the methadone treatment facility and the psychotherapy study was considered to be an integral part of ongoing treatment services. The time between entrance into the methadone program and the beginning of the psychotherapy study was an average of 3 to 4 weeks in Philadelphia.

Fourth, with the low rate of recruitment in New Haven, the group who sought treatment was highly select, consisting partly of those patients who were highly motivated for treatment and largely of those who were heavily encouraged by methadone clinic staff to become involved in it because of their having extraordinarily severe clinical problems. This low recruitment rate and the attempt to identify a more treatment-resistant patient population may have resulted in the selection of a population with a comparatively poor prognosis. The Philadelphia study had more successful client recruitment, with at least 25% of the eligible clinic population participating in the study at a given time. However, that study indicated that psychotherapy, while helpful, was not a necessary adjunct for those clients in the low psychiatric severity range. These clients, it was found, could benefit as much from the services offered by the methadone treatment program. It was those clients in the high psychiatric severity range that benefited from psychotherapy. It was estimated that 15% of the clinic population met the criteria for high severity.

IPT Compared With Relapse Prevention in Ambulatory Cocaine-Abusing Patients

In this study (Carroll et al. 1992), IPT adapted for use with patients who abused cocaine was contrasted with a cognitive-behavioral approach emphasizing relapse prevention (Marlatt and Gordon 1985). This study evaluated the efficacy of 12 sessions of weekly individual psychotherapy without adjunctive pharmacotherapy as the sole initial treatment for 42 subjects who were randomly assigned to receive IPT or relapse-prevention approaches.

Rates of attrition were significantly higher in IPT than in relapse prevention, with only 38% of those in IPT versus 66% of those in relapse prevention completing a 12-week course of treatment. On most measures of outcome, significant differences by treatment type were not seen, but did emerge when subjects were stratified by pretreatment severity of cocaine abuse. Among the subgroups of more severe users, subjects who received relapse prevention were significantly more likely to achieve abstinence than subjects in IPT (54% vs. 9%, respectively), whereas subjects with lower levels of severity improved regardless of treatment received. A similar pattern was seen when subjects were stratified by pretreatment severity of psychological symptoms: for those subjects high in psychopathology, those in the relapse-prevention group were more likely to become abstinent than those in IPT (58% versus 14%, respectively). In parallel to Woody et al.'s findings with opiate-addicted patients, cocaine-abusing patients with concurrent depressive disorders tended to improve regardless of treatment received, while those with antisocial personality disorder were significantly more likely to drop out of, and thus benefited little from, treatment.

Regarding the utility of IPT in the treatment of cocaine-abusing patients, it should be noted that outcome was comparable and favorable for both treatment types for subjects with lower severity of substance abuse. However, patients with more severe abuse may require the greater structure and direction offered by the relapse-prevention approach, which emphasized learning and rehearsal of specific strategies to interrupt and control cocaine use.

Enhancing the Efficacy of Interpersonal Psychotherapy With Drug-Abusing Patients

The efficacy findings based on clinical trials of IPT with drug-abusing patients are clearly less promising than those with ambulatory depressed patients. To understand the differences in apparent efficacy with IPT for drug abuse and for depression, we point to, first, administrative issues and, second, differences in clinical issues faced by drug-abusing patients and depressed patients.

Administrative Issues in Delivering
Psychotherapy to Drug-Abusing Patients

Regarding administrative issues, we believe that the lack of differential improvement in the IPT methadone study was largely accounted for by adverse aspects of the implementation of this psychotherapy within the New Haven methadone program. To maximize the efficacy of IPT or other adjunctive professional psychotherapy within methadone treatment, we recommend the following:

1. Make sure that therapists are physically and emotionally integrated into the methadone program.
2. Require coordination and cooperation between therapists and the program counselor.
3. Pay close attention to patient compliance, especially around attendance, and remind patients of appointment times.
4. Start patients in therapy shortly after they enter the program.
5. Offer treatment shortly after problems arise rather than reserving psychotherapy only for those patients who have been refractory to other treatment interventions.
6. Offer psychotherapy primarily to those patients who are found to have comparatively severe psychiatric symptoms. In the Philadelphia study these patients comprised 15% of the methadone program population, and psychiatric severity was rated using an instrument that can be easily administered by paraprofessional counselors, the Addiction Severity Index (McLellan et al. 1980). Agencies can use this instrument as a screening device to detect the addicted individuals who are most likely to benefit from psychotherapy.

Clinical Differences Between Drug-Abusing Patients
and Depressed Patients

Regarding clinical differences between drug-abusing patients and depressed patients, our clinical experience from applying IPT to both groups suggests two important differences: the severity of symptomatology and the greater importance of behavior control in drug-abusing patients. Although both depressed patients and drug-abusing patients apply to treatment with syndromes ranging widely in severity, our impression is that the latter experience a higher level of problems *before* seeking treatment. The typical drug-abusing patient seeks treatment after at least several years of regular use of the abused substance. In part this is due to the gratifying nature of the drug abuse itself, which is in marked contrast to the painful nature of depressive symptomatology that often leads patients to seek treatment earlier in the course of the disorder. Because of the relatively protracted course of drug abuse prior to drug-abusing patients' first seeking treatment, they often present to treatment with impairments in multiple areas (McLellan et al. 1981; Rounsaville et al. 1982a) and with relatively entrenched habitual drug use that they have typically attempted several times to curtail without treatment.

The typical drug-abusing patient seeking treatment has frequently come to organize his or her entire life around drug use. Before the patient can have the energy and concentration to engage in the work of psychotherapy, it is often necessary for drug use to be curtailed, at least temporarily. This contrasts with depression, in which useful clinical work can proceed while mild or moderate symptoms continue. Given the problem severity of drug-abusing patients and the need for effective behavior control, IPT is unlikely to be seen as the sole treatment for most patients who abuse drugs, although it is likely to be effective when used as one component in the armamentarium of many treatments that can be administered to meet these patients' individual needs.

Uses for IPT With Patients Who Abuse Drugs

On the basis of our clinical experience in providing IPT to drug-abusing patients, we suggest that this form of therapy may have the following uses: 1) to introduce drug-abusing patients into treatment, 2) to treat patients with low levels of drug dependence, 3) to treat patients who did not benefit from other modalities, 4) to complement other ongoing treatment modalities for selected patients, and 5) to help patients solidify gains following achievement of stable abstinence.

IPT as an Introduction to Treatment

As noted above, a key advantage of individual therapy is the privacy and confidentiality that it affords. This aspect may make individual therapy or counseling an ideal setting to clarify the treatment needs of patients who are at early stages (i.e., contemplation, precontemplation) of thinking about changing their drug-use habits. For individuals with severe dependence or severe drug-related problems who deny the seriousness of their drug involvement, a course of individual therapy in which the patient is guided to a clear recognition of the problem may be an essential first step toward more intensive approaches such as residential treatment or methadone maintenance. An important part of this process may involve allowing the patient to fail one or more times at strategies that have a low probability of success such as attempting to cut down on drug use without stopping or attempting outpatient detoxification. A general principle underlying this process is the successive use of treatments that involve greater expense and/or patient involvement only after less intensive approaches have been shown to fail. Hence, brief individual treatment can serve a cost-effective triage function.

IPT For Patients Who Are Mildly or Moderately Dependent on Drugs

Although less studied with nonalcoholic drug-abusing patients, the drug dependence syndrome concept (Edwards 1986) has received considerable attention in the study of alcoholism. This concept, first described by Edwards and Gross (1976), suggests that drug dependence is best understood as a constellation of cognitions, behaviors, and physical symptoms that underlie a pattern of progressively diminished control over drug use. This dependence syndrome is conceived of as being arrayed along a continuum of severity, with higher levels of severity associated with poorer prognosis and the need for more intensive treatment and lower levels of severity requiring less intensive interventions.

The dependence syndrome construct has generated a large empirical literature suggesting its validity with alcoholic patients (Edwards 1986). Moreover, several scales have been developed for gauging severity of alcohol dependence (Chick 1980; Skinner 1981), although similar instruments are not yet available for other drugs of abuse. Generally, however, measures of quantity and frequency of alcohol use are highly correlated with dependence severity, and similar quantity and frequency indices for other drugs of abuse may be an adequate gauge of dependence severity. Evidence from studies of individuals who are mildly or moderately dependent on alcohol has indicated that a brief course of psychotherapy is sufficient for many to achieve substantial reduction or abstinence from drinking (Edwards 1986; Miller and Heather 1986; Sanchez-Craig and Wilkinson 1986–1987). These findings, although they have yet to be replicated with other types of substance-abusing individuals, are likely to be generalizable.

Failures From Other Modalities

Although numerous predictors of treatment outcome for drug-abusing patients have been identified (Luborsky and McLellan 1978; McLellan 1983), few are robust and still fewer have been evaluated regarding the issue of matching patients to treatment (McLellan 1983). As a result, choice of treatments involves an amount of trial and error. Each type of treatment has its strengths and weaknesses that may have an idiosyncratic appeal to particular patients. Thus, for example, individual therapy is more expensive but more private than group therapy, more enduring and less disruptive to normal routine than residential treatment, and less troubled by side effects and medical contraindications than pharmacotherapies. Each of these advantages may be crucial for a patient who has responded poorly to alternative treatments.

Psychotherapy as Ancillary Treatment

In thinking of the place of psychotherapy as part of an ongoing comprehensive program of treatment, it is useful to distinguish between treatment of opioid addiction for which powerful pharmacological approaches are available and treatment of other drugs of abuse for which strong alternatives to psychosocial treatments are unavailable. For opioid abuse, the modal approach is methadone maintenance, and this approach is used with the vast majority of those individuals in treatment. An alternative pharmacotherapy, naltrexone, is also highly potent for the minority who choose this approach. Given the powerful and specific pharmacological effects of these agents either to satisfy the need for opioids or to prevent illicit opioids from yielding their desired effect, these agents can be all that is needed, with only minimal ancillary counseling for many opioid-addicted patients. The choice of those patients who might benefit from individual psychotherapy can be guided by the unique but robust empirical findings of Woody et al. (1984, 1985) and McLellan et al. (1983), which suggest that psychotherapy is most likely to be of benefit for those opioid-addicted individuals with high levels of psychiatric symptoms as measured by the Addiction Severity Index (McLellan et al. 1980) or with a diagnosis of major depression, as defined in DSM-III or DSM-III-R (American Psychiatric Association 1987). Because benefits of psychotherapy may be maximized when instituted relatively soon after treatment admission, screening instruments such as the Addiction Severity Index or the Beck Depression Inventory could be used to quickly identify an individual with psychopathology or depression, alerting staff to the need to refer the client to psychotherapy.

For drugs of abuse other than opioids, an active search for effective pharmacotherapies is currently underway, and some agents have been shown to be promising for treating cocaine abuse (Gawin and Kleber 1986). However, most of the evidence to date is based on open studies or unreplicated reports from randomized clinical trials (Kosten 1989). Thus, the mainstay of treatment for non-opioid drugs of abuse remains some form of psychosocial treatment offered in a group, family, residential, or individual setting. In the absence of empirically validated guidelines, the choice of an individual form of psychotherapy for this population can then be based on such factors as expense, logistical considerations, patient preference, or the clinical "fit" between the patient's presenting picture and the treatment modality (e.g., family therapy being ruled out for those without families).

Psychotherapy Following Achievement of Sustained Abstinence

As noted above, a drug-abusing patient who is experiencing frequent relapses or who is only tenuously holding on to abstinence may be a poor candidate for certain types of psychotherapy, particularly those that involve bringing into focus painful and anxiety-provoking clinical material as an inevitable part of helping the patient to master dysphoric affects or to avoid recurrent failures in establishing enduring intimate relationships. In fact, some arousal of anxiety or frustration can be a concomitant of most types of psychotherapy, even those that are conceived of as being primarily supportive. Because of this, individual psychotherapy may be most effective for many individuals only after they have achieved abstinence using some other method such as residential treatment, methadone maintenance, or group therapy. Given the vulnerability to relapse that can extend over a lifetime and the frequency with which dysphoric affects of interpersonal conflict are noted as precipitants of relapse, individual psychotherapy may be especially indicated for those patients whose psychopathology or disturbed interpersonal functioning is found to endure following the achievement of abstinence. Psychotherapy aimed at these enduring issues can be helpful not only for these problems independent of their relationship to drug use but also as a form of insurance against the likelihood that these continuing problems will eventually lead to relapse of drug abuse.

References

Adams EH, Gfroerer JC, Rouse BA, et al: Trends in prevalence and consequences of cocaine use. Adv Alcohol Subst Abuse 6:49–71, 1986

American Psychiatric Association: Diagnostic and Statistical Manual of Mental Disorders, 3rd Edition. Washington, DC, American Psychiatric Association, 1980

American Psychiatric Association: Diagnostic and Statistical Manual of Mental Disorders, 3rd Edition, Revised. Washington, DC, American Psychiatric Association, 1987

Brill L: The treatment of drug abuse: evolution of a perspective. Am J Psychiatry 134:157–160, 1977

Brunswick AF: Black youth and drug use behavior, in Youth Drug Abuse. Edited by Friedman AS. Lexington, MA, Lexington Books, 1979, pp 305–331

Carroll KM, Rounsaville BJ, Gawin FH: A comparative trial of psychotherapies for ambulatory cocaine abusers: relapse prevention and interpersonal psychotherapy. Am J Drug Alcohol Abuse 17:229–247, 1992

Chick J: Alcohol dependence: methodological issues in its measurement: reliability of the criteria. Br J Addict 75:175–186, 1980

Colliver J: A Decade of DAWN: Cocaine-Related Cases, 1976–1985. Washington, DC, National Institute on Drug Abuse, Division of Epidemiological and Statistical Publications, 1987

Cummings N: Turning bread into stones: our modern anti-miracle. Am Psychol 34:1119–1129, 1979

Edwards G: The alcohol dependence syndrome: a concept as stimulus to enquiry. Br J Addict 81:171–183, 1986

Edwards G, Gross MM: Alcohol dependence: provisional description of a clinical syndrome. BMJ 1:1058–1061, 1976

Fuller R, Branchey L, Brightwell D, et al: Disulfiram treatment of alcoholism: a Veteran's Administration cooperative study. JAMA 256:1449–1455, 1986

Gawin FH, Kleber HD: Pharmacological treatment of cocaine abuse. Psychiatr Clin North Am 9:573–583, 1986

Gawin FH, Kleber HD, Byck R, et al: Desipramine facilitation of initial cocaine abstinence. Arch Gen Psychiatry 46:117–121, 1989

Hubbard RL, Rachal JV, Craddock SG, et al: Treatment Outcome Prospective Study (TOPS): client characteristics and behaviors before, during, and after treatment, in Improving Drug Abuse Treatment (NIDA Research Monogr Ser No 51). Edited by Tims FM, Ludford JP. Rockville, MD, National Institute on Drug Abuse, 1984, pp 7–15

Jaffe JH, Kleber HD: Opioids: general issues and detoxification, in Treatments of Psychiatric Disorders, Vol 2. Washington, DC, American Psychiatric Association, 1989, pp 1309–1332

Kaufman E, Blaine GB: Full services in methadone treatment. Am J Drug Alcohol Abuse 1:213–231, 1974

Kleber HD (ed): Psychoactive substance use disorders (not alcohol), in Treatments of Psychiatric Disorders, Vol 2. Washington, DC, American Psychiatric Association, 1989, pp 1181–1482

Kleber HD, Gawin FH: Cocaine abuse: a review of current and experimental treatments, in Cocaine: Pharmacology, Effects, and Treatment of Abuse (NIDA Research Monogr Ser No 50). Edited by Grabowski J. Rockville, MD, National Institute on Drug Abuse, 1984, pp 37–50

Kleber HD, Kosten TR: Naltrexone induction: psychologic and pharmacologic strategies. J Clin Psychiatry 45:29, 1984

Klerman GL, Weissman MM, Rounsaville BJ, et al: The Theory and Practice of Interpersonal Psychotherapy for Depression. New York, Basic Books, 1984

Kosten TR: Pharmacotherapeutic interventions for cocaine abuse: matching patients to treatment. J Nerv Ment Dis 177:379–389, 1989

Luborsky L, McLellan AT: Our surprising inability to predict the outcomes of psychological treatments with special reference to treatments for drug abuse. Am J Drug Alcohol Abuse 5:387–398, 1978

Marlatt GA, Gordon JR: Relapse Prevention: Maintenance Strategies in the Treatment of Addictive Behaviors. New York, Guilford, 1985

McLellan AT: Patient characteristics associated with outcome, in Research on the Treatment of Narcotic Addiction: State of the Art (DHHS Publ No ADM-83-1281). Edited by Cooper JR, Altman F, Brown BS. Rockville, MD, National Institute on Drug Abuse, 1983

McLellan AT, Luborsky L, O'Brien CP, et al: An improved diagnostic evaluation instrument for substance abuse patients: the Addiction Severity Index. J Nerv Ment Dis 168:26–33, 1980

McLellan AT, Luborsky L, Woody GE, et al: Are the "addiction related" problems of substance abusers really related? J Nerv Ment Dis 169:232–239, 1981

McLellan AT, Luborsky L, Woody GE, et al: Predicting response to alcohol and drug abuse treatments. Arch Gen Psychiatry 40:620–625, 1983

Miller WE, Heather N (eds): Treating Addictive Behaviors. New York, Plenum, 1986

O'Brien CP, Woody GE: Antagonist treatment: naltrexone, in Treatments of Psychiatric Disorders, Vol 2. Washington, DC, American Psychiatric Association, 1989, pp 1332–1341

O'Donnell JA: Narcotic addicts in Kentucky (USPHS Publ No 1981). Washington, DC, U.S. Government Printing Office, 1969

O'Donnell JA, Voss HL, Clayton RR, et al: Young men and drugs: a nationwide survey (NIDA Res Monogr Ser No 5). Washington, DC, U.S. Government Printing Office, 1976

Rawson RA, Obert JL, McCann MJ, et al: Cocaine treatment outcome: cocaine use following inpatient, outpatient, and no treatment, in Problems of Drug Dependence, 1985 (NIDA Res Monogr Ser No 67). Edited by Harris LS. Rockville, MD, National Institute on Drug Abuse, 1986

Robins LN: Addicts' careers, in Handbook on Drug Abuse. Edited by Dupont RI, Goldstein A, O'Donnell J, et al. Rockville, MD, National Institute on Drug Abuse, 1979

Robins LN, Davis DH: How permanent was Vietnam drug addiction? Am J Public Health 64(suppl):38–43, 1974

Ross HE, Glaser FB, Germanson T: The prevalence of psychiatric disorders in patients with alcohol and other drug problems. Arch Gen Psychiatry 45:1023–1031, 1988

Rounsaville BJ, Tierney T, Crits-Christoph K, et al: Predictors of outcome in treatment of opiate addicts: evidence for the multi-dimensional nature of addicts' problems. Compr Psychiatry 23:462–478, 1982a

Rounsaville BJ, Weissman MM, Kleber HD, et al: Heterogeneity of psychiatric diagnosis in treated opiate addicts. Arch Gen Psychiatry 39:161–166, 1982b

Rounsaville BJ, Glazer W, Wilber CH, et al: Short-term interpersonal psychotherapy in methadone-maintained opiate addicts. Arch Gen Psychiatry 40:629–636, 1983

Rounsaville BJ, Kosten TR, Weissman MM, et al: Evaluating and Treating Depressive Disorders in Opiate Addicts. Baltimore, MD, National Institute on Drug Abuse, 1985

Rounsaville BJ, Anton SF, Carroll K, et al: Psychiatric diagnoses of treatment-seeking cocaine abusers. Arch Gen Psychiatry 48:43–51, 1991

Sanchez-Craig M, Wilkinson DA: Treating problem drinkers who are not severely dependent on alcohol. Drugs and Society 1(2/3):39–67, 1986–1987

Senay EC: Methadone maintenance, in Treatments of Psychiatric Disorders, Vol 2. Washington, DC, American Psychiatric Association, 1989, pp 1342–1359

Shapiro D: Neurotic Styles. New York, Basic Books, 1965

Simpson DD, Joe GW, Bracy SA: Six-year follow-up of opioid addicts after admission to treatment. Arch Gen Psychiatry 39:1318–1326, 1982

Skinner HA: Primary syndromes of alcohol abuse: their management and correlates. Br J Addict 76:63–76, 1981

Spitzer RL, Endicott J, Robins E: Research Diagnostic Criteria: rationale and reliability. Arch Gen Psychiatry 23:41–55, 1978

Valliant GE: Twelve-year follow-up of New York addicts. Am J Psychiatry 122:727–737, 1966

Washton AM, Gold MS, Pottash AC: Treatment outcome in cocaine abusers, in Problems of Drug Dependence, 1985 (NIDA Res Monogr Ser No 67). Edited by Harris LS. Rockville, MD, National Institute on Drug Abuse, 1986, pp 279–291

Weiss RD, Mirin SM, Michael JL, et al: Psychopathology in chronic cocaine abusers. Am J Drug Alcohol Abuse 12:17–29, 1986

Woody GE, Luborsky L, McLellan AT, et al: Psychotherapy for opiate addicts: does it help? Arch Gen Psychiatry 40:639–645, 1983

Woody GE, McLellan AT, Luborsky L, et al: Severity of psychiatric symptoms as a prediction of benefits from psychotherapy: the Veterans Administration–Penn Study. Am J Psychiatry 141:1172–1177, 1984

Woody GE, McLellan AT, Luborsky, L, et al: Sociopathy and psychotherapy outcome. Arch Gen Psychiatry 42:1081–1086, 1985

Interpersonal Psychotherapy for Bulimia Nervosa

Christopher G. Fairburn, M.D.

Bulimia nervosa is a major source of morbidity among young adult women, and it is the most common eating disorder encountered in psychiatric practice. Studies of its prevalence suggest a rate among women ages 16 to 35 of between 1% and 2% (Fairburn and Beglin 1990), although this is likely to be an underestimate (Beglin and Fairburn 1992). There are many more subthreshold cases and "partial syndromes," but their clinical significance is not clear. The disorder is not common among men.

Clinical Features

Patients with bulimia nervosa complain of loss of control over eating. They describe recurrent episodes of uncontrolled overeating (commonly referred to as "binges"), many of which involve the consumption of truly large amounts of food. The food eaten generally consists of energy-rich

I wish to acknowledge the major contribution made by the colleagues who worked with me as therapists in the two Oxford trials. Not only were they excellent therapists, but they contributed actively to development and refinement of the form of treatment described in this chapter. Thanks are due to Tony Hope, M.D., Rosemary Jones, Ph.D., Robert Peveler, M.D., Joan Kirk, Ph.D., Ruth Solomon, M.D., and Sally Carr, Ph.D. I am also grateful to Phillipa Hay for her comments on an earlier version of the chapter. The first Oxford study was supported by a grant from the Medical Research Council and the second by a grant from the Wellcome Trust. The author is a Wellcome Trust Senior Lecturer.

items that the patient is attempting to avoid because they are viewed as fattening. Most of these patients compensate for the overeating by inducing vomiting or abusing purgatives, or both, and almost all restrict their food intake between the episodes of overeating. Accompanying the behavioral disturbance is a characteristic set of attitudes toward shape and weight that resemble those found in anorexia nervosa, and their presence is required to make either diagnosis. Recognized by clinicians of widely different theoretical orientations, these attitudes have been described as a "morbid fear of fatness" (Russell 1979) or, in DSM-III-R (American Psychiatric Association 1987, p. 67), as a "persistent overconcern with body shape and weight." The core feature is the tendency to judge self-worth largely or exclusively in terms of shape or weight (Fairburn and Garner 1988). It has been argued that these attitudes are likely to play a major role in the maintenance of anorexia and bulimia nervosa (Fairburn et al. 1986a).

Patients with bulimia nervosa show other features. Typically there is a wide range of depressive and anxiety symptoms, with pathological guilt and poor concentration being particularly common. Interpersonal functioning is also often impaired. For example, many patients are socially isolated. Factors contributing to the social isolation include the secrecy that surrounds the repeated episodes of overeating and these patients' acute sensitivity to being seen eating in public. Isolation is often compounded by other less specific social anxieties as well as long-standing low self-esteem. One aspect of functioning—performance at work—tends to be spared, however. Most patients with bulimia nervosa are perfectionistic, setting themselves demanding standards that they do their utmost to meet. As a result, they are often successful at work despite their difficulties in other spheres. There is a small subgroup of patients who show a pervasive disturbance in social functioning. This heterogeneous group of patients show features such as impetuosity, lability of mood, substance abuse, self-harm, and an inability to form or sustain lasting relationships. Some of these patients fulfill criteria for borderline personality disorder.

The course of bulimia nervosa has not been well studied. It appears to be varied. Community-based studies suggest that some cases are transitory and resolve of their own accord, whereas clinical experience suggests that the disorder often runs a chronic, unremitting course. The history of disturbed eating almost always stretches back into adolescence, starting with a period of extreme dietary restriction. In about a third of cases this restriction is so severe that the patient eventually meets criteria for anorexia nervosa. After a variable length of time, control over eating breaks down and episodes of overeating emerge. As a result, body weight gradually increases to near normal levels. Other patterns of onset are observed, with obesity or overeating, for example, being the initial feature.

Research on Treatment

Given that bulimia nervosa has only recently been described, it is remarkable how much has been learned about its treatment. Over 25 controlled trials have been completed, and more are in progress. (See Fairburn et al. 1992 for an account of the work to date.) It is clear from this research that the great majority of patients may be managed on an outpatient basis. If hospitalization is indicated, it should usually be brief, possibly on a day-patient basis, and regarded as a preliminary to outpatient treatment.

With regard to outpatient care, the choice lies between drug treatment and the use of various specific forms of psychotherapy. The drug treatment studies have mostly focused on the effects of antidepressant drugs. Other drugs have been studied, including appetite suppressants, opiate antagonists, antiepileptic drugs, and lithium, but none seems promising and their use is not recommended. In contrast, it is clear that antidepressant drugs have an effect on bulimia nervosa, at least in the short term.

Three groups of findings have emerged. First, antidepressant drugs are superior to placebo at reducing many of the features of bulimia nervosa. There is a marked reduction in the frequency of overeating and self-induced vomiting, and this is accompanied by an enhanced sense of control over eating. At the same time the degree of general psychiatric disturbance lessens substantially. However, the high level of dietary restraint appears not to be affected. The effect of the drugs on these patients' attitudes toward shape and weight has not been adequately studied. Second, the rapidity of the time course resembles that seen in the treatment of depression. It has been suggested that the dose required is also similar, but systematic dose-response studies have yet to be conducted. Third, no consistent predictors of response can be identified. The level of depressive symptoms prior to treatment does not seem to predict outcome.

Maintenance of change following treatment with antidepressant drugs has received remarkably little attention. This is a serious gap in knowledge given that bulimia nervosa tends to run a chronic course. The findings of two recent studies suggest that maintenance is poor, whether or not the patient stays on the drug (Pyle et al. 1990; Walsh et al. 1991).

The main focus of the psychological treatment studies has been on a form of cognitive-behavior therapy (CBT) designed specifically for patients with bulimia nervosa (Fairburn 1981, 1985). This approach has been compared with being on a waiting list, antidepressant drug treatment, supportive psychotherapy, focal psychotherapy, a purely behavioral version of the treatment, and exposure with response prevention. With few exceptions, most notably focal psychotherapy, CBT has been shown to be superior in its effects. It is at least as effective as antidepressant drug treatment at reducing the frequency of overeating and vomiting, and it appears to have a much greater effect on the level of dietary restraint, which may explain why maintenance of change seems good.

The research on the treatment of bulimia nervosa indicates, therefore, that the approach of choice is CBT. If clinicians are to use one single form of treatment, this is the one to adopt. However, CBT is neither necessary nor sufficient for all patients with bulimia nervosa. For some patients it probably constitutes overtreatment. For these patients simpler and briefer treatments are likely to be as effective. For example, there is evidence that both brief educational programs and expert dietary advice can be helpful (Laessle et al. 1991; Olmsted et al. 1991). On the other hand there are patients for whom CBT is not effective. Thus, there is a need to develop and evaluate new treatment approaches. It is in this context that interpersonal psychotherapy (IPT) merits particular attention.

The Status of Interpersonal Psychotherapy as a Treatment for Bulimia Nervosa

Two studies, both conducted at Oxford, are of relevance to IPT and bulimia nervosa.

In the first, Fairburn et al. (1986b) compared CBT with a specific form of focal psychotherapy—adapted from Rosen's method of structured brief psychotherapy (Rosen 1979)—designed to be a credible alternative to CBT. The adaptation was primarily based upon Bruch's writings about psychotherapy for patients with anorexia nervosa (Bruch 1973) and on Stunkard's psychotherapeutic approach to the treatment of overweight persons who binge-eat (Stunkard 1976, 1980). Central to the treatment was the notion that eating problems constitute a maladaptive solution for other "underlying difficulties." The major aim of treatment was therefore to help patients to recognize and address these difficulties, and to understand how the eating problem had served to disguise—and, in some instances, to perpetuate—the difficulties.

There were four main adaptations to Rosen's method. First, particular note was taken of the events and feelings that provoked the patients' episodes of overeating. According to Stunkard, bulimic episodes can serve as markers of difficulties that might otherwise remain undetected. To facilitate recall and discussion of these episodes, patients were asked to record their eating habits and the circumstances under which overeating occurred. Second, the therapists adopted Bruch's noninterpretative fact-finding style of psychotherapy in which particular emphasis is placed upon helping patients recognize and develop confidence in their own opinions, feelings, and needs. Third, information was given on body weight regulation, dieting, and the adverse effects of using self-induced vomiting or purgatives as a means of weight control. Lastly, the treatment was structured to match CBT in the pattern and number of appointments (i.e., 19 sessions over 18 weeks).

In the first stage of treatment, "underlying difficulties" were identified both from a detailed review of the patients' past and from examination of the circumstances under which overeating tended to occur. Once identified, these difficulties became the focus of treatment. Most were interpersonal in character. Toward the end of treatment, when the subject of termination became a major additional issue, the therapists attempted to instill hope for the future. With the exception of the self-monitoring of eating habits, none of the behavioral or cognitive techniques characteristic of CBT were employed.

The results were unexpected. Both treatment groups improved substantially, with the changes being well maintained over a 12-month treatment-free follow-up period. While some findings favored CBT, it was clear that the focal psychotherapy had a major impact on the disorder. However, the inclusion in the treatment of self-monitoring and education about eating, shape, and weight made it impossible to conclude with certainty that the effective ingredients differed from those of CBT.

The second Oxford study (Fairburn et al. 1991, in press) was designed to replicate and extend the findings of the earlier trial using a larger sample size. On this occasion 75 patients were randomized to three treatments: CBT, behavior therapy (BT), and IPT. BT was a dismantled version of CBT consisting solely of those behavioral procedures directed at normalizing eating. IPT was chosen as the comparison psychotherapy condition for several reasons. First, like Rosen's method, it seemed a credible alternative to CBT given the disturbed interpersonal functioning of patients with bulimia nervosa. Second, it had been used in previous treatment studies, albeit of depression, and was in the process of being compared with CBT in the National Institute of Mental Health Treatment of Depression Collaborative Research Program. Third, a detailed treatment manual was available (Klerman et al. 1984). Fourth, the resemblance between IPT and Rosen's method was striking. In this study, care was specifically taken to minimize potential overlap between CBT and the focal psychotherapeutic treatment by excluding both self-monitoring and education about eating, shape, and weight. (The treatment procedure is described in full detail in the next section.)

The findings indicated that all three treatments had a significant effect on the disorder. By 12-month follow-up, however, almost half those in the BT condition had either dropped out or been withdrawn because of their poor progress. In contrast, those who received CBT or IPT did well. CBT was more rapid in its effects, with almost all the changes occurring during treatment itself, whereas with IPT improvement continued during follow-up. The impact of IPT on eating habits and on attitudes toward shape and weight was particularly striking given that these issues were not addressed in treatment.

Taken together, the findings of these two studies indicate that bulimia nervosa responds to treatments that are not cognitive-behavioral in character. This is not to say, however, that bulimia nervosa responds to any form of psychotherapy. It is common clinical experience that many patients referred for treatment have received psychotherapy in the past with limited or transitory benefit, and the studies of supportive psychotherapies and family therapy do not support their use in treatment of this disorder

(Fairburn et al. 1992). What the findings of the two Oxford studies suggest is that short-term focal psychotherapies with an emphasis on current interpersonal problems are a promising alternative to CBT.

Interpersonal Psychotherapy for Bulimia Nervosa: Treatment Procedure

Described below is the form of IPT that was used in the second Oxford trial. This treatment closely resembles IPT for depression. In this account the focus is on the differences between the two approaches. It assumes that the reader is familiar with IPT for depression, as specified in the manual by Klerman and colleagues (1984).

The differences between IPT for depression and IPT for bulimia nervosa (as used in the second Oxford trial) stem from two sources: 1) differences between the two disorders, particularly with respect to their course; and 2) the constraints of the study itself. The latter necessitated that there be a fixed number and pattern of sessions: 19 sessions over 18 weeks, with the first 8 sessions being twice weekly, the following 8 sessions being weekly, and the final 3 sessions being at 2-week intervals. In addition, the study design required that little or no reference be made in the IPT condition to the patient's eating disorder other than during the assessment stage of treatment, and that no use be made of behavioral or cognitive procedures of the type employed in CBT. In all other respects this form of IPT was very similar to IPT that is used in the treatment of depression. The treatment had equivalent stages, strategies and techniques, and therapeutic style.

Stage One: Assessment

There were three related aims in our use of IPT in the treatment of bulimia nervosa. Our first aim was to establish a sound therapeutic relationship; to effect this, IPT guidelines were followed. Our second aim was to orient the patient to this specific form of treatment. Our third aim was to identify the patient's major problem areas in order to establish a treatment contract. Both the second and third aims necessitated adaptations to IPT for depression, as specified below.

Orienting the Patient to IPT

Treatment rationale.   First, a general account was obtained of the patient's current problems and their development. Then, the therapist outlined the treatment rationale, adapting the explanation to suit the patient. In general, it was emphasized that although tackling the eating problem directly (i.e., addressing the disturbed eating habits and attitudes) usually produces benefits, there remains a risk of relapse. Instead, the therapist explained that we wish to modify certain factors that we believe play a major role in maintaining eating disorders, thereby hopefully reducing the risk of relapse. Patients were also told that we thought that this form of treatment might benefit those who did not respond to other approaches. It was explained that we had conducted one previous study of this type and had obtained promising findings with a similar form of treatment.

To justify further the focus on maintaining factors, the following additional information was given. It was explained to patients that although many teenage girls diet to an extreme degree, and binge-eating and self-induced vomiting are also not uncommon, few people become "trapped" in the behavior characteristic of bulimia nervosa. Instead, their behavior is usually transitory. What is of importance, therefore, in understanding patients' eating disorders and in achieving enduring change is the identification and modification of those factors that have resulted in the persistence of their eating difficulties. The patients were told that this was the primary aim of this form of treatment. It was explained that it usually emerged that the key "underlying" problems were interpersonal in character. For this reason treatment tended to focus on these issues, although it was adapted to suit each patient's particular needs. Patients were also told that it usually emerged that the factors that had led up to the development of their eating problem in the first instance—the average duration of eating disorder in the sample was 4.4 years (95% confidence interval = 3.4 to 5.3 years)—were often found to be no longer operating or relevant.

This focus on maintaining factors and processes differs from that in IPT for depression, in which the emphasis is on the problems associated with the onset of the current episode. This difference reflects the respective courses of the two disorders, with depression tending to be episodic, and bulimia nervosa of clinical severity typically running a chronic, unremitting course.

In our previous study some patients were unhappy at the suggestion that they might have difficulties other than their eating problem. In this study we encountered this problem less often: patients seemed to accept the arguments presented above, particularly the need to identify why the problem had persisted. With the few patients who remained dissatisfied with the focus of treatment, we found it helpful to explain how eating problems tend to disguise other difficulties and thereby give the misleading impression that all would be well were control over eating established.

Likely outcome.   Patients were told that on the basis of the findings of our previous study we expected that the majority would overcome their eating problem and that the improvements would be maintained. However, two qualifications were added. The first was that it was usual for patients to still have problems with eating at the end of treatment, but that it was equally usual for there to be continuing improvement over the following 4 to 8 months. Treatment was designed to help the patient recognize and modify relevant interpersonal problems, but it took time for new patterns of interpersonal behavior to get established and for these to have an impact on the eating disorder itself. The second point was that patients should not expect to be "cured" in the conventional sense: disturbed eating was likely to remain their reaction at times of stress, but between such times it should not be a problem. Nevertheless, in our experience, patients tended to remain more sensitive than the average person about food, eating, shape, and weight.

Treatment structure.   It was made clear that the treatment we were using had a predetermined beginning and end. It was explained that it was our view that better results were obtained if treatment was time-limited rather than open-ended, possibly because it "concentrated the mind" of the patient and therapist, thereby making both work harder. The frequency of sessions was specified. Patients were told that each session would begin on time and that sessions would never extend beyond the allocated 50 minutes.

The three stages in treatment were outlined. It was explained that the first stage (up to Session 5 or thereabouts) would be concerned with the identification of key problem areas. These would then become the focus of the remainder of treatment. In the final stage preparations for the future would also be discussed.

Style of treatment. The style of treatment was explained. Patients were told that treatment required their full commitment and should be given priority. The more effort that was put into treatment, the greater the rewards were likely to be. Treatment required hard work both during and between the sessions. It was particularly important for the patient to be committed to making changes. During treatment, problematic behaviors and attitudes might well come to light. It was essential that patients consider alternative ways of behaving and experiment with them. Such attempts at change were fundamental to the success of this treatment approach.

It was also explained that during the first stage of treatment, when problem areas were being identified, the therapist would be more directive and active than in the later stages, when patients would be responsible for taking the lead in choosing topics for discussion.

Identifying Major Problem Areas

Identification of major problem areas is a critical aspect of treatment and one that is likely to be therapeutic in its own right. In our study, this process was generally started in Session 2 and took three or four sessions to complete.

To identify major problem areas, three procedures were used: 1) a detailed review of the patient's past; 2) an assessment of the quality of the patient's current interpersonal functioning; and 3) identification of the precipitants of individual episodes of overeating. Finally, conclusions were drawn.

Reviewing the past. The aim of this procedure was to gain an understanding of the context in which the eating disorder had developed and been maintained, with particular reference being made to interpersonal issues. The following topics were assessed one at a time:

1. The history of the eating problem (and changes in weight)
2. The patient's interpersonal functioning prior to and since the development of the eating problem
3. The occurrence of major life events
4. Problems with self-esteem and depression

The order in which these topics were discussed did not seem to be important and varied from patient to patient. With those patients who had doubts about the suitability of IPT, we generally started with the history of the eating problem. The history-taking was thorough and the patient was given ample time to describe events and identify associated feelings, and was encouraged to think further between sessions. Often topics would be discussed again at subsequent sessions. To enhance recall, patients were encouraged to go through diaries and old photographs. The latter are of particular interest when evaluating patients with eating disorders because such disorders can be apparent at particular times in the patients' lives.

The aim was to identify relationships among interpersonal functioning, self-esteem and mood, the occurrence of life events, and the onset and maintenance of the eating problem. Usually these relationships became obvious to both therapist and patient during history-taking. To help identify these relationships, patients were asked to construct a "life-chart" in which a horizontal line (representing time) was devoted to each of the four aspects of the history.

Assessing the quality of the patient's current interpersonal functioning. Each patient's current social network was assessed in detail. This included a review of work contacts, nonintimate acquaintances, family, friends, partners, and confidants. Every relationship was reviewed in terms of frequency of contact, intimacy, reciprocity, expectations, and satisfying and unsatisfying aspects.

Identifying precipitants of episodes of overeating. As noted earlier, episodes of overeating can serve as "markers" of difficulties that might otherwise remain undetected. Therefore, the context in which the patient overeats is of relevance to the identification of problem areas.

At some point during each of the assessment sessions the therapist inquired generally about the patient's eating and, if there had been episodes of overeating, explored the context in which these episodes had occurred. There was particular emphasis on understanding interpersonal precipitants. These inquiries were designed not to interrupt the flow of the sessions or to alter their style. Instead, they were timed to complement the assessment of problem areas, and the information gained was discussed from this perspective. Apart from these inquiries, no reference was made to the patients' eating, shape, or weight.

Drawing Conclusions and Establishing a Treatment Contract

This information-gathering phase culminated in the identification of one or more major problem areas. These were classified using the same scheme as that used in IPT for depression—that is, as grief, interpersonal disputes, role transitions, and interpersonal deficits. In most cases the problem areas were obvious to both therapist and patient, especially when these problems involved a specific ongoing relationship. In some cases, however, the problem was less immediate and therefore less obvious to the patient (e.g., an unresolved grief reaction). In other cases the problem was subtle and long-standing, involving an established unsatisfactory pattern of interpersonal behavior such as being too unassertive in relationships, repeatedly choosing unsatisfactory partners (often with characteristics in common), or sabotaging potentially intimate relationships at a particular stage in their development. No problems were put aside because they seemed too difficult to address in the time available. Our view was that we needed to determine empirically what types of problems could, and could not, be successfully addressed with this type of treatment.

With most patients there was no difficulty agreeing on the problem areas. In several cases the therapist identified a problem but the patient did not recognize it. Usually these were the more long-standing problems. In such cases it was sometimes necessary to agree to differ but to agree nevertheless to address the problem in treatment. There was no instance of the patient identifying a problem and the therapist disagreeing, although on occasions problems were reformulated.

Once the problem areas had been agreed upon, a specific treatment "contract" was formulated. It was made clear that the focus of treatment would be on the identified current problem areas, and that from now on the patient should take the lead in treatment sessions, the aim being to examine further the problem areas, their causes, and possible means of change. Patients were given clear guidelines—the same as those used in IPT for depression—as to their role in the remaining therapy sessions.

Stage Two: The Intermediate Sessions

The intermediate sessions constitute the core of IPT. From Session 8 onward, appointments were weekly and treatment was exactly as in the IPT manual with one exception—no use was made of role-playing or problem solving because of potential overlap with CBT.

Perhaps surprisingly, few problems arose as a result of the focus on interpersonal issues rather than the eating disorder. It was easy for therapists to forget at times that the patient had presented with an eating problem, because the topics of eating, shape, and weight rarely arose. If these topics were raised, the therapists' tactic was to shift the focus almost immediately onto the identified problem areas. For example, if a patient opened a session by saying that her eating had been terrible, the therapist would reply along the following lines, "It is important that we understand why this has happened. . . . Can you relate it to any of the issues we have been talking about?"

Stage Three: Termination and Preparation for the Future

The IPT manual was closely followed. At regular intervals during the final five sessions the issue of termination was raised and its implications were discussed.

Toward the end of treatment it was not uncommon for patients to start referring to their eating problem. If it was still troublesome, therapists would remind patients that it was our experience that improvements in eating usually followed changes in the identified interpersonal problem areas and that often it took some months for the effects of these changes to be felt. Patients were also reminded that it was usual for the eating problem to continue to improve over the course of the year following treatment. It was pointed out that in our view it is important for patients to see that this continuing improvement is the result of changes that they themselves have made, whereas had they remained in treatment their natural tendency would have been to attribute the improvement to ongoing therapy. Some patients nevertheless insisted that they were not ready for discharge. They were told that people almost invariably feel that they need more treatment, but some weeks or months later most recognize that discharge was the right thing.

In contrast with these reassurances, patients were also reminded that the eating problem would in all likelihood remain an Achilles heel. They were asked to consider how they envisaged tackling future (or continuing) problems. They were encouraged to identify early warning signals (e.g., feelings of depression, episodes of overeating) and to formulate possible plans of action.

During this final stage of treatment, the treatment contract was also reviewed. Patients were asked to consider what remained to be done, either during the remaining few weeks of treatment or afterward. Whenever possible, progress was attributed to patients' own efforts rather than to treatment itself.

Interpersonal Problem Areas of Patients With Bulimia Nervosa

There was considerable overlap in the problem areas identified in the Oxford sample (Fairburn et al., in press). The most common difficulties were role disputes, which were present in 64% (16 out of 25) of the subjects. In the majority of cases the dispute was marital, and it was usually entrenched. Often it was combined with relative social isolation and lack of social support. Treatment followed IPT for depression and was often successful in resolving, or at least reducing, the problem.

Difficulty with a "role transition" was next most common, being present in 36% (9 out of 25) of the subjects. It usually took the form of problems disengaging from parents and adjusting to life away from home. Often a major part of the difficulty was an "enmeshed" relationship between the patient and her mother. Other problems in this category included difficulties adjusting to marriage or motherhood. IPT seemed well suited to the treatment of these problems.

The two other IPT problem areas were encountered less often. In three cases (12%) grief was a major unresolved issue. Treatment went well in each case. In contrast, treatment of interpersonal deficits, which were identified in four patients (16%), was less successful. In each case there was a long history of an inability to form or maintain intimate relationships coupled with low self-esteem. Only one of these patients did well (see next section below for description of her treatment). One of the others dropped out midway through treatment, as she had done in previous attempts at treatment. She has since moved away from the Oxford area and has had further treatment but to no avail. The two others did not benefit from IPT and, after having further treatment, remain highly symptomatic.

An Illustrative Case History

Assessment Stage (Sessions 1–5)

Ms. B. was 21 years old when she was referred for treatment. Although she had a long-standing eating problem, she had only confided in her doctor 6 weeks earlier. Alarmed at her degree of distress and the severity of laxative abuse, the doctor had promptly referred her on for specialist treatment. This was her first contact with psychiatric services.

Ms. B. complained of having lost control over eating. She said that the binges were "destroying her" by taking over more and more of her life. In addition, she described a range of depressive and anxiety symptoms. She denied having other problems, although she acknowledged that her relationship with her boyfriend was "turbulent." She was adamant that all she needed was help regaining control over eating. Not surprisingly, following assessment she was not pleased to learn that she had been randomized to receive IPT. Nevertheless, she agreed to become involved in the study, persuaded in part by the findings of the first Oxford trial.

The review of the past began in the second session. The therapist started by taking a history of the eating disorder. Ms. B. was 15 years old when she started to diet shortly after moving to a new school. She had liked her previous school, but the family had been obliged to move from the area because of her father's recent redundancy, and, in any case, they could no longer afford the school fees. Within weeks of arriving at the new school Ms. B. became self-conscious about her appearance. Dieting was endemic among the girls, and for the first time she felt "fat." Her weight and appearance were unremarkable at the time. (This was corroborated by family photographs.) She proved to be a good dieter and recalled vividly the sense of achievement that came from dieting and losing weight. After about 3 months her parents became concerned about her weight loss. Mealtimes became progressively more tense. Soon she gave in to her parents' insistence that she increase her food intake, but to compensate she began to vomit in secret after each meal. Over the following year her weight increased due to a gradual, but progressive, loss of control over eating. By the time she left school at the age of 18 she was binge-eating and vomiting almost every day and her weight had returned to its previous level.

Over the following 7 years this pattern of binge-eating and vomiting persisted despite many changes in her life. There would be fluctuations in the frequency of binge-eating, but the longest period that she could remember being free of this behavior was for 10 days while on holiday 2 years earlier. Over the 6 months prior to referral she had become increasingly desperate about her eating. On five occasions, following a binge, she had taken large quantities of laxatives (about 50 tablets) to "punish" herself.

After leaving school, Ms. B. moved to another part of the country and received training in sales. She was good at her work, and at the time of presentation she led a force of 20 traveling salespersons. The job suited her because she enjoyed the driving and freedom to make her own schedule. She also enjoyed negotiating sales. However, the nature of the job meant that it was easy for her to overeat and vomit during working hours.

The history of her relationships revealed that she was excellent at striking up superficial relationships, particularly with men. Indeed, she thought that this skill had contributed to her success at work. However, on only two occasions had she developed a more intimate relationship with a man, once with a client who was married, and about 4 months ago with a school teacher. It was the latter relationship that she had described as turbulent. She had little contact with her family apart from the occasional telephone call on birthdays. She had never been close to women: indeed, she said that she was unpopular with women because of her "success" with men.

No major life events were identified other than the change in schools when Ms. B. was 15 and the occasional change of job. The review of depressive symptoms and self-esteem suggested that she had felt insecure as a child: she attributed this feeling to her parent's social isolation and her lack of friends. She reported that they lived in an expensive neighborhood and were probably living beyond their means. They were not accepted by the neighbors. She sensed that her father's redundancy and her move away from the local private school were welcomed by those who lived around them. Ms. B. gave no history of depressive features prior to the onset of the eating problem. She had been unhappy around the time of her change of school, but clinically significant depressive symptoms did not emerge until she was about 20. For most of the 2 years prior to referral she had experienced a range of depressive features including depressed mood, pathological guilt, hopelessness, occasional suicidal thoughts, and feelings of worthlessness. Examination of the content of the depressive symptoms and the factors that influenced them suggested that they were probably a secondary psychological response to the eating disorder. There was no history of obesity, substance abuse, self-harm (other than the laxative abuse), or sexual abuse. There was no family history of obesity or psychiatric disorder.

The review of Ms. B.'s current interpersonal functioning revealed that she had no confidants or friends. She had numerous nonintimate social acquaintances, all of whom were men she had met either through work or at the local pub. The relationship with her boyfriend was problematic. She had known him for 4 months, and they had rapidly established a sexual relationship. Ms. B. noted that this was the only satisfactory aspect of their relationship. In all other respects he was a difficult partner. He drank heavily and was violent at times. He was also unpredictable. Often he would fail to appear at prearranged times and would subsequently refuse to explain why. On two occasions he had unexpectedly appeared at her house in the middle of the night insisting on being let in. Ms. B. was clear that this was not the type of relationship that she wanted, but she was reluctant to break it off, partly through fear and partly because "something is better than nothing."

Analysis of the precipitants of overeating added little to what had already been learned. Many of the episodes were by now habitual; for example, she always overate and vomited in midafternoon. More telling were the occasional "additional binges" that were usually preceded by feelings of loneliness or by anger over her boyfriend's behavior.

The assessment was completed in the fifth session. By this point Ms. B. was clear that her relationships were a problem and that they needed attention in their own right. She was less clear that doing so would result in any improvement in the eating problem. The therapist had some doubts over how best to view the case from an IPT perspective. Certainly the relationship with the boyfriend constituted an interpersonal role dispute and was identified by her as an area of concern, but more striking was her inability to form or sustain lasting intimate relationships. The therapist decided that the latter problem must also be addressed in treatment if lasting changes were to be made. Ms. B. was interested in this proposal but doubted whether anything could be done, saying, "Leopards don't change their spots." Nevertheless, she agreed to this dual focus.

Intermediate Stage (Sessions 6–16)

The sixth session began with Ms. B. saying that she did not see how she could make any progress while she was still seeing her boyfriend. The previous evening he had stood her up again. She had already decided to telephone him after the session and break off the relationship. This she did. Part of each of the following six sessions was devoted to the repercussions of this decision. The boyfriend rejected the idea of separation and came round to her house at unpredictable hours, pleading with her to change her mind. He was at times drunk and physically aggressive. Much of the work of these sessions was devoted to helping Ms. B. determine what she wanted from this relationship and ensuring that she retain a long-term rather than short-term perspective. As her boyfriend's behavior became more extreme, so did Ms. B.'s views crystallize: the boyfriend came to represent the bad aspects of her past. In Session 12 Ms. B. announced that she thought that the relationship was finally over. She had received an abusive note saying that he had found someone else while at a meeting abroad and that he was glad to be rid of her. This was the last she was to hear of him.

The therapist made sure that in each of these sessions time was also devoted to the second problem area. Ms. B. thought that an issue which had to be tackled was her lack of female friends. At first she was at a loss as to how to make progress on this front because she hardly met any women. The solution emerged when she recalled that she used to enjoy tennis but had not played since leaving school. She decided to join a local sports club. This proved to be a crucial step. There she was not known, and therefore no reputation preceded her. Joining the club gave her an opportunity to try a new style of relating. By Session 14 it was apparent to both Ms. B. and the therapist that she was becoming accepted in the club, particularly by a small group of women who were passionate about sports. Over this time her evenings and weekends had changed from being centered around the local pub to joining in the activities of the sports club.

Although Ms. B. was making important changes, and her depressive symptoms had lifted, the therapist had become concerned by Session 14 that insufficient attention was being paid to certain other aspects of her interpersonal functioning. Two areas seemed to merit particular attention: how she related to male colleagues and clients, and how she related to men outside work. The therapist ensured that both these areas were addressed in each of the subsequent sessions. Progress was made in the former but not the latter. Ms. B. decided that she was flirtatious with male colleagues and clients and, although she saw no harm in this and it was probably a factor in her success at negotiating sales, she viewed it as "unhealthy" and not how she wished to behave. Changing the way she related to new clients proved not to be difficult: simply being businesslike seemed to be as effective. However, changing established relationships with clients and colleagues proved much more of a problem. Ms. B. showed no inclination to work on the other area of concern: her relationships with men outside work.

Final Stage (Sessions 17–19)

The main focus was on work that remained to be done. Ms. B. was congratulated by the therapist on the changes that had been made, particularly ending the relationship with the boyfriend and making female friends at the sports club. It was also noted that she was starting to conduct her work in a different manner. However, the therapist pointed out that there were still important issues outstanding. Ms. B. thought it would be impossible to change established relationships with male clients and colleagues and that the only solution was to change jobs. As it happened it was an appropriate time for her to seek promotion elsewhere. It was therefore left that she would look for a new post.

Ms. B. was less willing to review her relationships with men outside work. The therapist suggested that little or no progress had been made on this front and that the issue merited thought because treatment was shortly to end. Ms. B. replied, "All in good time."

In Session 18, the therapist inquired about the state of the eating problem. The topic had not been mentioned for at least 10 sessions. Ms. B. reported that things were much better, but there were still problems. The "additional binges" had long since gone, and she had ceased to abuse laxatives. However, she was still overeating and vomiting at least two afternoons a week. She was unable to identify specific precipitants to these episodes—she regarded them as "a bad habit." The therapist reminded Ms.

B. that her eating was likely to improve over the following months but that she should think further about the precipitants of the remaining episodes. It was stressed that it was important that she continue to deal with difficulties that might be masked by the eating disorder. It was also emphasized that the eating problem was likely to be an Achilles heel and that any future deterioration in her eating habits might signify the emergence of other problems. Treatment ended on an optimistic note.

Five months after ending treatment Ms. B. obtained a new job. About the same time she started going out with a man she met at the sports club. This relationship lasted almost a year and had many good qualities. Now, 4 years after treatment, Ms. B. is married and continues to work in sales. She does not regard herself as having an eating problem, although once or twice a year she makes herself sick if she feels she has overeaten. She no longer has "binges." She still carefully monitors her weight, but it rarely changes. She has had no further treatment.

Mechanism of Action
of Interpersonal Psychotherapy

Neither of the two Oxford studies was designed to examine the mechanisms of action of the treatments being studied. Given that in the second Oxford study there were no differences at 12-month follow-up between CBT and IPT in their effects on the eating disorder or psychosocial functioning, it might seem reasonable to conclude that these approaches operated through the same mechanism. However, this seems unlikely given the temporal differences in the pattern of response to IPT and CBT (Fairburn et al., in press). At the end of treatment, although the patients receiving IPT had improved to the same degree as the CBT patients with respect to frequency of overeating and psychosocial adjustment, they were faring less well with respect to self-induced vomiting, intensity of dieting, and degree of concern with shape and weight. By 4-month follow-up this difference between IPT and CBT was no longer present. Thus, in IPT the changes in overeating and psychosocial adjustment occurred as rapidly as in CBT, whereas the changes in the other aspects of the disorder took longer to be established.

Our clinical observations as therapists are relevant to understanding the mechanism of action of IPT. We observed repeated instances of patients making major positive changes in their relationships, particularly with respect to parents, partners, peers, and employers. Often these changes set in train other positive changes, many of which were still evolving at the end of treatment. It seemed as if successful IPT often operated by bringing about "fresh-start" events (Brown et al. 1988). While the precise relationship between interpersonal events and changes in symptomatology was not assessed, and could not be gauged by the therapists because they were ignorant of the state of the eating problem, it is possible to envisage how improved interpersonal functioning might have affected the eating disorder. At least five processes could have been operating:

1. Patients' realization that they were capable of bringing about changes in what were often entrenched problems might have enhanced their self-efficacy with respect to other areas of difficulty including control over eating.
2. Improved self-confidence and mood might have lessened concerns about appearance and weight, resulting in a decreased tendency to diet.
3. Reduction in the level of depressive symptoms might have reduced vulnerability to overeating.
4. Enhanced interpersonal functioning might have resulted in a reduction in the frequency and severity of interpersonal stressors, in part by increasing social support, thereby affecting a common precipitant of episodes of overeating.
5. Increased social activity might have resulted in a decrease in the amount of unstructured time, thereby decreasing vulnerability to overeating.

Through the operation of processes of this type, it is not difficult to see how the eating problem could have been progressively eroded. It is also easy to see how the effects of IPT on the eating disorder itself might take longer to be expressed than those produced by CBT, because the latter treatment presumably operates directly through its focus on eating habits and attitudes to shape and weight. In CBT it is possibly the changes in these areas that result in improved psychosocial functioning. This postulated difference between IPT and CBT is illustrated in Figure 13–1. If correct, it is an illustration of the importance of Hollon and colleagues' (1987) distinction between *causal* and *consequential* specificity—namely, that different treatments may have the same outcome but operate through different mediating mechanisms.

Interpersonal Psychotherapy in Clinical Practice

Interpersonal psychotherapy has yet to be established as a treatment for bulimia nervosa. Its merits relative to CBT need to be studied in more detail. It may be that IPT is more effective than CBT with certain types of patients, although as therapists we were unable to form a picture of the type of patient best suited to IPT. Some patients disliked the focus of IPT on problems other than eating. This difficulty could usually be overcome even with those patients with few apparent interpersonal difficulties. For others, IPT was an attractive alternative to CBT because it was seen as not "simply" symptom focused, although such patients were not necessarily better off receiving IPT than CBT.

Should IPT and CBT be somehow combined? In practice, this would be difficult, if not impossible, because their style and focus are so different. There would be a risk that rather than the combination being more potent than either treatment alone, it would be a watered down and less effective version of both. This is not to say that the IPT therapist should avoid discussing eating habits and attitudes, as in the Oxford study. Nor is it an argument against combining IPT with a psychoeducational element, possi-

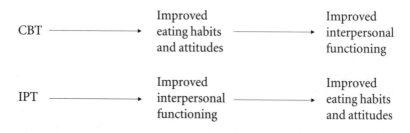

Figure 13–1. Postulated temporal differences between interpersonal psychotherapy (IPT) and cognitive-behavior therapy (CBT) in their effects on psychosocial adjustment and on eating habits and attitudes.

bly along the lines developed by Olmsted and colleagues (1991).

In a study of a notoriously difficult patient group—those with both bulimia nervosa and insulin-dependent diabetes mellitus—we found IPT to be a useful adjunct to CBT (Peveler and Fairburn, in press). Some such patients react unusually poorly to CBT, particularly to the detailed self-monitoring of eating habits. With several of these patients we found that switching over to IPT for 10 or more sessions engaged them in treatment and resulted in significant improvement. We then returned to CBT to address the remaining difficulties. In general, however, we would not advocate this practice: instead, it is our impression that it is better to persevere with CBT or IPT than to chop and change treatment approach.

The form of IPT used in the Oxford study could be adapted in other ways. For example, rather than having a fixed number of sessions, the length of treatment could be tailored to suit the presumed needs of each patient. We have some reservations about this more flexible approach because, as discussed earlier, a fixed number of sessions tends to intensify the treatment process, and a subsequent treatment-free period gives the patient and therapist an opportunity to evaluate longer-term gains.

Two other adaptations merit consideration: 1) conducting IPT in a group setting and 2) using IPT and antidepressant drugs together. Group treatment for bulimia nervosa has several attractions: first, it directly addresses many patients' concern that they are the only one with an eating problem of this type and severity; second, it should facilitate the identification of problems common to many patients; and, third, it may be a cost-effective alternative to individual treatment. Against these advantages must be set the general impression that group treatment is not acceptable to many patients with bulimia nervosa and that there are therefore higher refusal and drop-out rates. Combining IPT and antidepressant drugs has yet to be tried: it seems, however, that little is gained by combining CBT and antidepressant drugs (Pyle et al. 1990; Walsh et al. 1991).

At this stage IPT should be regarded as a promising new approach to the treatment of bulimia nervosa. For clinicians it is worth considering as an alternative to CBT in the treatment of established cases. For research workers the next step must be a further comparison of IPT with CBT, and preferably one that is designed both to identify predictors of outcome and to illuminate the respective mechanisms of action of the two treatments.

Addendum

At the time this book was going to press, a new multisite study on the treatment of bulimia nervosa was funded. The study has four specific aims:

1. To probe the nature of bulimia nervosa by determining whether effective treatment must necessarily focus on the modification of eating attitudes and behavior, or if it suffices to focus solely on the interpersonal aspects of the disorder.
2. To compare the relative efficacy of CBT and IPT to determine, in part, whether they have comparable effects on all measures (the "common factors" position) or mode-specific effects (the "specificity hypothesis").
3. To investigate whether CBT and IPT have different effects on different features of bulimia nervosa, and at different times. Comparing the time-courses of these two treatments is a necessary first step toward identifying their mechanisms of action.
4. To identify predictors of clinical response to CBT and IPT. The goal is to determine whether subgroups of patients with identifiable characteristics respond differentially to the two conceptually and procedurally distinct treatments.

Two hundred women with bulimia nervosa will be randomized to receive individual treatment with either CBT or IPT at two sites (Stanford [W. S. Agras] and Columbia [B. T. Walsh]), with training and evaluation of the quality of therapy and assessment being the task of C. G. Fairburn at Oxford. Doctoral-level therapists will administer both treatments using detailed manuals. Binge eating, purging, and other features of bulimia nervosa will be comprehensively assessed before treatment, at the midpoint of treatment, post-treatment (after 5 months of therapy), and at 4-, 8-, and 12-month follow-up.

References

American Psychiatric Association: Diagnostic and Statistical Manual of Mental Disorders, 3rd Edition, Revised. Washington, DC, American Psychiatric Association, 1987

Beglin SJ, Fairburn CG: Women who choose not to participate in surveys on eating disorders. International Journal of Eating Disorders 12:113–116, 1992

Brown GW, Adler Z, Bifulco A: Life events, difficulties and recovery from chronic depression. Br J Psychiatry 152:487–498, 1988

Bruch H: Eating Disorders: Obesity, Anorexia Nervosa and the Person Within. New York, Basic Books, 1973

Fairburn CG: A cognitive behavioral approach to the management of bulimia. Psychol Med 11:707–711, 1981

Fairburn CG: Cognitive-behavioral treatment for bulimia, in Handbook of Psychotherapy for Anorexia Nervosa and Bulimia. Edited by Garner DM, Garfinkel PE. New York, Guilford, 1985, pp 160–192

Fairburn CG, Beglin SJ: Studies of the epidemiology of bulimia nervosa. Am J Psychiatry 147:401–408, 1990

Fairburn CG, Garner DM: Diagnostic criteria for anorexia nervosa and bulimia nervosa: the importance of attitudes to shape and weight, in Diagnostic Issues in Anorexia Nervosa and Bulimia Nervosa. Edited by Garner DM, Garfinkel PE. New York, Brunner/Mazel, 1988, pp 36–55

Fairburn CG, Cooper Z, Cooper PJ: The clinical features and maintenance of bulimia nervosa, in Handbook of Eating Disorders: Physiology, Psychology and Treatment of Obesity, Anorexia and Bulimia. Edited by Brownell KD, Foreyt JP. New York, Basic Books, 1986a, pp 389–404

Fairburn CG, Kirk J, O'Connor M, et al: A comparison of two psychological treatments for bulimia nervosa. Behav Res Ther 24:629–643, 1986b

Fairburn CG, Jones R, Peveler RC, et al: Three psychological treatments for bulimia nervosa: a comparative trial. Arch Gen Psychiatry 48:463–469, 1991

Fairburn CG, Agras WS, Wilson GT: The research on the treatment of bulimia nervosa: practical and theoretical implications, in The Biology of Feast and Famine: Relevance to Eating Disorders. Edited by Anderson GH, Kennedy SH. New York, Academic, 1992, pp 318–340

Fairburn CG, Peveler RC, Jones R, et al: Psychotherapy and bulimia nervosa: the long-term effects of interpersonal psychotherapy, behavior therapy, and cognitive-behavior therapy. Arch Gen Psychiatry (in press)

Hollon SD, DeRubeis RJ, Evans MD: Causal mediation of change in treatment for depression: discriminating between nonspecificity and noncausality. Psychol Bull 102:139–149, 1987

Klerman GL, Weissman MM, Rounsaville BJ, et al: Interpersonal Psychotherapy of Depression. New York, Basic Books, 1984

Laessle RG, Beumont PJV, Butow P, et al: A comparison of nutritional management with stress management in the treatment of bulimia nervosa. Br J Psychiatry 159:250–261, 1991

Olmsted MP, Davis R, Garner DM, et al: Efficacy of a brief group psychoeducational intervention for bulimia nervosa. Behav Res Ther 29:71–83, 1991

Peveler RC, Fairburn CG: The treament of bulimia nervosa in patients with diabetes mellitus. International Journal of Eating Disorders (in press)

Pyle RL, Mitchell JE, Eckert ED, et al: Maintenance treatment and 6-month outcome for bulimic patients who respond to initial treatment. Am J Psychiatry 147:871–875, 1990

Rosen B: A method of structured brief psychotherapy. Br J Med Psychol 52:157–162, 1979

Russell GFM: Bulimia nervosa: an ominous variant of anorexia nervosa. Psychol Med 9:429–448, 1979

Stunkard AJ: The Pain of Obesity. Palo Alto, CA, Bull, 1976

Stunkard AJ: Psychoanalysis and psychotherapy, in Obesity. Edited by Stunkard AJ. Philadelphia, PA, WB Saunders, 1980, pp 355–368

Walsh BT, Hadigan CM, Devlin MJ, et al: Long-term outcome of antidepressant treatment for bulimia nervosa. Am J Psychiatry 148:1206–1212, 1991

Index

Page numbers printed in **boldface type** *refer to tables or figures.*

E

Psychotherapy Research Review
Committee, 54

Q

Quality of life, 43–44

R

Rand Medical Outcomes Study
(MOS), 44
Recall, 233
Recurrences and relapses of
depression, 4, 75–79, 235
in adolescents, 153–154
maintenance treatment for, 8, 12,
21. *See also* Maintenance
interpersonal
psychotherapy;
Maintenance treatment
interpersonal psychotherapy,
21–22, 75–100
prognosis for patients with, 76
in victimized women, 99
warning signs of, 91–92
Rejection, fear of, in dysthymic
patients, 234, 244, 246
Relapses, of substance abuse,
336–337
Relaxation training, for
adolescents, 136
Research
on conjoint interpersonal
psychotherapy for
depressed patients with
marital disputes, 120–124
on depression treatment in

primary care patients,
269–272
on drug treatments, 46
Harvard Community Health
Plan study of
interpersonal counseling,
297, 308–315
on interpersonal psychotherapy
for acute depression, 15–18
evaluating quality of
psychotherapists, 18
selection of psychotherapists,
16–17
specification of treatment by
manual, 15–16
training of psychotherapists,
17–18
on interpersonal psychotherapy
for drug-abusing patients,
339–343
ambulatory cocaine-abusing
patients, 342–343
opioid-addicted patients on
methadone
maintenance, 339–342
on interpersonal psychotherapy
for dysthymia, 254–261
on interpersonal psychotherapy
for HIV-seropositive
depressed patients,
221–222
NIMH Treatment of
Depression Collaborative
Research Program, 16–18,
20–21, 23
on psychotherapy, 54–59
humanistic critique of, 59